AF574333

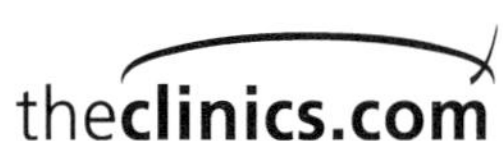

Robert A. Smith, DVM, MS
CONSULTING EDITOR

VETERINARY CLINICS OF NORTH AMERICA

Food Animal Practice

Barnyard Epidemiology and Performance Assessment

GUEST EDITOR
Pamela L. Ruegg, DVM, MPVM

March 2006 • Volume 22 • Number 1

SAUNDERS

An Imprint of Elsevier, Inc.
PHILADELPHIA LONDON TORONTO MONTREAL SYDNEY TOKYO

W.B. SAUNDERS COMPANY
A Division of Elsevier Inc.

Elsevier, Inc., 1600 John F. Kennedy Blvd., Suite 1800, Philadelphia, PA 19103-2899

http://www.vetfood.theclinics.com

VETERINARY CLINICS OF NORTH AMERICA: FOOD ANIMAL PRACTICE
March 2006
Editor: John Vassallo

Volume 22, Number 1
ISSN 0749-0720
ISBN 1-4160-3581-8

Veterinary Clinics of North America: Food Animal Practice (ISSN 0749-0720) is published in March, July, and November by W.B. Saunders, 360 Park Avenue South, New York, NY 10010-1710. Business and Editorial Offices: 1600 John F. Kennedy Blvd., Suite 1800, Philadelphia, PA 19103-2899. Accounting and Circulation Offices: 6277 Sea Harbor Drive, Orlando, FL 32887-4800. Periodicals postage paid at New York, NY and additional mailing offices. Subscription prices are $120.00 per year for US individuals, $195.00 per year for US institutions, $60.00 per year for US students and residents, $140.00 per year for Canadian individuals, $250.00 per year for Canadian institutions, $165.00 per year for international individuals, $250.00 per year for international institutions and $85.00 per year for Canadian and foreign students/residents. To receive student/resident rate, orders must be accompained by name of affiliated institution, date of term, and the *signature* of program/residency coordinator on institution letterhead. Orders will be billed at individual rate until proof of status is received. Foreign air speed delivery is included in all *Clinics* subscription prices. All prices are subject to change without notice. POSTMASTER: Send address changes to *Veterinary Clinics of North America: Food Animal Practice*, Elsevier Periodicals Customer Service, 6277 Sea Harbor Drive, Orlando, FL 32887-4800, USA; phone: (+1) (877) 839-7126 [toll free number for US customers], or (+1) (407) 345-4020 [customers outside US]; fax: (+1) (407) 363-1354; e-mail: usjcs@elsevier.com.

Reprints. For copies of 100 or more, of articles in this publication, please contact the Commercial Reprints Department, Elsevier Inc., 360 Park Avenue South, New York, New York 10010-1710. Tel.: (212) 633-3813; Fax: (212) 462-1935; e-mail: Reprints@elsevier.com.

Veterinary Clinics of North America: Food Animal Practice is covered in *Current Contents/Agriculture, Biology and Environmental Sciences, Index Medicus, and Excerpta Medica.*

Printed in the United States of America.

CONSULTING EDITOR

ROBERT A. SMITH, DVM, MS, Diplomate, American Board of Veterinary Practitioners; Veterinary Research and Consulting Services, LLC, Greeley, Colorado

GUEST EDITOR

PAMELA L. RUEGG, DVM, MPVM, Diplomate, American Board of Veterinary Practitioners (Dairy); Associate Professor, Department of Dairy Science, University of Wisconsin, Madison, Wisconsin

CONTRIBUTORS

JOHN R. CAMPBELL, DVM, DVSc, Professor, Department of Large Animal Clinical Sciences, Western College of Veterinary Medicine, University of Saskatchewan, Saskatoon, Saskatchewan, Canada

MARILYN J. CORBIN, DVM, MS, PhD, Staff Veterinarian, Central States Research Centre, Inc., Oakland, Nebraska

IAN R. DOHOO, DVM, PhD, Professor, Department of Health Management, Atlantic Veterinary College, University of Prince Edward Island, Charlottetown, Prince Edward Island, Canada

DAVID GALLIGAN, VMD, MBA, Professor of Animal Health Economics, Center for Animal Health and Productivity, School of Veterinary Medicine, University of Pennsylvania, Kennett Square, Pennsylvania

JOHN M. GAY, DVM, PhD, Associate Professor of Epidemiology, Department of Veterinary Clinical Sciences, AAHP Field Disease Investigation Unit, College of Veterinary Medicine, Washington State University, Pullman, Washington

DEE GRIFFIN, DVM, MS, Professor, University of Nebraska, Great Plains Veterinary Educational Center, Clay Center, Nebraska

DAVID F. KELTON, DVM, MSc, PhD, Associate Professor, Department of Population Medicine, Ontario Veterinary College, University of Guelph, Guelph, Ontario, Canada

JOANNA LUKAS, MS, PhD Candidate, Dairy Production Systems, Department of Animal Science, University of Minnesota, St. Paul, Minnesota

SHAWN L. B. McKENNA, DVM, PhD, Assistant Professor, Department of Health Management, Atlantic Veterinary College, University of Prince Edward Island, Charlottetown, Prince Edward Island, Canada

D. OWEN RAE, DVM, MPVM, Associate Professor, Department of Large Animal Clinical Sciences, College of Veterinary Medicine, University of Florida, Gainesville, Florida

JEFFREY K. RENEAU, DVM, MS, Professor, Dairy Management, Department of Animal Science, University of Minnesota, St. Paul, Minnesota

PAMELA L. RUEGG, DVM, MPVM, Diplomate, American Board of Veterinary Practitioners (Dairy); Associate Professor, Department of Dairy Science, University of Wisconsin, Madison, Wisconsin

MICHAEL W. SANDERSON, DVM, MS, Diplomate, American College of Veterinary Preventive Medicine (Epidemiology Specialty); Diplomate, American College of Theriogenologists; Associate Professor, Department of Clinical Sciences, Kansas State University, Manhattan, Kansas

YNTE H. SCHUKKEN, DVM, PhD, Director, Quality Milk Production Services, Professor of Epidemiology and Herd Health, Department of Population Medicine and Diagnostic Sciences, College of Veterinary Medicine, Cornell University, Ithaca, New York

BARRETT D. SLENNING, MS, DVM, MPVM, Associate Professor of Dairy Production Medicine, Epidemiology, and Economics, College of Veterinary Medicine, North Carolina State University, Raleigh, North Carolina

CHERYL L. WALDNER, DVM, PhD, Associate Professor, Department of Large Animal Clinical Sciences, Western College of Veterinary Medicine, University of Saskatchewan, Saskatoon, Saskatchewan, Canada

RUTH N. ZADOKS, DVM, PhD, Research Associate, Quality Milk Production Services, Director, Quality Milk Molecular Laboratory, College of Veterinary Medicine, Cornell University, Ithaca, New York

CONTENTS

GOAL STATEMENT

The goal of the *Veterinary Clinics of North America: Food Animal Practice* is to keep practicing veterinarians up to date with current clinical practice in food animal medicine by providing timely articles reviewing the state of the art in food animal care.

ACCREDITATION

The *Veterinary Clinics of North America: Food Animal Practice* offers continuing education credits, awarded by Cummings School of Veterinary Medicine at Tufts University, Office of Continuing Education.

Cummings School of Veterinary Medicine at Tufts University is a designated provider of continuing veterinary medical education. Veterinarians participating in this learning activity may earn up to 6 credits per issue up to a maximum of 18 credits per year. Credits awarded may not apply toward license renewal in all states. It is the responsibility of each participant to verify the requirements of their state licensing board.

Credit can be earned by reading the text material, taking the examination online at ***http://www.theclinics.com/home/cme***, and completing the program evaluation. Following your completion of the test and program evaluation, and review of any and all incorrect answers, you may print your certificate.

TO ENROLL

To enroll in the *Veterinary Clinics of North America: Food Animal Practice* Continuing Veterinary Medical Education Program, call customer service at 1-800-654-2452 or sign up online at ***http://www.theclinics.com/home/cme***. The CVME program is now available at a special introductory rate of $49.95 for a year's subscription.

FORTHCOMING ISSUES

July 2006

Stocker Cattle Management
Mark F. Spire, DVM, MS, and
Robert A. Smith, DVM, MS, *Guest Editors*

November 2006

Parasitology
Lora R. Ballweber, DVM, MS, *Guest Editor*

RECENT ISSUES

November 2005

Emergency Medicine and Critical Care of Cattle
Sheila M. McGuirk, DVM, PhD, and
Simon F. Peek, BVSc, MRCVS, PhD
Guest Editors

July 2005

Bovine Theriogenology
Grant S. Frazer, BVSc, MS, MBA, *Guest Editor*

March 2005

Update in Soft Tissue Surgery
André Desrochers, DMV, MS, *Guest Editor*

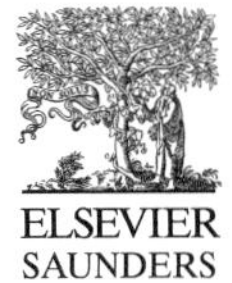

ELSEVIER
SAUNDERS

VETERINARY
CLINICS
Food Animal Practice

Vet Clin Food Anim 22 (2006) xi–xii

Preface

Barnyard Epidemiology and Performance Assessment

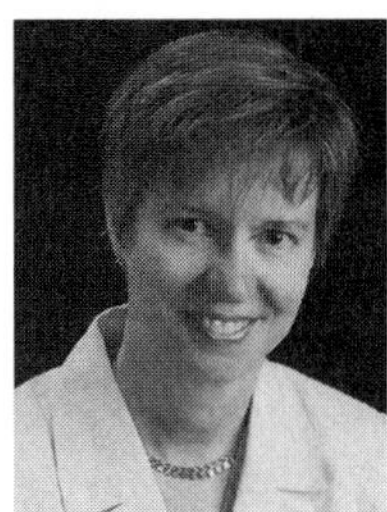

Pamela L. Ruegg, DVM, MPVM
Guest Editor

Veterinarians who serve animal agriculture are working in an exciting environment that is experiencing rapid change. Over the past 2 decades, livestock farms have evolved from small, isolated units where animal health was provided based on reactive care of individual animals to larger, consolidated units where most animal health care is proactively provided based on management of animal groups. In this environment, it is vitally important that veterinarians possess strong quantitative skills that are based on sound epidemiologic principles. The objective of this issue of the *Veterinary Clinics of North America: Food Animal Practice* is to provide a concise volume that describes the practical application of veterinary epidemiology across the spectrum of livestock enterprises.

The authors of the articles included in this issue are veterinarians who combine a broad background of practical experience within specific livestock commodity areas with well-recognized scholarship in veterinary epidemiology. Many practical examples of the uses of epidemiology are included within this volume. Several commodity-specific articles review the use of essential epidemiologic concepts in monitoring animal health and performance. Other articles are more broadly written on specific topics such as on-farm trials, investigation of disease outbreaks, evaluation of diagnostic test outcomes, economic assessment of performance, determination of causality, and the use of simple statistical tools. Newer concepts such as the use

0749-0720/06/$ - see front matter
doi:10.1016/j.cvfa.2005.12.005

of process control to evaluate performance and the uses of molecular epidemiology in veterinary practice are included.

Throughout the editorial process, I have been continually impressed with the enthusiasm that the authors brought to this project and am indebted to them for their excellent work. It has been my privilege to have the honor of reading these articles first and I hope that the readers will gain as much from this volume as I have.

Pamela L. Ruegg, DVM, MPVM
Department of Dairy Science
College of Agricultural & Life Sciences
University of Wisconsin
281 Animal Science Building
1675 Observatory Drive
Madison, WI 53706-1284, USA

E-mail address: plruegg@wisc.edu

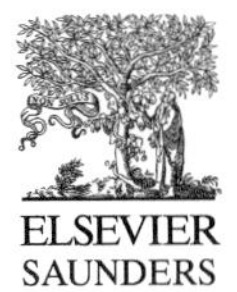

ELSEVIER
SAUNDERS

Vet Clin Food Anim 22 (2006) 1–19

VETERINARY
CLINICS
Food Animal Practice

Basic Epidemiologic Concepts Related to Assessment of Animal Health and Performance

Pamela L. Ruegg, DVM, MPVM

Department of Dairy Science, University of Wisconsin, 1675 Observatory Drive, Madison, WI 53706, USA

Modern animal production systems are increasingly complex. Sustaining long-term performance on these farms depends on the ability of the farm manager to manage many assets, including people, animals, money, machinery, and land. Veterinarians have an important role as experts about animal health and performance. They depend on various types of data to monitor animal health, assure animal well-being, and assess farm profitability. Critical control points for farm profitability include the level of production and quality of the specific commodity (eg, meat or milk), management of animal health, animal comfort, reproductive management, and oversight of the replacement and nutritional programs. A variety of data sources is available to help assess these critical control points. Data sources range from notes written on calendars to sophisticated on-farm computer systems and external industry sources, such as Dairy Herd Improvement Association (DHIA) records and Cattle-Fax. Data sources used for farm analyses vary, depending on the size of the production unit and the technical ability of the farm owner. For example, a recent survey of 587 Wisconsin dairy producers asked managers about the use of computerized records to track antibiotic treatments. The survey found that <4% of those farms with ≤100 lactating cows used computerized records while 65% of Wisconsin dairy producers with >200 lactating cows used computers to track treatments. On small farms, handwritten records may be sufficient for assessing many key performance indicators. However, analysis requires a system designed to be easily accessible. On larger farms, analysis of data can be time-consuming and is unlikely to be performed on a regular basis unless the farm manager or consultant is highly motivated and the data are collected in a manner that allows for easy

E-mail address: plruegg@wisc.edu

doi:10.1016/j.cvfa.2005.12.002 **vetfood.theclinics.com**

summarization. An unsuitable form of data collection can make herd performance problems hard to recognize. On some operations, regardless of herd size, data may be collected on paper but never entered into a computer or collected in a manner that accommodates easy summarization (Fig. 1). This type of data has limited value because it can't easily be analyzed to determine trends or summarized in a fashion that guides management decisions.

Veterinarians are important advisors. They help farmers make sound decisions based upon valid interpretation of data. The identification of key indicators of animal performance and the ability to differentiate between values that reflect normal biologic variation and those that require intervention can be challenging. As part of this advisory role, the veterinary consultant must understand the strengths and weaknesses of data, accurately assess production trends, and evaluate the results of management changes. This article describes some basic epidemiologic concepts about animal performance data. These concepts equip veterinary practitioners with the tools they need to give the best advice. More complex use of data is described in other articles in this volume.

General concepts of epidemiology relevant to animal agriculture

Epidemiology concerns the assessment and control of disease in populations of humans and animals. The related terms "epizootiology" and

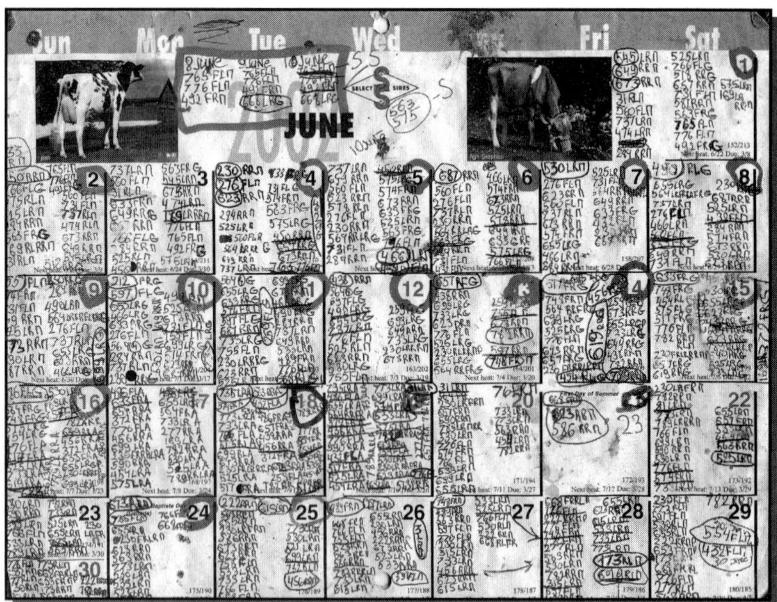

Fig. 1. Calendar obtained from a commercial dairy farm. Data collected in this way is virtually unusable.

"epizootic" were once used to refer specifically to diseases occurring in animal populations. However, these terms are now considered outdated. The term "veterinary epidemiology" is generally preferred because many diseases can affect both animals and humans. Populations can consist of communities, distinct geographical areas, defined production units (eg, farms), or subunits (eg, pens). Many epidemiologic methods were initially developed to control highly infectious diseases that could rapidly spread through regional populations and that often resulted in devastating outcomes, such as decimation of entire animal populations. The characterization and role of infectious agents in transmission of disease is generally termed "qualitative epidemiology." The term quantitative epidemiology commonly refers to the use of epidemiologic methods to measure the amount of disease and the use of comparative observational studies and statistical techniques to evaluate disease and the impact of risk factors on the occurrence of disease. Methods used in quantitative veterinary epidemiology have often originated from national policy programs used to control diseases of public health significance (eg, tuberculosis or brucellosis). Many of these methods are highly relevant for veterinarians involved in modern animal agriculture. Animal agriculture has evolved rapidly from small, isolated herds and flocks, where management was based on individual animals, to larger entities, where management is based on groups of animals. This trend has increased the necessity for veterinarians to develop quantitative skills. Likewise, many food animal veterinarians intuitively perform some type of qualitative epidemiology daily. The challenge for veterinarians is to identify inherent biases in data and to be able to accurately synthesize various data sources to arrive at sound recommendations for their clients.

Understanding performance and disease data

The practitioner should consider the following questions before beginning an assessment of animal health and production data:

- What type of data is available and what are the inherent characteristics of that data?
- What is the best way to summarize this data and arrive at solid conclusions about performance?
- What management decisions will I make based on this data?

Type of management decisions

In some herds, considerable collected information is rarely used for making decisions. Examples of such data include routine reports generated by herd management software or performance monitoring programs, such as DHIA. Often, this data have potential value for making daily decisions but are overlooked because of producer apathy, the perception that data are inaccurate, the complex analysis required to properly use the data, or insufficient time to assess herd performance. When data are routinely collected and not used, that data may become steadily less reliable because the people gathering the data perceive that their efforts are not valued. As data become unreliable a cycle is generated. The data are not used because the information is considered unreliable. Because the information is not used, data collectors become more careless, making data even less reliable. A typical example of unreliable data is the analysis of reasons for culling dairy cows. Many dairy herds record just one reason why each cow is sold. That reason could be, for example, low production, mastitis, or infertility. Analysis of this data often results in misleading conclusions because, while just one reason may be recorded, the decision to replace a dairy cow is generally based several reasons. A more complex assessment of the data could increase the value of the data and ultimately result in more accurate and complete recording of culling reasons. A small volume of accurate data is more useful than large volumes of unreliable data. Veterinary consultants should discourage the collection of data that are rarely used. Efforts at collecting rarely used data should be redirected to efforts at summarizing data that contribute to a decision-making process.

Thresholds versus averages

Before data are summarized, their underlying characteristics and expected use should be considered. Some management decisions are based on identification of animals that meet or exceed a specific threshold. Other decisions may require the determination of a population average. The analysis of nutritional programs by using body condition scores (BCSs) is an excellent example of when thresholds are more useful than population means. Body condition scoring is often performed for beef cattle using a scale of 1 to 9. A BCS of 5 to 6 is considered ideal for cows throughout the production cycle. However, BCSs are used to assess the adequacy of the nutritional program. Thus, the key management decision is based on identification of animals that are either too thin (ie, scores 1–3) or too fat (ie, scores 8–9). The use of an average score can lead to inaccurate decisions because important management decisions are based on an assessment of how many animals fall outside the desired BCS range rather than an assessment of a population average for BCS (Fig. 2). Unless the scores are all extreme, the average BCS of a group will rarely result in a defined management outcome.

Types of data

In general, data are considered either qualitative or quantitative. Qualitative data has to do with characteristics (eg, breed, gender), or yes-or-no data (eg, pregnancy, disease status). Sometimes, qualitative data are called categorical data. This type of data may be the result of a measurement but the

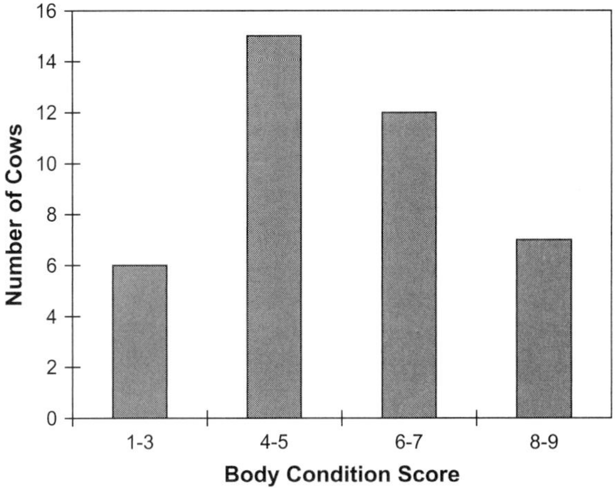

Fig. 2. BCS histogram obtained from beef cattle. This data has an average BCS of 5.4, but 33% of the scores are in unacceptable ranges. (The ideal BCS for all type of cattle is approximately 4–5 [1].)

measurement is used to place the animal within a category. For example, body temperature may be routinely measured on a group of cattle with the objective of categorizing the animals as healthy or febrile, depending on whether or not an animal's temperature exceeds a predetermined threshold, such as 102.5°F. Obviously, measuring the average body temperature of a pen of cattle would be meaningless. What is meaningful is determining how many animals exceed a certain standard for temperature. That determination can be made only by measuring each animal's temperature against that standard. Qualitative data can be referred to as nominal, which normally corresponds to a name or word (eg, breed, gender, pregnancy status). Quantitative data can also be referred to as ordinal, and is used if there is a comparative and progressive basis to the categories (ie, baby calf, heifer, adult). For example, fecal consistency of calves may be assessed using a score of 0 = normal; 1 = semiformed or pasty; 2 = loose but with enough consistency to stay on bedding; and 3 = watery. An increasing score on an ordinal scale will generally be associated with a trend such as deterioration or improvement. Analysis of all types of qualitative data is based on counting events. The data are best summarized by frequency distributions or rates. Generally, the categories have a clearly defined qualitative basis (Table 1). In production agriculture, qualitative data are often useful to set herd goals for animal performance. See related articles in this volume for commodity specific goals. The veterinarian comparing herd data against performance goals should thoroughly understand the context of industry goals. Many data sets used to create performance goals may have inherent biases. Also, the data may be obsolete because of changes in the industry.

Table 1
Frequency of udder hygiene scores for a dairy herd

Udder hygiene score	Frequency	Relative frequency
1: Very clean	40	9.7%
2: Clean	228	55.3%
3: Dirty	105	25.5%
4: Very dirty	39	9.5%
Total	412	100.0%

Quantitative data are based on actual measurements with numerical meaning. When measurements can take any value in a range, the data are termed "continuous." Examples include data on age at weaning, pounds of milk produced, number of pigs weaned, daily weight gain from birth to weaning, and scrotal circumference. When gaps occur between values, the data are referred to as "discrete." Examples include data on BCS, locomotion score, and parity. Some inherently discrete data are commonly summarized using averages. Examples of this kind of data include data on serum antibody titers and minimum inhibitory concentrations of antibiotics. For most discrete data, the most expeditious use is summarization using categories. When categories are used to group continuous data (eg, breeding intervals or percent linear score 0–4), the data are treated as though they were discrete. When clearly defined categories are meaningful, frequency distributions, rates, and ratios are often used to summarize discrete quantitative data (Table 2).

Quantitative data that are truly continuous are summarized by measures of central tendency and measures of dispersion. The objective of these summary statistics is to characterize group performance. Most continuous herd-performance data are summarized using averages. However, measures of variation are often omitted. This oversight can misrepresent group performance, especially the performance of small herds, and may result in incorrect management decisions. For example, assume hypothetical Group A consists of 100 cows. In this group, 50 of the cows produce 40 lbs of milk and 50 of the cows produce 60 lbs of milk. The population mean milk production for Group A would be 50 lbs per cow with a standard deviation of

Table 2
Categorization of continuous data for linear somatic cell score from a 172-cow Ohio dairy farm

	No. of cows			Percentage of cows		
Parity	LSCS 0–3	LSCS 4–6	LSCS $\geq$ 7	LSCS 0–3	LSCS 4–6	LSCS $\geq$ 7
1	41	15	7	68	25	7
2	26	8	3	70	22	8
3+	31	18	9	53	31	16
Total	98	41	16	63	26	10

Abbreviation: LSCS, linear somatic cell score.

10.1 lbs. The performance of Group A is generally consistent and the overall performance may be judged as poor or good, depending on group performance goals. In contrast, consider hypothetical Group B, also consisting of 100 cows. In Group B, 50 of the cows produce 10 lbs of milk and 50 produce 90 lbs of milk. The population mean milk production for Group B is identical to that of Group A (ie, 50 lbs per cow) but the standard deviation is 40.2 lbs/cow. The performance of Group B is highly variable and clearly some problem needs to be addressed. This hypothetical example is obviously extreme. However, it does illustrate the problem of relying solely on group averages. See the article by Reneau and Lukas elsewhere in this volume for more on the importance of understanding the role of variation in identifying changes in animal performance.

The difference between qualitative and quantitative data may be confusing because qualitative data are nonnumeric in nature but are summarized by counts. Another source of confusion is the tendency to categorize quantitative data. An example of assigning categories to quantitative data is when a dairy farm groups "low producers" as cows with daily milk yields of <50 lbs; "average producers" as cows with daily milk yields of 51 to 85 lbs; and "high producers" as cows with daily milk yields >85 lbs. The resulting categories are analyzed as qualitative data. The value of information is considered greatest for continuous data and progressively less valuable for discrete, ordinal, and nominal data, respectively.

Rates, ratios and proportions

Analysis of qualitative and discrete data is based on counting defined events and dividing by the appropriate population (eg, animals at risk for the event) within a specified time period. The most commonly used descriptive statistics for this type of data are proportions, rates, and ratios. Proportions relate the frequency of the animals with the condition of interest to the larger population to which they belong (eg, herd or flock). The numerator is always included in the denominator and the denominator is always the population at risk. For example, to characterize pinkeye treatments in a cow-calf herd at a point in time, the following proportion could be used:

Number of animals treated for pinkeye ÷ number of animals in the herd

In contrast to a proportion, the essential features of a rate are that the numerator is included in the denominator and a time period of observation is specified. Rates can be used to describe changes in the condition of interest over time. Animals included in the numerator are always limited to the same time period as the denominator. When the rate refers to the population in general, rather than a specific subpopulation, it is referred to as a crude rate. To calculate the crude rate of pinkeye treatments, the proportion described above would be changed as follows:

Number of animals treated for pinkeye in June ÷
average number of animals in the herd in June

The determination of which animals to include in the denominator depends on the rigor needed in the analysis. In most instances, when the population of the group is relatively stable, a simple average of the population is sufficient. The average in this case is determined by adding the number of animals present in the herd at the beginning of the time period to the number of animals present at the end the time period and dividing by 2. In other instances, more rigor may be required or the population may be very dynamic and the use of incidence-density (described below) may be more appropriate.

Ratios are used to compare the frequency of two different outcomes and are useful to describe conditions when determining an accurate denominator is difficult. The numerator is not necessarily part of the denominator. An example of a ratio would be one used to describe abortion patterns:

Number of cows that aborted ÷ number of cows with confirmed pregnancies

Not all pregnant animals would have been confirmed. Therefore, animals that aborted but had not yet been confirmed pregnant could be included in the numerator but would not be included in the denominator.

Defining rates

Defining the parameter of interest

Numerous rates are routinely calculated to monitor animal performance. These statistics may be calculated by herd management software, industry programs, or by hand. Often, the indices determined using different programs do not agree. Thus, the veterinary consultant must understand the underlying formulas used in the calculations.

The initial step is to define the population. Which animals should be included and, more importantly, which animals should be excluded? Definitions for both the numerator and the denominator need to be carefully considered. For the numerator, the key issue is defining the disease or production target of interest. For the denominator, the key issue is to define the population at risk. For many diseases, risk varies depending on stage of production cycle or age. The veterinarian may want to define the at-risk population narrowly to ensure that changes can be recognized. The incidence of postparturient paresis (ie, milk fever) in dairy cattle provides an excellent example of differential risk. Milk fever can occur in any age of animal or during any stage of lactation, but the risk of this disease is considerably higher in mature periparturient cows than it is for either first lactation animals or cows in the later stages of lactation. While all animals are technically at risk, the inclusion of the entire population of lactating cows in the denominator may hamper detection of important changes in disease incidence (Table 3).

The numerator should include animals that have experienced the event of interest. These events may be based on the occurrence of symptoms (eg, diarrhea, abnormal milk, retained placenta) or events (eg, twin births, failure to reach a performance target). Detection bias can be a significant problem on many farms. In many instances, treatments, rather than detection of disease or symptoms, are recorded in computerized software. This means that animals that exhibit mild signs of disease but are not treated may not be noted. The veterinarian should ensure that personnel responsible for recording events understand what to look for with each disease or event of interest. Practicing veterinarians should not feel constrained by technical "rules" related to the development of rates, but should feel free to evaluate herds based on useful definitions of populations at risk and diagnostic criteria for events of interest pertinent to making farm decisions.

Defining the time span

A critical step in the calculation of rates is to define the time span. A basic rule of rates is that each animal should only experience the event of interest once during a time period. Therefore, the time period should be defined so that it encompasses a unit that is meaningful to the production unit and the disease. Typically, rates are calculated using one of three methods. The first is the rolling time frame or rolling method. The second is the cohort approach. The third is the current-data method. When the rolling method is used, all of the herd's animals that fit the defined population criteria are included in the statistic for every time period regardless of when the event

Table 3
Different populations at risk of disease in a hypothetical 500-cow dairy herd

Population at risk used in calculation	Number of animals calved in time period	Number of cases of milk fever	Estimated incidence
All lactating cows (n = 500)	NA	4	4/500 = 0.008 or < 1%
All cows that calved in the time period	80	4	4/80 = 0.05 or 5%
Only multiparous cows that calved in the time period[a]	40	4	4/40 = 0.10 or 10%

Abbreviation: NA, not applicable.
[a] These cows are at the highest risk for the disease.

occurred. With this method, computation is easy. However, the method is very slow to demonstrate changes in recent performance and may not be useful for evaluating recent management changes.

The cohort method is calculated by following a cohort of animals defined by some characteristic. For example, reproductive performance, production, or somatic cell count could be followed for cohorts of cows defined by month of calving. This method can be more abstract to interpret because it may require calculations involving the same statistics for several cohorts. The method is often useful for retrospective analyses but can be unwieldy and require complex interpretation.

The current-data method is calculated by including a cohort of only animals with the most current data in the index. Using this approach, peak milk production would be calculated only for the cohort of animals that were peaking. For example, peak milk could be defined as the test-day milk for animals that were 40 to 70 days in milk at the last test. Another use for the current method is in calculating days to first service for a cohort of cows that received a first service in the specified time period (eg, 1 month). This method has the advantage of being very current and reflecting the current herd situation. However, this method can be misleading if there are few animals that meet the criteria of the cohort. Table 4 illustrates differences for several management parameters calculated using each of three approaches in one herd. Each of the methods can be used successfully, provided the assessor is aware of the underlying definitions and populations.

Common morbidity rates

Morbidity rates describe the level of disease in a population (Table 5). Crude rates specify neither disease nor host characteristics and differ depending upon whether new cases or existing cases are of interest. Incidence rates describe the probability of a new case developing during a stated time interval. For most diseases, incidence rates are the most important measures for monitoring the success (or failure) of disease control strategies. Cases

Table 4
Management indices in one herd using three methods of determining the population

Parameter	Rolling[a] (n)	Cohort[b] (n)	Current[c] (n)
Peak milk (lb.)	110 (84)	102 (12)	113 (10)
Days to first service	79 (102)	54 (2)	80 (4)
Somatic cell count	NC	291 (20)	286 (148)

Abbreviations: N, number of cows; NC, not calculated.

[a] Data included for all lactating cows with non-zero values.

[b] Data included for cows that calved in January.

[c] Data for peak milk includes cows that were 40–70 days in milk at the last test date. Data for days to first service includes cows that received their first breeding in March; Somatic cell count data included for all cows that had somatic cell count values at the last test date.

Table 5
Rate of pneumonia treatments for calves (n = 10)

	Week 1								Week 2							
Calf	1	2	3	4	5	6	7	DAR	8	9	10	11	12	13	14	DAR
1	H	H	H	H	H	H	H	7	H	H	H	H	H	H	H	7
2	H	H	H	H	**RX**	RX	RX	4	RX	H	H	H	H	H	H	6
3	H	H	H	H	H	H	H	7	**RX**	RX	RX	RX	H	H	H	3
4	H	H	H	H	H	H	H	7	D[b]							0
5	H	H	H	H	H	H	**RX**	6	RX	RX	RX	H	H	H	H	4
6	H	H	H	H	H	H	H	7	H	**RX**	RX	RX	RX	H	H	3
7	H	D						1								0
8	H	H	H	H	H	H	H	7	**RX**	RX	RX	RX	RX	RX	H	1
9	H	H	H	H	H	H	H	7	**RX**	RX	RX	RX	H	H	H	3
10	H	H	H	**RX**	RX	RX	RX	3	H	H	H	H	H	H	H	7
								56								34

	Week 1	Week 2
Average population at Risk	(10 + 9)/2 = 9.5	(8 + 8)/2 = 8
Days at risk	56 calf-days	34 calf-days
New treatments	3	4
Total treatments	3	6
Incidence of treatment[a]	3/10 = 30%	4/6 = 67%
Prevalence of treatment	3/9.5 = 32%	6/8 = 75%
Incidence density	3/56 = .054 (5.4 treatments per 100 calf days)	4/34 = .118 (11.8 treatments per 100 calf days)
Relative Risk of Treatment in week 2		11.8/5.4 = 2.2

Boldface indicates initial treatment.

Abbreviations: D, died of other cause; DAR, days at risk in time period; H, healthy; RX, treatment.

[a] Denominator is animals at risk at the begining of the time period.

that exist at the beginning of the time period are not included. The denominator of an incidence rate is usually the population at risk at the beginning of the time period. The numerator is the number of animals that develop the attribute or disease during the time period. Animals that have the condition at the beginning of the time period are not included in either the numerator or the denominator. For example, the incidence of lameness could be calculated as:

Number of cows that became lame during June ÷
average number of cows in the herd in the beginning of June

It can be more difficult to define denominators when the risk period is not as clearly defined or when the disease exists in a subclinical state for long periods of time.

Incidence-density is a more precise measure of incidence and is calculated using the same numerator as above. The denominator is calculated by adding together all the days at risk for each individual in the population at risk. An animal ceases to be at risk once it develops the disease. The unit is therefore the number of cases, treatments, or events per animal-day at risk (Table 5). This figure is especially useful when used in large populations. However, collecting data for this method requires excellent record-keeping to monitor dynamic animal populations.

Prevalence rate is a static measure of disease frequency. It is the fraction of the population that is diseased or possesses the attribute at any one point in time. The point in time can be a single day or may be a defined time period, such as a month (period prevalence). Both new and existing cases are counted. For example, the monthly prevalence of lame cows would be calculated as:

Number of lame cows in June ÷ average number of cows in the herd in June

Obviously, for rates related to morbidity to be reliable, they must be based on precise definition and accurate detection of disease. For many diseases, the difference between a new case and an existing case may be subtle and depend on meticulous detection methods.

Chronic diseases can have higher prevalence than incidence, as the number of animals at risk will steadily decrease as more animals become diseased. The prevalence of disease within a herd is a function of incidence and duration. This relationship can be demonstrated by using hospital pen populations in animal production units to represent prevalence. Consider a hypothetical dairy herd containing 1000 lactating cows. This herd experiences one new case of clinical mastitis per day. To calculate incidence, the numerator would be 30 and the denominator 1000. Monthly incidence is thus 3%. The sick-pen population would represent prevalence. That is, the number of cows sick per 1000 cows per day. If the duration in the sick pen were 1 day, one cow would enter and leave the sick pen each day, so the prevalence of clinical mastitis would always be one case per 1000 cows per day. If the incidence doubled to two new cases per day but the duration in the sick pen remained 1 day, the sick-pen population (prevalence) would also double and would be stable at two cases per 1000 cows per day. Alternatively, if the incidence of mastitis remained stable at one case per day, but the duration of time in the sick pen doubled to 2 days, the prevalence (sick-pen population) would also increase to two cases per 1000 cows per day. Incidence is generally strongly influenced by herd control strategies. Duration can be influenced by such factors as death, culling, and treatment efficacy. These factors can have a strong influence on estimates of disease prevalence within a herd (Table 5).

Summarizing quantitative data

Computerized herd management programs and industry reports are filled with quantitative data. Interpretation of the data depends on an understanding of the underlying distributions of the population and the typical characteristics of the specific values.

Distributions

Data that are normally distributed form a bell shaped curve and have a mean, median, and mode that are approximately equal (Fig. 3). The mean, median, and mode for the mature equivalent milk yield data shown in Fig. 3 are 26,655, 26,690 and 26,333 lbs, respectively. Continuous data that have a wide range of values usually follow a normal distribution pattern. Most direct production and performance parameters are, to at least some degree, normally distributed.

Data that are not normally distributed are termed "skewed" (Fig. 4). Compared to the mean and the mode, the median is generally more representative of the central tendency of skewed data because it indicates the midpoint of the number of pieces of data and is unaffected by the underlying value of the parameter. The mean, median and mode for the somatic cell count data shown in Fig. 4 are 181,190, 65,000 and 11,000 cells per mL, respectively.

Measures of central tendency

Often, continuous quantitative data are used to characterize animal performance. Three basic measures of central tendency are used to analyze continuous quantitative data. Arithmetic means (ie, averages) are the most commonly used statistic. Means are simple to calculate and appear to be easily understandable. They have an important disadvantage in that they are easily influenced by extreme values, especially in small herds or flocks.

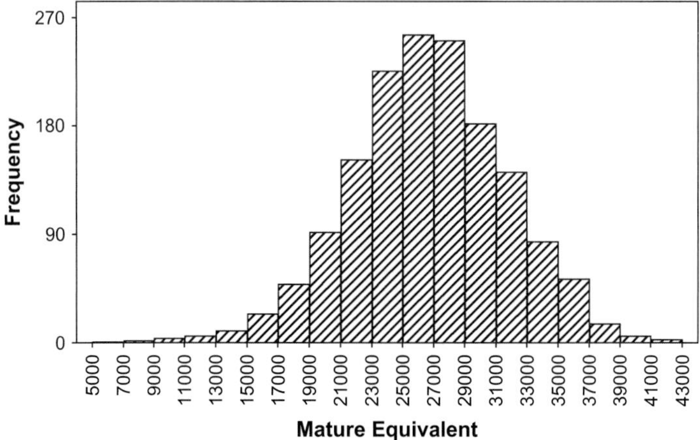

Fig. 3. Frequency histogram of mature equivalent milk yield that approximates a normal distribution on a dairy farm with 1600 cows.

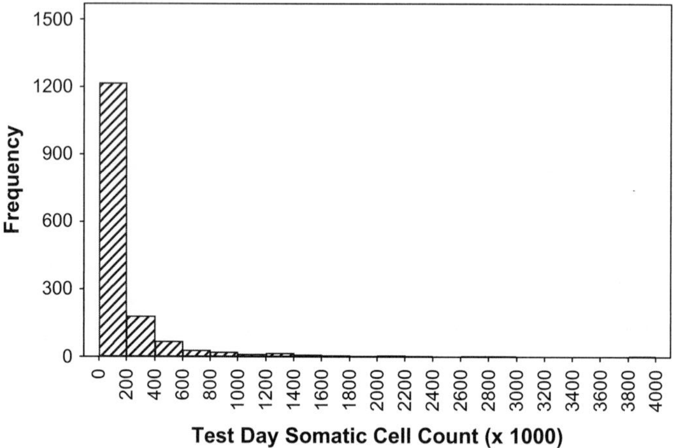

Fig. 4. Frequency histogram of somatic cell count data from a dairy herd with 1600 cows.

This disadvantage is especially important when data are not normally distributed or when few numbers contribute to the average.

When comparing averages over time, rolling averages, such as rolling herd averages, can help smooth out fluctuations stemming from small numbers or isolated extreme values. However, data used to compile rolling averages occurred retrospectively. Thus, rolling averages exhibit considerable lag for determination of herd performance problems. This means that rolling averages may not be as useful as other measures in recognizing and responding to immediate problems (Fig. 5).

Weighted averages are used for some statistics to ensure that each animal contributes equally to a statistic. Similarly, weighted averages may be useful for monitoring statistics on small subsets of animals where the number of animals contributing varies between measurement periods. For example,

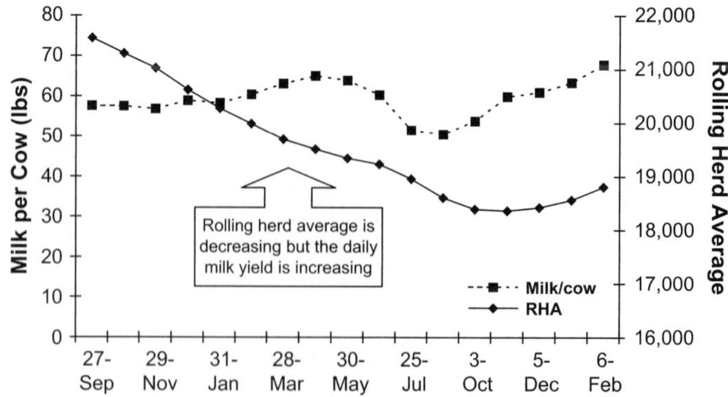

Fig. 5. Rolling herd average versus test-day milk from a 220-cow Indiana dairy.

a farm manager monitoring age at first calving for cows that calved during a specified time period in a small herd (< 100 cows) may find widely varying numbers of animals that contribute to the statistic each month (Table 6). By using a weighted rolling average, variation due to the individual unit (eg, animals, month) is minimized.

Medians (ie, 50th percentile) are an underused statistic. They are independent of the value of the underlying measurement and are not routinely found on most performance reports. A median is simply the midpoint of an ordered range of values. Any time that data is grouped by percentiles or ranked, a median can be estimated. In the field, medians can be easily calculated from data charted on histogram-type forms (Table 7). Medians are not affected by extreme values and are especially useful when data are not normally distributed. Many of the values routinely examined to assess animal performance are not normally distributed and are better represented by medians.

The mode is simply the most frequently occurring value. The mode is rarely used but may be useful if one value makes up a large portion of the data set. A disadvantage of using mode as a measure of central tendency is that there can be several different modes in any individual data set. Modes are not generally calculated in sources available to veterinarians.

Measures of dispersion

The standard deviation is one measure of variability. The standard deviation defines the width of a normal distribution. In a normal distribution, 65% of values are within one standard deviation of the mean, 95% of values are within two standard deviations of a mean, and 99% are within three

Table 6
Calculation of age at first calving using various methods

Month	N	Average days to first calving[a]	Four-month weighted rolling average[b]	Four-month rolling average[c]
July	4	754	NA	NA
August	1	735	NA	NA
September	3	763	NA	NA
October	1	784	758	759
November	5	769	765	763
December	8	746	758	766
January	8	756	767	764
February	9	755	755	757
March	2	725	750	746
Mean		754	754	

Abbreviations: N, number of cows calving for first time; NA, not applicable.

[a] Calculated as a simple average of the number of animals contributing each month.

[b] Calculated over 4 months by weighting each month by the number of animals contributing. For example for October: [(4 × 754) + (1 × 735) + (3 × 763) + (1 × 784)] ÷ 9.

[c] Calculated by adding 7 months of averages and dividing by 4.

Table 7
Body condition scoring form GROUP: CLOSE UP DRY DATE: Jan 2006 SCORER: PLR

	Number of cows																								
BCS	1	2	3	4	5	6	7	8	9	10	11	12	13	14	15	16	17	18	19	20	21	22	23	24	25
>4.00	X	X	X	X	X	X	X	X																	
4.00	X	X	X	X	X	X	X	X	X																
3.75	X	X	X																						
3.50	X	X																							
3.25																									
3.00																									
2.75																									
2.50																									
2.25																									
2.00																									
<2.00																									

Median = 4.00.

standard deviations. The coefficient of variation is the standard deviation divided by the mean. One rule of thumb asserts that a coefficient of variation of more than 30 (ie, the standard deviation greater than 30% of the mean) indicates a great deal of variability in the data. The standard deviation is an important component of statistical control process analysis. See the related chapter in this issue by Reneau and Lukas about statistical control process analysis. Herd problems, as opposed to individual animal problems, can be identified by comparing the mean value to the standard deviation. In Table 8, the mean age at first calving for both farms is too old, but the standard deviation for Farm 1 indicates that the performance at that farm is consistently poor, as demonstrated by the relatively small standard deviation, in comparison with the highly variable performance of Farm 2. Probably Farm 2 has a small number of animals influencing the average while the performance of most animals may be acceptable. Many recommendations for herd management are directed at increasing uniformity of performance. Decreases in the standard deviation for a herd parameter may be a good indication that overall management of that area has improved.

Variability in data can make it difficult to interpret averages. The standard deviation of an average is called the standard error. Standard errors are calculated by dividing the standard deviation by the square root of the number of pieces of data in the average (N). A rough approximation of the standard error can be estimated for small data sets (ie, <15 data points) by dividing the range, which is the difference between the largest

Table 8
Age at first calving for two herds

Farm	No. of cows	Mean age at first calving (days)	Standard deviation (days)
1	39	1043	316
2	36	1192	710

and the smallest value, by N, the number of pieces of data. Obviously, the standard error decreases as N increases and this is why analysts can be more confident of the population means of larger data sets. Confidence intervals are calculated using standard errors. An average plus or minus approximately two standard errors will account for 95% of the possible values of that average. Confidence intervals can be used to differentiate a mean from a previous level. A value outside of the confidence interval is significantly different from the average. A value that is different than the average but within the confidence interval may be the result of chance. See the article by Slenning in this volume for more information about comparing averages. Understanding the influence of variation is important in interpreting responses to management change.

A large amount of variability in a performance parameter can make it difficult to determine if differences are due to management changes or other influences. For example, Table 9 demonstrates every-other-day milk shipments for one dairy with 100 cows for two separate months. Due to heat stress, milk shipments varied considerably more in August than in January. In this herd, a 500-lb increase above the average shipped in the bulk tank in August would still fall within the 95% confidence interval. By comparison, the same increase in January would exceed the upper bound of the 95% confidence interval. In other words, the response to a small management change will be easier to detect in January than in August because normal daily production variations are smaller in January.

As noted above, standard error is calculated by dividing the standard deviation by the square of the number of pieces of data. It is important to recognize that confidence intervals decrease as the sample size (ie, population or subpopulations included in the calculation) increases. This means that management indices are more useful for measuring change related to large herds than small herds because the effect of individual cow variations is minimized when many pieces of data are included in the calculation. An adequate sample size is especially important for parameters with more variations.

Confounders of production

When evaluating the relationship between two factors, such as between nutritional management and milk produced per cow per day, other

Table 9
Every-other-day milk shipments for one dairy in August and January

Parameter	August	January
Average milk shipped (lbs)	13,541	15,005
Standard deviation	1,701	503
Standard error	439	130
95% Confidence interval	12,680–14,402	14,751–15,260
Coefficient of variation	13%	3%

Table 10
Conception rate by artificial insemination technician

Technician	No. bred	No. conceived	Conception rate
A	360	198	0.55
B	200	88	0.44
Total	560	286	

extraneous factors may affect the relationship that is being studied. The epidemiologic term for factors that influence outcome variables, such as milk production, is "confounder". Confounders are risk factors associated with both the outcome variable being assessed and the risk factor being considered. Essentially, a confounder is a factor that when controlled may reduce or eliminate the effect of the variable being studied.

Many factors can confuse interpretation of production values associated with animal performance. In the dairy industry, confounders for milk production may include stage of lactation, number of times milked, percent of herd in first lactation, fat percentage, breed, culling patterns, and season. Other confounders exist for other animal production systems. When assessing management changes, the effects of these confounders must be considered. In the dairy industry, for example, if most of the herd is in early lactation when instituting a management change, production will naturally decrease as the herd average days-in-milk increases. Unless the confounder is recognized, the management change might be interpreted as detrimental rather than beneficial. Adjusted performance measures may be used to offset the bias stemming from confounders. A special type of confounding can occur when an unrecognized confounder can actually reverse the direction of an association. This type of confounding is referred to as Simpson's paradox. Simpson's paradox can be demonstrated by a hypothetical comparison of conception rates involving two artificial insemination technicians. A

Table 11
Conception rate by artificial insemination technician for repeat breeders

Technician	No. bred	No. conceived	Conception rate
A	120	18	0.15
B	120	24	0.20
Total	240	42	

Table 12
Conception rate by artificial insemination technician for first services

Technician	No. bred	No. conceived	Conception rate
A	240	180	0.75
B	80	64	0.80
Total	320	244	

practitioner reviewing such data in Table 10 may feel compelled to send Technician B back to breeding school. The practitioner would be wise, however, to explore the data in more depth before proceeding (Tables 11 and 12). The type of animal being bred is confounding the relationship between technician and conception rate. In this example, Technician B had a higher conception rate for both repeat breeders and first services. Technician A however, bred more first services. When the data was combined, the resulting conception rate was misleading.

Summary

Veterinarians have an important role in advising clients regarding the use of farm management data. An understanding of the basic concepts of veterinary epidemiology is important for accurate assessment of animal health and performance. Data collected should be used on a regular basis and evaluated in a simple fashion that properly characterizes the group, herd, or individual animal.

Further readings

Dohoo I, Martin W, Stryhm H. Veterinary epidemiologic research. Charlottetown (Canada): AVC Inc.; 2003.

Martin SW, Meek AW, Willeberg P. Veterinary epidemiology. Ames (IA): Iowa State University Press; 1987.

Noordhuizen JPTM, Frankena K, Thrusfield MV, et al. Application of quantitative methods in veterinary epidemiology. Wageningen (The Netherlands): Wageningen Press; 2001.

Schwabe CW, Riemann HP, Franti CE. Epidemiology in veterinary practice. Philadelphia: Lea and Febiger; 1977.

Smith RD. Veterinary clinical epidemiology. Boston: Butterworths; 1991.

Van Belle G. Statistical rules of thumb. New York: John Wiley and Sons; 2002.

Reference

[1] Browne MF, Hall JB, et al. Body condition scoring beef cows. Virginia Cooperative Extension. Available at: http://www.ext.vt.edu/pubs/beef/400-795/400-795.html. Accessed December 11, 2005.

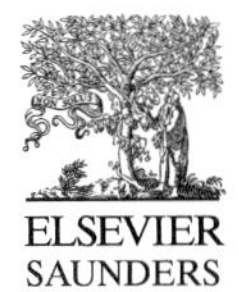

ELSEVIER
SAUNDERS

Vet Clin Food Anim 22 (2006) 21–33

VETERINARY
CLINICS
Food Animal Practice

Epidemiology: A Foundation for Dairy Production Medicine

David F. Kelton, DVM, MSc, PhD

Department of Population Medicine, Ontario Veterinary College, University of Guelph, Guelph, Ontario, Canada N1G 2W1

Epidemiology is defined as the study of the frequency, distribution, and determinants of health and disease in populations [1]. The essence of that definition is the basis of dairy production medicine, whereby we strive to optimize production through the elimination and control of disease and the implementation of management practices that promote animal health, welfare, productivity, and profitability. To be successful, health management programs must be built on a solid foundation of health and production records that can be used to define the frequency and distribution of events within the herd and used in aggregate to identify and investigate important risk factors, or causes, for these health and disease events.

Epidemiology has traditionally been seen as a fairly narrow discipline, with a focus on public health and food safety applications; however, in the last decade or so, the role of the discipline in veterinary medicine has broadened significantly to include many aspects directly applicable to clinical and preventive medicine. These aspects include the evaluation and interpretation of tests, outbreak investigation, critical appraisal of scientific literature, and the design and evaluation of clinical trials. A number of textbooks on veterinary clinical epidemiology and food animal production medicine have large sections devoted to the principles of epidemiology and their application to the practice of clinical and production medicine [2–5].

Health management programs are developed through an iterative process that has become known as the health management cycle [5]. In its simplest form, this cycle includes the setting of performance goals, the gathering of data to assess current performance relative to those goals, the development and implementation of actions to move the herd closer to the goals in instances where they are not being met, and the continued assessment of continuously available data to verify that progress is being made. Goals for

E-mail address: dkelton@uoguelph.ca

doi:10.1016/j.cvfa.2005.12.003 ***vetfood.theclinics.com***

performance parameters must be SMART: specific, measurable, attainable, realistic, and timely [5]. As each individual target is met, the goals can be enhanced or reinforced, depending on the overall management goals of the dairy unit.

Epidemiology is a broad discipline that encompasses many inter-related areas of activity. At least three of these areas have a direct application to dairy production medicine and are explored in some detail in this article. The first area is quantitative epidemiology and includes a range of activities, from counting clinical cases to the development of complex hierarchic decision models. The monitoring component of dairy production medicine is based on these quantitative principles. The second area is the evaluation and interpretation of "tests" that are applied at various levels of the health management cycle and that serve as the basis for diagnostic and monitoring systems. The third area is the critical evaluation of the published scientific literature in the practice of evidence-based veterinary medicine. Evaluating the strengths and weaknesses of evidence facilitates the appropriate use of knowledge in support of health management decisions.

Monitoring dairy herd performance

Measuring the current performance of a dairy herd is an integral part of the health management cycle. Monitoring has been defined as the systematic, consistent, and regular use of records to evaluate health and performance and to aid in the development of interventions [6,7].

Monitoring requires readily available data that are appropriate to the hierarchic level for the parameter of interest. For instance, mastitis can be attributed at the quarter level or the cow level, and although there is value in knowing which quarter is infected with which pathogen, for monitoring purposes, it is generally most useful to know which cows are infected.

To be performed regularly, the act of monitoring must be performed quickly. Few veterinarians are financially compensated for time spent evaluating records but are generally well compensated for on-farm activities. Hence, a good monitoring program makes efficient use of records to quickly identify areas of concern and generates and refines "questions" pertaining to these areas that are best addressed at the farm while interacting with the owner/manager and observing the animals and their environment.

Sources of dairy herd data

Dairy veterinarians generally have access to a broad range of health and performance data, although some types of data are clearly more plentiful than other types. Dairy herd data can be grouped into three categories based on their availability. At the first level (most plentiful), most dairy producers can provide some data pertaining to animal inventories and milk production. Milk production data may be available at the aggregate group level (volume of milk produced by the herd or group on a given day), periodically at the cow level (milk per cow per day available monthly through Dairy Herd Improvement [DHI] programs), or continuously at the cow level (milk per cow per milking available through computer software linked to electronic milking parlors with individual-cow identification). Second-level data (less plentiful) include somatic cell counts (SCC) and reproductive records (breedings and breeding outcomes) for individual cows. SCC data are usually available for herds enrolled in milk recording programs, whereas reproductive records are maintained but are not always in a readily accessible form. Third-level data (least plentiful) are records of disease and management events (vaccination, deworming, and so forth). Although many dairy producers record disease events of interest/importance for their herd and their interests, there is tremendous variability in the rigor and consistency of disease recording [8]. Variability in disease definitions and reporting continues to present challenges to potential third-party users.

Data vary hierarchically in how they are collected and how they are used. Lameness and mastitis events can be recorded at the leg/quarter level or the animal level but are often used at the management-group, parity, stage-of-lactation, or herd level. Data also vary in where they are stored, from paper records to computerized herd management programs. Although the former can be quite meticulous and detailed, they are not easily summarized for monitoring purposes. Computerized systems offer the capacity to store large volumes of data and tools to quickly manipulate the data. Computer-based record systems have not yet been widely adopted by all dairy producers: many larger dairy farms use computer-based systems, but for the most part, smaller producers still tend to rely on paper record systems. It is fortunate, however, that many herds enrolled in milk recording through DHI organizations have electronic production, health, and management data available even the farm owner/manager is not a computer user.

Summarizing dairy production and health data

Dairy health and production data are generally of two distinct types: continuous data and categoric data. Continuous data include most measures of milk production, SCC, time intervals such as days open, and animal heights and weights. Although their central tendencies and variability are often summarized using means (averages) and SD, many are not normally distributed and should more appropriately be represented by medians and interquartile ranges. In some specific cases, such as SCC, which are usually right-skewed, logarithmic transformations are used to produce more normally distributed linear scores, which can then be averaged.

Categoric data include the reproductive attributes of open, bred, or pregnant, and the binary conditions of diseased or not diseased. These data are predominantly count data and often summarized as incidence risk (eg, conception risk being the number of pregnancies divided by the number of breedings in a defined time period) or incidence rate (eg, annual mastitis incidence rate being number of cases of mastitis during the year divided by the number of cow years at risk) [1,9]. It may be worthwhile to note that many dairy performance parameters are incorrectly called "rates" rather than 'risk." The aforementioned conception risk is more commonly referred to as conception rate, even though there is no specified time component to the parameter. It is likely that discussion about risk versus rate is of interest to only a limited audience and is not pursued further at this stage.

Data analysis activities should be driven by specific questions rather than by a nontargeted scanning of available data. In that context, the choice of the appropriate way to report or display a summary parameter depends on the question to be answered. One can report a mean or median value to represent the central tendency of a group of observations; the minimum, maximum, or extreme percentiles to describe the range of those observations; or the SD, variance, interquartile range, or confidence interval to describe the variability within the group of observations. Beyond numeric representations, one can view data graphically as histograms, scatter plots, or survival curves. A histogram of a reproductive parameter such as days open for pregnant cows is often much more informative than a simple mean because it is the variability around the mean that often drives the economic loss, through cows conceiving too early or too late relative the production profile of the herd. Scatter plots of SCC or linear scores from two successive DHI tests are often used to evaluate the change in subclinical mastitis from one test date to the next. Although a 2 × 2 table can be used to present the same information, the visual graphic allows the interpreter to account for cases in which a cow moves from just below the cut-point to just above as being attributable to normal variation. Finally, survival curves provide a very effective way of assessing reproductive parameters such as days to first service, especially in herds using complete herd heat synchronization programs; the steep drop in percentage of cows not bred at the target days in milk is a much better measure of adherence to the program than the mean of the parameter.

Monitoring parameters are often examined over time, with one time period being compared with another. It needs to be recognized that although calendar time is the most commonly used time scale, it is not the only one. Realigning data based on animal age (parity) or stage of lactation is common practice in dairy production medicine and often proves more useful than calendar time in identifying patterns of interest. For example, plotting clinical mastitis cases caused by environmental pathogens by days in milk at diagnosis may help distinguish between a problem caused by environmental streptococci and coliform bacteria based on their underlying epidemiologic patterns.

Challenges of using dairy data

There are many challenges to using data from dairy herds for assessing health and productivity. Small herd or group sizes, inaccurate or inconsistent disease definitions, missing or incomplete data, and moderate to large variability among individual members of the herd or group can produce meaningless or erroneous summary parameters.

News versus history

To be of most value, monitoring parameters should represent current events in the herd or group. To that end, it is most useful to select monitoring parameters that minimize the lag between the management event and the measured outcome [10]. For instance, it is clearly more useful to monitor the days to conception rather than the days to calving if one is interested in assessing the breeding program for replacement heifers. Some parameters of interest will have a lag that is unavoidable, such as the delay between a breeding event and the determination of its success; however, we generally strive to keep this lag as short as possible. We must also recognize that efforts to shorten the lag too much may not be ideal. Although ultrasonography facilitates the diagnosis of bovine pregnancy as early as 25 to 30 days after breeding, the recognition that an associated "normal" pregnancy loss of up to 10% by day 40 postbreeding may adversely effect the utility of the early pregnancy diagnosis, unless there is a subsequent verification at some point after 40 days.

Statistical and biologic significance

Summary parameters can cover various periods of time, from weeks to years, depending on the density of the observations and the frequency of the monitoring activity. Herd or group size becomes a consideration, particularly in small herds (less than 100 cows) in which the frequency of some events generates very small to insignificant summary values. Changes to one or more monitoring parameters from month to month are of interest, although we are often frustrated by the inability to determine whether what appears to be a biologically significant change is statistically different or merely a result of normal variation. There is often a temptation to extend the period of observation by creating parameters such as rolling averages to capture enough events or observations to produce statistically significant results. The problem with this approach is that by expanding the time frame, we are including more and more historical data and giving the parameter of interest far too much momentum [10]. At the end of the day, we often have to accept that we may not be able to wait until we have statistically significant changes in a parameter before we act, especially in small herds. This is part of the reality of practicing production medicine and clinical epidemiology in dairy herds. A possible solution to this dilemma may be the application of techniques such as the statistical process control methodology to dairy herd health and production data [11]. This topic is addressed in detail elsewhere in this issue.

Consistent disease definition

A major challenge to summarizing disease events at the farm, practice, regional, or national level is the lack of consistent definitions for diseases of interest and performance parameters. This issue has been addressed on a number of occasions [8,12]. At the farm level, as herd size increases and the number of persons (owners, managers, farm workers) involved in identifying and recording animal events increases, the variability in disease definition also increases. Even simple diseases such as mastitis, lameness, or ketosis can be recognized at various levels, but are usually recorded simply as present or absent. For example, ketosis can manifest clinically or subclinically, may be primary or secondary to another disease, might be identified by way of an active or passive monitoring program, and could be defined by a "positive" result from any of a number of tests, from olfactory detection of ketone odor to the application of powders, tablets, or sticks to milk, urine, or blood. Each of these detection methods is a test with its own sensitivity and specificity [13]. It follows that depending on the detection method, the estimated prevalence or incidence of ketosis may vary considerably, even among the same group of animals. Although it may be unrealistic to expect uniformity of disease definition across herds, the within-herd (and possibly the within–veterinary practice) standardization of disease definition should be considered.

Missing data—or not?

Missing data can have a profound impact on the inference drawn from health or performance data. Missing data can be of two varieties: animals intentionally removed from the herd and excluded from consideration or animals, observations, or events that occurred but did not get recorded. Animals that have been removed from the herd (culled) or that have been designated for removal could be included or excluded in the calculation of many monitoring parameters. For instance, the inclusion of cows culled during the preceding 12 months because they did not get pregnant by some stage of lactation increases the herd average days open (pessimist's parameter), whereas their exclusion decreases it (optimist's parameter). In reality, it is likely that the truth lies somewhere in between and that both options may be biased [10]. It is likely unreasonable to expect that all bias should or could be removed from monitoring parameters, but those who use the information should understand how the parameter was constructed, which individuals were included or excluded, and thus, in which direction the potential bias will drive the parameter.

Missing data that result from incomplete event records are more problematic because they often are not verifiable. A missing milk weight or SCC for an individual cow on a DHI test date for which all other cows in the herd have a milk weight can be readily identified as a true missing piece of information; however, the absence of a displaced abomasum event from the record of a third-lactation cow could mean that the cow did not have a displacement, that she had a displacement that was not identified, or that she had a displacement that was identified but not recorded. The frustration with these missing events is that they are virtually impossible to verify unless one has access to veterinary invoices/records that are sufficiently detailed to attribute specific disease diagnoses to individual cows. Even under circumstances in which veterinary records are complete and detailed, however, disease events that are not diagnosed or treated by a veterinarian may not be verifiable.

Diagnosis of animal and herd "disease"

Dairy production medicine is ultimately concerned with identifying problems or bottlenecks on dairy farms and developing strategies to relieve those bottlenecks. A major part of that process involves making diagnoses at the individual-animal level or at the group level. The hypothetico-deductive diagnostic process [14] involves developing a finite list of possible diagnoses for a particular problem or condition and narrowing that list through the application of activities or actions that rule-in or rule-out members of the list. Invariably, this process involves the application of a number of "tests," with test defined in its broadest sense as something that is used to differentiate, classify, or categorize individuals.

In the context of dairy production medicine, the detailed analysis of records is an important part of the herd-level diagnostic process. Although routine monitoring of certain parameters can point to areas that are in need of attention, a second level of more thorough records analysis is often used to narrow the list of causes for the problem. For instance, routine monitoring activities may uncover an elevation in the herd average SCC or an increase in clinical mastitis cases over a defined period of time, signaling a mastitis problem. This finding should illicit an examination of a series of second-order herd parameters aimed at better defining the mastitis problem and directing the veterinarian's on-farm activities to pinpoint the source of the problem. Examination of SCC or clinical case records for subsets of the herd, based on parity, stage of lactation, or management group, should help to define the problem as involving primarily the lactating herd or a recently fresh cohort. The culturing of frozen stored milk samples may help narrow the search if there is a predominant pathogenic organism involved. Ultimately, the search should lead to a farm visit and an interactive outbreak investigation whereby the veterinarian collects and analyzes additional data.

The aforementioned investigation activity is in reality an outbreak investigation, a process based on the fundamental principles of epidemiology. Defining the problem, identifying the source, removing the inciting cause or causes, and implementing a preventive program to decrease the likelihood of reoccurrence are its major components. Although dairy practitioners may not recognize it as such, they are confronted by "outbreaks" of mastitis, calf diarrhea, and lameness on a regular basis. Although they seldom use the terms "attack rate" and "epidemic curve" to describe their approach to investigating these problems, the principles are clearly employed.

An examination of the approach to diagnosis would be incomplete without a discussion of the application and interpretation of tests. By definition, tests are used to classify or categorize individuals or groups. As such, tests include everything from rectal palpation of the reproductive tract to detect pregnancy, to measures of SCC and rectal temperatures, to laboratory tests for pathogen-specific antigen or antibody [15,16]. All tests have inherent characteristics—namely, sensitivity (the proportion of diseased individuals classified as diseased by the test) and specificity (the proportion of nondiseased classified as such by the test). A complete understanding of how these characteristics, together with the underlying prevalence of disease, impact the predictive values and diagnostic utility of each test is important. A more thorough examination of test characteristics appears elsewhere in this issue. It is important to understand that test results are rarely absolute (there are few, if any, tests with 100% sensitivity and specificity) and that they generate probabilities of disease that move us toward or away from one or more possibilities on our list of rule-outs [17,18]. It is also important to appreciate that a change in the cut-point at which a continuous test result is considered positive will change the test itself, generating new sensitivity and specificity parameters with unique predictive values. Furthermore, changes in the prevalence of disease in a herd, even when the test remains the same, can profoundly influence the predictive value of the test. For instance, we generally use a cut-point of 200,000 to 250,000 somatic cells per milliliter to identify cows with subclinical mastitis. At this cut-point, the test has a sensitivity of 73% and a specificity of 86% for prevalent infections caused by major and minor pathogens [19]. In a low-prevalence herd (<10% of cows with subclinical mastitis), the predictive value of a positive test would be about 37%, suggesting that a cow exceeding the threshold has a 37% probability of being infected. On the other hand, the same cut-point applied to a cow in a high-prevalence herd (50% of cows infected) would have a positive predictive value of 84%, indicating a much greater probability of being infected.

One of the greatest challenges in test interpretation for dairy practitioners is explaining test results to producer clients. Experience with serum and milk ELISA tests for Johne's disease, which have poor sensitivities and specificities at best [20–22], has taught many of us that producers expect test results to be absolute. Changing that expectation and convincing a dairyman that a negative test result does not necessarily mean that the subject animal is disease-free or, conversely, that a positive test may be a false-positive, can be a taxing exercise.

Traditionally, we have interpreted continuous test results using a single cut-point, above which the result is considered positive and below which it is considered negative. More recently, the introduction of likelihood ratios to the interpretation of diagnostic tests has added value in two ways. First, likelihood ratios do not change with changes in disease prevalence, so that unlike positive and negative predictive values, they are easier to interpret. Second, the likelihood ratio approach allows for the incorporation of multiple cut-points in the application of test results. The notion that an animal with more antibody is more likely to be disease positive can be quantified and expressed using likelihood ratios. The interpretation of cowside tests, such as milk test strips for β-hydroxybutyrate, is based on the likelihood ratio approach [23]. As the color of the reagent strip intensifies, the probability that the level of β-hydroxybutyrate indicated by the test strip came from a subclinically ketotic rather than a nonketotic cow increases. This probability is expressed qualitatively or quantitatively on the interpretative color chart.

Given the uncertainty inherent in many of the tests we use, there are important questions concerning how many animals to test and how often to repeat the test. Depending on whether one wishes to rule-in or rule-out disease or estimate the prevalence or incidence of an endemic disease, the answers to these questions vary considerably. If one wants to demonstrate that a herd is free of disease, then depending on the sensitivity of the test, one may need to test the entire herd or a sufficient proportion of the herd to be assured that the prevalence is below a predetermined and acceptable level [23,24]. Alternately, if one is monitoring an endemic disease and the objective is to identify a significant change in the prevalence, then sample size calculations are driven by the expected prevalence, desired precision of the estimate, and characteristics of the test being used.

The interpretation of tests at the individual animal level is relatively easy, given that the test sensitivity, specificity, and disease prevalence are known. At the herd level, however, the application of imperfect tests presents some diagnostic challenges [25]. With tests that are less than 100% specific, as the number of individuals tested increases, so does the probability of at least one false-positive result and the herd apparent prevalence. Therefore, as herd size increases, so does the probability that the herd will be classified as positive (at least one animal will test positive) for any disease of interest. The difficulty lies in sorting out whether this is the truth (the herd may have expanded and the disease of interest may been have introduced through the purchase of animals) or whether it is merely a result of the application of an imperfect test to a larger number of individuals.

Deciding whether, when, and how to intervene

As veterinarians, we are ultimately judged not on how well we identify problems on dairy farms, but on how well we resolve those problems. Our clients are generally more willing to pay for our advice and our actions when they are directed toward the resolution of a significant problem. To this end, our ability to identify, understand, interpret, and apply existing and new knowledge in the areas of animal health and productivity is what sets us apart as professionals. A major part of this skill set is the ability to critically appraise the information that is presented to us from various sources. This information includes everything from scientific material from refereed journals and professional conferences to glossy advertising material for new drugs, vaccines, and other products. By being able to distinguish good information from bad and by being able to identify strengths and weaknesses in scientific arguments, we strive to practice evidence-based veterinary medicine for the benefit of our dairy clients [26]. Although there is not always strong scientific evidence to back up each of our actions or recommendations, it behooves us to recognize when we have the backing of strong evidence and when we are acting based on our best guess.

Although some of the advice we give to our clients with respect to dairy herd management is based on opinion and observation (recommendations for stall design and specifications in free-stall barns comes to mind), other advice is based on sound scientific evidence. A strength-of-evidence hierarchy exists that includes well-executed observational studies and clinical field trials at the top of the list. Although many of the journals that we rely on for our evidence have rigorous review processes, the reviews are not perfect and the review process is limited by the time, expertise, and availability of qualified individuals to participate in the review process. Given the limitations of peer reviewed and refereed journals to cover all of the intricate aspects of each submitted publication, some articles are published with serious flaws in design, execution, or interpretation. The ability of the veterinary practitioner to critically appraise a scientific journal article is an important skill that needs to be developed and practiced. This critical appraisal process is part of the practice of evidence-based veterinary medicine [27–32], a paradigm that has its roots in human medicine and clinical epidemiology [14].

The critical appraisal process involves the careful scrutiny of the methodologic detail of observational studies, experiments, and clinical trials. The process has been described in detail [29–31,33], with modifications of the basic approach applied to each study type. One of the most resounding demonstrations of the power of critical appraisal was presented by Perino and Hunsaker [34] at the 1997 meeting of the American Association of Bovine Practitioners. These investigators reported their experience in critically reviewing 183 articles published over a 24-year period that pertained to field trials of vaccines against bovine respiratory disease agents. They concluded that only 22 of the articles met their minimum quality standards and, thus, could be relied on for providing evidence of reasonable quality regarding vaccine efficacy under field conditions. The remainder of the articles did not address efficacy under conditions compatible with the "real world" field experience or had fatal flaws. Although it is beyond the scope of this manuscript to cover the approach to critical appraisal of the scientific literature, there are a number of outstanding resources that can help guide the practicing veterinarian through this process [26–32].

Our understanding of the dynamics of health and disease in populations and the multifactorial cause of most important diseases have been critical in our development of preventive and control programs. The contribution of high-quality observational studies, which include data from large numbers of animals in many herds with varying demographic and management characteristics, has created the foundation for much of this knowledge. Although few dairy practitioners initiate observational studies, they are increasingly being asked to collaborate with veterinary college faculty in the execution of these studies. Furthermore, large-scale clinical trials involving private practitioners and their clients' herds are becoming more common and offer a supplementary source of income to both parties. Dairy practitioners who wish to take advantage of these collaborative opportunities need to become more knowledgeable about how these observational studies and field trials are conducted, not only as readers of scientific literature but as participants in applied field-based research.

Summary

Twelve years ago, Dohoo [35] challenged us to take the principles of epidemiology and apply them to the practice of veterinary herd medicine. Although at times we seem to shy away from the "*E* word," as a profession, I believe we have made strong inroads to meeting that challenge. Our use of quantitative epidemiologic techniques in our herd health and performance monitoring programs, our acceptance of the imperfection of tests and the ability to communicate the concept to our dairy producer clients, and our application of evidence-based veterinary medicine at the animal and herd level support that assertion. It is hoped that this article has served to lay the framework for the application of epidemiology to dairy production medicine on which the more detailed discussion of its various aspects found in the following articles can be built.

References

[1] Martin SW, Meek AH, Willeberg P. Epidemiologic concepts. In: Veterinary epidemiology: principles and methods. Ames (IA): Iowa State University Press; 1987. p. 3–21.

[2] Smith RD. Veterinary clinicial epidemiology: a problem-oriented approach. 2nd edition. Boca Raton (FL): CRC Press; 1995.

[3] Brand A, Hoordhuizen JPTM, Schukken YH. Herd health and production management in dairy practice. Wageningen, The Netherlands: Wageningen Press; 1996.

[4] Cockcroft P, Holmes M. Handbook of evidence-based veterinary medicine. Cambridge, United Kingdom: Blackwell Publishing; 2003.

[5] Radostits O. Herd health: food animal production medicine. 3rd edition. Philadelphia: WB Saunders Co.; 2001.

[6] Fetrow J, Harrington B, Henry ET, et al. Dairy herd health monitoring. Part 1. Description of monitoring systems and sources of data. Comp Cont Ed Pract Vet 1987;9:F390–8.

[7] Fetrow J. Dairy production medicine and herd monitoring. Bovine Pract 1990;22:95–111.

[8] Kelton DF, Lissemore KD, Martin RE. Recommendation for recording and calculating the incidence of selected clinical diseases of dairy cattle. J Dairy Sci 1998;81:2502–9.
[9] Thurmond MC. Epidemiologic approaches for measuring and understanding abortion in dairy cows. In: Proceedings of the 37th Annual Convention of the American Association of Bovine Practitioners. Fort Worth (TX): American Association of Bovine Practitioners; 2004. p. 83–9.
[10] Stewart S, Fetrow J, Eicker S. Analysis of current performance on commercial dairies. Comp Cont Ed Pract Vet 1994;16(8):1099–103.
[11] Niza-Ribeiro J, Noordhuizen JPTM, Menezes JC. Capability index—a statistical process control tool to aid in udder health control in dairy herds. J Dairy Sci 2004;87:2459–67.
[12] Fetrow F, McClary D, Harman R, et al. Calculating selected reproductive indices: recommendations of the American Association of Bovine Practitioners. J Dairy Sci 1990;73: 78–90.
[13] Geishauser T, Leslie K, Tenhag J, et al. Evaluation of eight cow-side ketone tests in milk for detection of subclinical ketosis in dairy cows. J Dairy Sci 2000;83:296–9.
[14] Sackett DL, Haynes RB, Guyatt GH, et al. The interpretation of diagnostic data. In: Clinical epidemiology: a basic science for clinical medicine. 2nd edition. Boston: Little, Brown and Co.; 1991. p. 119–39.
[15] Kelton DF, Leslie KE, Etherington WG, et al. Accuracy of rectal palpation and of a rapid milk progesterone enzyme immunoassay for determining the presence of a functional corpus luteum in subestrous dairy cows. Can Vet J 1991;32:286–91.
[16] Wenz JR, Barrington GM, Garry FB, et al. Use of systemic disease signs to assess disease severity in dairy cows with acute coliform mastitis. J Am Vet Med Assoc 2001;218(4):567–72.
[17] Ruegg PL. Use of basic epidmiologic principles in dairy production medicine. Part I. Assessing production. Comp Cont Ed Vet Pract 1992;14(11):1535–55.
[18] Ruegg PL. Use of basic epidemiologic principles in dairy production medicine. Part II. Investigating herd problems. Comp Cont Ed Vet Pract 1993;15(2):309–13.
[19] Dohoo IR, Leslie KE. Evaluation of changes in somatic cell counts as indicators of new intramammary infections. Prev Vet Med 1991;10:225–37.
[20] Hendrick SH, Duffield TF, Kelton DF, et al. Evaluation of enzyme-linked immunosorbent assays performed on milk and serum samples for detection of paratuberculosis in lactating dairy cows. J Am Vet Med Assoc 2005;226(3):424–8.
[21] Wells SJ, Godden SM, Lindeman CJ, et al. Evaluation of bacteriologic culture of individual and pooled fecal samples for detection of *Mycobacterium paratuberculosis* in dairy cattle herds. J Am Vet Med Assoc 2003;223(7):1022–5.
[22] Wells SJ, Whitlock RH, Wagner BA, et al. Sensitivity of test strategies used in the Voluntary Johne's Disease Herd Status Program for detection of *Mycobacterium paratuberculosis* in dairy cattle herds. J Am Vet Med Assoc 2002;220(7):1053–7.
[23] Geishauser T, Leslie K, Kelton D, et al. Evaluation of five cowside tests for use with milk to detect subclinical ketosis in dairy cows. J Dairy Sci 1998;81:438–43.
[24] DiGiacomo RF, Koepsell TD. Sampling for detection of infection or disease in animal populations. J Am Vet Med Assoc 1986;189(1):22–3.
[25] Martin SW, Shoukri M, Thorburn MA. Evaluating the health status of herds based on tests applied to individuals. Prev Vet Med 1992;14:33–43.
[26] Holmes M, Cockcroft P. Evidence-based veterinary medicine. 1. Why is it important and what skills are needed? In Pract 2004;26(1):28–33.
[27] Holmes M, Cockcroft P. Evidence-based veterinary medicine. 2. Identifying information needs and finding evidence. In Pract 2004;26(2):96–102.
[28] Holmes M, Cockcroft P. Evidence-based veterinary medicine. 3. Appraising the evidence. In Pract 2004;26(3):154–64.
[29] Dohoo IR, Waltner-Toews D. Interpreting clinical research. Part I. General considerations. Comp Cont Ed Vet Pract 1985;7(8):S473–8.

[30] Dohoo IR, Waltner-Toews D. Interpreting clinical research. Part II. Descriptive and experimental studies. Comp Cont Ed Vet Pract 1985;7(9):S513–9.
[31] Dohoo IR, Waltner-Toews D. Interpreting clinical research. Part III. Observational studies and interpretation of results. Comp Cont Ed Vet Pract 1985;7(10):S605–13.
[32] Hancock D. Critical reading of the scientific literature. In: Proceedings of the 24th Annual Convention of the American Association of Bovine Practitioners. Orlando (FL): American Association of Bovine Practitioners; 1992. p. 29–38.
[33] Ribble CS. Assessing vaccine efficacy. Can Vet J 1990;31:679–81.
[34] Perino LJ, Hunsaker BD. A review of bovine respiratory disease vaccine field efficacy. Bovine Pract 1997;31(1):59–66.
[35] Dohoo IR. Monitoring livestock health and production: service—epidemiology's last frontier? Prev Vet Med 1993;18:43–52.

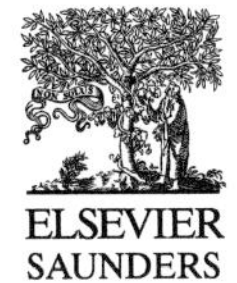

ELSEVIER
SAUNDERS

Vet Clin Food Anim 22 (2006) 35–51

VETERINARY
CLINICS
Food Animal Practice

Assessing Performance of Feedlot Operations Using Epidemiology

Marilyn J. Corbin, DVM, MS, PhD[a],
Dee Griffin, DVM, MS[b,*]

[a]*Central States Research Centre, Inc., 1443½ Hwy 77, Oakland, NE 68045, USA*
[b]*University of Nebraska, Great Plains Veterinary Educational Center, P.O. Box 148, State Spur 18D, Clay Center, NE 68933, USA*

Traditionally, beef feedlots were small, family-oriented operations; however, current feedlots are large, intensively managed, economically based businesses. Today the feedlot industry is dynamic, changing, and adapting to new technologies, public concerns, and economic constraints. As such, the progressive feedlot veterinarian must be well versed in not only individual production animal medicine but also population-based medicine. The successful feedlot veterinarian understands interactions among health, nutrition, and performance and has the ability to monitor and analyze parameters directly related to each of these components.

Monitoring parameters

Feedlot health programs must be goal oriented. Goals should include (1) reducing losses due to disease, (2) minimizing disease outbreaks, (3) taking steps to enhance performance, and (4) providing professional assistance in health and production management [1,2]. Goal evaluation is accomplished through diligent use of record systems that measure production changes and resultant economic effects, coupled with analytic evaluation of these record systems. Recognition of the importance of achieving balance between the complexity and the clarity of record systems foregoes pitfalls of compiling reams of records that are not easily analyzed.

* Corresponding author.
E-mail address: dgriffin@gpvec.unl.edu (D. Griffin).

doi:10.1016/j.cvfa.2005.11.003 ***vetfood.theclinics.com***

Health monitoring parameters

Accurate records that detail descriptive parameters, preventative health measures, and treatment administrations are the basis of a sound record system. Collection of descriptive parameters such as pay weight, weight on arrival, sex, source (miles transported), background, and type of cattle/breed (Dee Griffin, DVM, MS, personal communication, 2000) allows for multiple categorizations, allowing examination of relevant outcomes.

The most widely used epidemiologic health outcomes used in the feeding industry are measures of incidence or prevalence. Incidence rates describe the probability or risk of a new case developing during a specifically stated time interval and are a dynamic measure of disease occurrence [3]. The general formula for incidence is the number of animals developing the disease during the time period divided by the number of animals in the group at the beginning of the time period. Recognizing that the number of animals in the group at the beginning of the time period may not be the same as the number of animals in the group at the end of the time period, an average of the beginning and ending numbers may be used for the denominator. Prevalence is the fraction of the population that is diseased at a given point in time and, as such, is a static measure [3]. The general formula for prevalence is the number of animals in the population with the disease at a certain point of time divided by the total number of animals in the population at that certain point of time. In contrast to incidence, prevalence includes old and new cases and may be affected by the length of disease duration. Defining the time frame is important. For example, a veterinarian may visit a feedyard and be informed of a "significant problem" with bovine respiratory disease. This disease may have a high prevalence on the day of the visit (a large number of animals pulled on the day of the visit) with a corresponding low incidence of disease over the entire feeding period, indicating a current disease outbreak. A significant problem with bovine respiratory disease, however, could also be defined as a low prevalence on the day of the visit with a corresponding high incidence of disease over the entire feeding period, indicating a constant, smoldering disease status. These two disease occurrence profiles indicate two very different management approaches.

Relevant outcomes or health production parameters commonly measured in the feedyard include morbidity, mortality, case fatality, re-treatment, repull, and nonresponder rates [2]. These outcomes can be measured as a prevalence (a measure of the event at a given point in time); however, they are more commonly measured as an incidence.

Crude morbidity rate represents the number of calves that become diseased during a time period divided by the number of calves in the group (population) during the time period. Establishing several different time periods (monthly, seasonally, or at time of close-out) may be necessary, and selecting the appropriate time period depends on how the outcome is intended to be used. Morbidity rates can be further categorized to describe specific rates based on pay weight, weight on arrival, sex, source (miles transported), background, and type of cattle/breed. This categorization allows for a more meaningful interpretation of the disease process or attributes of the population at risk. In addition, morbidity rates can be further classified by disease. Common disease morbidities evaluated are bovine respiratory disease, central nervous system disorders, and metabolic and lameness morbidities. Although many veterinarians monitor disease morbidities monthly, it is also important to evaluate some diseases on a seasonal basis. Identifying seasonal disease trends can provide management insight to help control diseases such as footrot, atypical interstitial pneumonia, and calving difficulties.

Crude mortality rate represents the number of calves that died during a time period divided by the number of calves in the group (population) during that time period. The number of calves in the group (population) during that time period is defined as the population at risk. There are numerous epidemiologic methods to help define the population at risk; however, the authors tend to use the number of cattle that arrived (per each lot of cattle or over the entire feedyard) as the population at risk. Mortality rates also can be further categorized similar to the categorization used for morbidity rates.

Case fatality rate is a measure of the mortality rate among calves with a specific disease. The formula for calculating case fatality rate is the number of calves that died divided by the number of calves that were diseased. Again, case fatality rate can be calculated for different disease categories. Case fatality rates are particularly useful for describing virulence and severity of the disease [3].

Re-treatment rate is the number of calves requiring a second treatment of the same disease for which they were previously treated divided by the number of calves receiving initial treatment of the disease during a specific time period. One minus the re-treatment rate multiplied by 100 will result in treatment efficacy. Bovine respiratory disease treatment efficacy can have a broad range; ideally, treatment efficacy should be 80% or higher. One must recognize that a broad range in efficacy could be due to not only choice of antibiotic treatments but also the effects of cattle sex, age, source, origin, and background.

Repull rate is the number of calves removed from the pen (pulled) for the same disease for which they were previously pulled divided by the number of calves initially pulled for the disease during a specific time period. Again, defining an ideal repull rate depends on the sex, age, source, origin, and background of the cattle. It should be recognized that feedyards that treat every calf pulled will have the same re-treatment and repull rates.

Calves that are salvaged due to poor performance (assessed visually or by body weight) or to a chronic disease process may be referred to as nonperformers and are thus constituents of the nonperformer rate. It is important to assign a separate measurement rate to nonperformers versus including them in the mortality rate because some economic benefit is realized with nonperformers. The formula for the nonperformer rate is the number of calves salvaged divided by the total number of calves in the group (population) during a time period.

Economic monitoring parameters

A sound record system should also capture economically significant parameters. Traditionally, financial assessments are summarized when the cattle are harvested and reported in the lot closeout. Several economic parameters are directly related to the health program and include processing costs and treatment costs. Processing costs can be calculated as total dollars spent per head. Treatment costs can be expressed two ways: treatment cost per each animal treated for a specific disease or total treatment cost per each animal received. Calculating treatment cost per each animal treated for a specific disease allows for identification of specific disease treatment protocols that result in treatment costs that are too high. Total treatment cost per each animal received allows for a pen-level basis to be established and for subsequent comparisons between pens of cattle. Calculation of total treatment costs also provides data to stimulate dialog between the veterinarian and the owner/manager of the feedyard as to the cost/benefit ratio of various treatments.

Total health and disease costs can also be calculated by including processing costs, treatment costs, and the value of dead calves. Health and disease cost can be expressed as percentage of the total costs per pound of body weight gain per day [4]. Economic monitoring parameters can also be calculated for multiple categorizations such as sex, source, background, and type of cattle/breed, allowing for further investigation of costs. For example, economic monitoring of health and disease cost may demonstrate that a feedyard possesses superior health capabilities in lightweight cattle but has less than ideal health capabilities in heavyweight cattle. This discovery may stimulate the feedyard to alter the type of cattle they receive and, in turn, lead to elevated economic returns.

Benchmarking of parameters

Collection of the health and economic parameters discussed previously should allow for a database of baseline parameters to be established for each feedyard. Although establishing baselines is an integral part of measuring progress, it should be recognized that when values diverge from the baseline, causality cannot always be ascertained. Changes that affect the feeding of cattle are multifaceted; therefore, attributing a change in baseline to a specific change in management is dangerous. Rather, baselines should be used to evaluate trends (yearly, monthly, seasonally, and categorically) and serve as a basis for discussion of implementing changes in the feeding process. Benchmarking of production parameters among feedyards is another useful tool. Veterinary consultants servicing multiple yards can establish monthly, yearly, or categoric baselines for each feedyard and confidentially share each feedyard's baselines with one another. The utmost care must be taken to assure that the specific feedyard is not identified when benchmarking, and confidentiality must always be assured. Benchmarking among feedyards allows for a more universal mean for each outcome to be established. In addition, production efficiency may increase because most yards have a competitive nature and strive to exceed other yards. It is imperative to understand and communicate to feedyards that baseline differences may be due to management differences between yards, such as differences in types of cattle, case definitions, nutritional programs, and sources of cattle.

Current obstacles in data management

Record systems are the foundation with which production changes and resultant economic effects are measured; however, understanding of the inherent weaknesses in record systems is necessary to avoid overinterpretation of the data. The industry has identified record systems as an integral portion of management; however, it has not constructed standardized, nationwide, query-friendly databases. This type of database is necessary to allow for meaningful industry-wide comparisons of health, nutrition, and economic parameters affecting the feeding industry.

Currently, to allow for meaningful comparisons, it is essential to establish case definitions for each feedyard. It must be recognized that variations of case definitions may exist between individual employees and the day of the week. Case definitions become even more important when using benchmarking among feedyards. Comparison of bovine respiratory disease morbidity rates among feedyards is more difficult to evaluate when a case is defined as (1) depression, removal from pen, lack of clinical signs suggestive of other disease process, and temperature of 104°F versus (2) depression, removal from pen, and lack of clinical signs suggestive of other disease process. Although comparisons among feedyards may have some agreement, it should not be assumed that the feedyards are identical [4]. The advent of computerized health systems has allowed services to generate national benchmarking tools. Although these benchmarks are valuable in establishing baseline parameters, practitioners must be diligent in evaluating outcomes, with recognition of differences in management protocols, environmental factors, and case definitions.

Feedyards traditionally began record systems for accounting or financial obligations, and as such, many of the systems measure input costs and the derived benefits and only minimally address health measurements. Validity of health data entered into financially driven record systems can be questionable. Often, health data that is valid and sufficient in regard to analysis and interpretation is nonexistent. Compounding this obstacle is the ability of the feedyard to record health events accurately and consistently. Although these obstacles should not be viewed as an excuse to forego record systems, they should be recognized as limitations within the current systems.

Using feedlot epidemiology in field investigations

Diligent use of record systems (measuring production changes and resultant economic effects), coupled with analytic evaluation of these record systems, allows monitoring of unexpected health, economic parameter changes, or both. Often, when these parameters have significant changes (defined as 2 SD from the mean) [3], steps are initiated to begin a field investigation or an outbreak investigation. The major objectives of the investigation are (1) halting the progress of the disease, (2) determining the reasons for the outbreak, (3) beginning corrective measures, and (4) establishing recommendations to reduce the risk of future outbreaks [3]. The successful completion of the four major objectives requires a sound, scientifically based, systematic approach to the problem. It is important to understand that the steps in the systematic approach are dynamic. Steps may be occurring concurrently and frequently and may need to be repeated when the knowledge base of the problem is further expanded or altered. The approach used by the FOCUS workgroup at the University of North Carolina School of Public Health serves as a template for the application of a systematic approach to field investigations [5].

Verify the problem and confirm the existence of the problem or outbreak

The foundation of a field investigation is to broadly define the problem and then determine whether the problem truly exists. To determine whether the problem truly exists, one must have access to health records, economic records, or both, preferably with adequate data to determine baseline parameters and evaluate whether changes from the mean have occurred.

Establish the etiologic agent involvement and define a case

In the face of an outbreak, it is tempting to skim over the part of the investigation that focuses on case definition and to proceed directly to potential risk factors. Although most of the investigative time cannot be consumed with determining the etiologic agent, one should judiciously allocate time to obtain a general history of the problem. General data collection should include but not be limited to calves affected and to health, nutritional, environmental, geographic, and management data. In addition to the general history, clinical examinations of those affected and postmortem examinations of those that have succumbed to the disease should be performed. Often, clinical examinations or postmortem examinations have already been conducted by those immediately involved with the problem. It is imperative to review these records thoroughly and to determine the validity of the observations. In many cases, it is wise to conduct the clinical and postmortem examinations oneself and obtain any potential samples. In the event of the uncertainty of the disease, one should collect a wide range of samples and retain the samples for future evaluations if needed. In some situations, clinical samples should also be collected from calves that are not afflicted with the disease to provide for a comparison group.

Synthesis of the history, clinical examinations, and postmortem examinations should provide a basis for establishing a case definition. Establishing an etiologic diagnosis is not always necessary when establishing a case definition; in some situations, the etiologic diagnosis does not further the establishment of control measures to reduce the disease. For example, determining *Mannheimia haemolytica* as the etiologic agent in an outbreak of bovine respiratory disease complex does not further the progress toward implementing control measures. Instead, the focus should be on the differences that existed that allowed these calves to be overwhelmed with bovine respiratory disease complex. After case definition, a review of any pertinent records should be conducted to determine whether any further animals are afflicted with the disease.

Tabulate and explore the data

One must remember, when beginning a field investigation, to tabulate and explore the objective data. Subjective data, perceptions, and opinions will abound. Although it is important to be cognizant of this type of data, it can often lead one astray. Therefore, the analysis must be based on scientifically sound, objective data. It should be recognized that subjective data may lead to some hypothesis formation; however, these data should be used with caution and be able to withstand scientific scrutiny.

Establishing an epidemiologic curve is one of the first steps to beginning a field investigation. An epidemiologic curve plots the frequency of new cases (vertical axis) over a certain time period (horizontal axis). The resultant curve will help to summarize a temporal pattern, incubation or exposure period, infectivity of pathogen, and the potential mode of transmission of the disease. After examination of the epidemic curve, one can generally classify the curve as a point source epidemic or a propagative epidemic (Figs. 1 and 2). Although this classification is somewhat academic, classifying the epidemic will assist in developing the steps to initiate for the

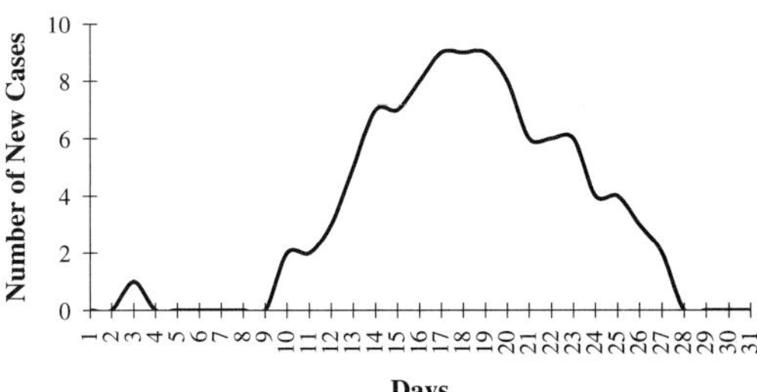

Fig. 1. Point source epidemic.

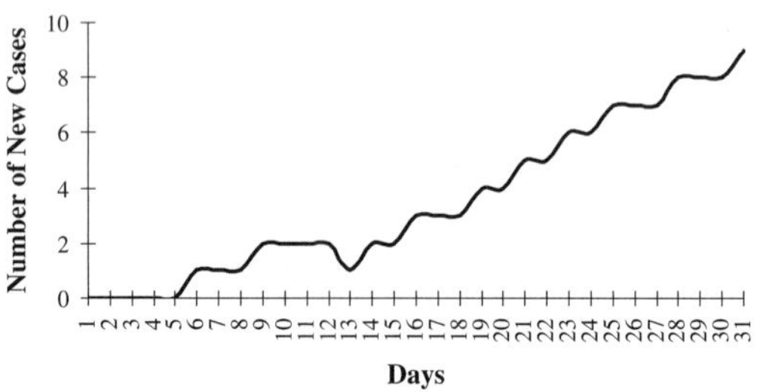

Fig. 2. Propagating epidemic.

field investigation. Point source epidemics tend to have a rapidly progressing number of cases, whereas propagated epidemics have a slower progression in the number of cases [3]. After constructing the epidemic curve, one should establish the index case or cases and the time frame of subsequent cases.

The second step in systematically conducting a field investigation is to determine whether a spatial pattern exists. Maps of the area, feedyard, or pens within a feedyard should be used to plot the location of animals at the time they became morbid or died. Generating plot maps to indicate cattle movements within the feedyard may also lead to identification of potential risk factors.

After determination of the case definition, one should assemble demographic data for the cases versus the noncases. Attention should be paid to similarities among cases and differences between cases and noncases. It is wise to remember that case definitions may not be 100% accurate, so some adjustments may need to be recognized and case definitions may evolve as more is learned about the outbreak.

Formulate and test hypothesis

Feedlot veterinarians are most likely to be asked for consultation when the number of cases is still increasing. As such, expeditiously executing the field investigation is crucial; however, the focus must still be scientific. Etiologic diagnosis of the disease may lead the investigator to potential risks; however, an etiologic diagnosis is not necessary to begin the investigation. It is also important to remember that epidemics are not necessarily linked to one or more specific pathogens but may be linked to environmental, nutritional, or managerial factors.

Armed with knowledge of the epidemic curve, spatial relationships, and demographic data, one can begin exploring the data to formulate hypotheses. Examination of the epidemic curve allows for hypothesis generation based on potential incubation periods, transmission factors, exposure periods, or a combination of these variables. Viewing the spatial maps can also generate hypotheses based on location of diseased or dead animals or on movements associated with diseased or dead animals. Attention should be paid to similarities among cases and differences between cases and noncases. One should begin to synthesize specific demographic information about potential risk factors such as background of cattle, date of arrival, sex, weight, animal movement (before arrival at the feedyard and within the feedyard), and nutrition with respect to cases and noncases. This information should be used to generate demographic hypotheses. At this point, some field investigations will show a strong link to a potential risk factor. For example, if all cases were exposed to risk factor A while none of the noncases were exposed to risk factor A, then it would be appropriate to initiate a control measure at this point, if the control measure would not be of any detriment to the operation. If potential detriments could result due to the control measure, however, one should not initiate the control measure until statistical analysis proves the risk factor is linked to the disease. After potential hypotheses are developed, each risk factor should be statistically evaluated for association with the disease. To statistically assess this, the relative risk is calculated. The relative risk measures the strength of the association between the risk factor and the disease [3]. It is calculated as the ratio between the rate of disease in the calves exposed to the risk factor and the rate of disease in the calves not exposed to the risk factor. To determine the statistical significance, the χ^2 test or the Fisher exact test is used. With some training, individuals can become adept at using Epi Info 2000 [6] to statistically evaluate risk factors. If not able to statistically evaluate risk factors on one's own, then the authors suggest contacting a university extension veterinarian for assistance.

Implement and evaluate control measures

After determining an association between the risk factor and the disease, one or more control measures should be discussed and implemented. It is important to monitor these control measures to assure that changes are adequately being applied. Follow-up monitoring should also evaluate whether the implemented control measures reduced the incidence of disease.

Example field investigation

During a routine monthly visit to a feedyard, the manager indicates that they have experienced an increased number of calves being diagnosed with diarrhea. After reviewing the records, it is determined the incidence of calves experiencing diarrhea has dramatically increased during the last month compared with the normal baseline incidence of diarrhea.

Information is gathered in regard to the feedyard's case definition of diarrhea. Clinical examinations of cattle afflicted with diarrhea are performed along with collecting clinical samples. Postmortem examination and sample collection are conducted on available calves. All samples are retained for further diagnostic work-up as time allows. A working case definition defines diarrhea as "any calf removed from the pen by the cowboy for watery, bloody, or loose stools."

An epidemiologic curve is plotted with the frequency of new cases over the time period of the previous 2 months (referred to as day 0 through day 60). The curve reveals (1) a point source epidemic with a potential index case on day 26, (2) that subsequent cases began occurring on day 28, and (3) that the number of new cases has been increasing steadily.

Feedyard spatial maps are constructed to visually indicate the home pens of the afflicted cattle. Spatial maps are also created to identify pen movements and individual animal movements for days 20 through 40. Spatial maps reveal cases to be sporadically spread throughout the feedyard, with most pens experiencing individual animal movements through the hospital, some pens experiencing individual animal movements to the nonperformer pen, and some pens experiencing pen movements through the processing facility for reimplanting.

Demographic data are collected. After comparing similarities and differences between cases and noncases, it is concluded that (1) most cases involve calves that have been on feed for less than 60 days, (2) the sex ratio is similar between cases and noncases, (3) the water source is similar between cases and noncases, (4) the background of calves is diverse among cases and noncases, (5) most cases were previously treated for respiratory disease, (6) pens experiencing cases are going through step-up ration, and (7) the processing protocol was similar for cases and noncases.

Based on the epidemic curve, spatial maps, and demographic data, two potential hypotheses are generated: starting ration is associated with diarrhea or respiratory disease is associated with diarrhea. Statistical analysis reveals that the starting ration is not associated with diarrhea; however, respiratory disease is associated with diarrhea. Spatial maps detailing cattle movement are reviewed again. It is determined that the index case was moved through the hospital facility for respiratory disease treatment on day 25 and then returned to his home pen. On day 26, he was again removed from his home pen for diarrhea, treated, and remained in the hospital facility. The next case of diarrhea was diagnosed in a different home pen on day 28. This calf had previously been moved to the hospital facility for treatment of respiratory disease on day 25. Subsequently, it is determined that calves that had been moved through the hospital facility were statistically more likely to have developed diarrhea. Further investigation determines heavy fecal contamination of equipment used to orally drench calves afflicted with respiratory disease, diarrhea, or both.

Control measures are implemented, including (1) thorough cleaning and disinfecting of the hospital facility and hospital pens; (2) thorough cleaning and disinfecting of all hospital equipment, particularly those with oral or rectal contact; (3) isolation of all diarrhea cases; and (4) cleaning, disinfectant, and zoonotic education of all personnel involved. Field investigation is followed up, and the reported incidence of diarrhea is declining rapidly.

Special applications in feedlot epidemiology

The responsibilities of the veterinarian in the feedlot have changed from the traditional role of diagnosis and treatment of individual morbid calves to that of a professional adviser [2,7]. Feedlot epidemiology has expanded its traditional confines and now uses several novel applications that are of sound scientific and economic value to the feeding industry. Although not every feedlot veterinarian has the desire or the time to implement each of these specialties, it is important to understand these epidemiologic concepts when evaluating literature and to be willing to employ these resources when appropriate.

Partial budget analysis

Basic budget analysis may be used to guide feedyard managers and veterinarians in evaluating decision choices. Partial budgets are a mechanism to organize data concerning inputs (costs), outputs (benefits), and the economic effect of each decision choice. The goal of partial budgeting is to estimate the change occurring in profit or loss of the operation due to a decision or change [8].

Partial budgets are useful tools to evaluate operational changes in agriculture, such as (1) expanding an enterprise, (2) an alternative enterprise, (3) different production practices, (4) hiring a custom operation rather than purchasing equipment, (5) making a capital improvement, and (6) buying new machinery to replace physical labor or older machinery [9]. Specifically, in the feeding industry, decisions concerning vaccine programs, processing programs, custom processing crews, custom maintenance crews, ration components, and other decisions can be evaluated using partial budgets.

Partial budgeting is based on the principle that a minor change in the operation will have one or more of the following effects: (1) eliminate or reduce some costs, (2) eliminate or reduce some returns, (3) cause additional costs to be incurred, or (4) cause additional returns to be received [9]. The summation of the effects will yield the net economic effects. By virtue of this principle, partial budgets allow realistic evaluation of operational changes without consulting complete financial records.

To construct a partial budget, each of these four effects is itemized (Box 1), which results in the categories of additional returns, reduced costs, additional costs, and reduced returns. Additional returns are defined as income or returns that are a result of the decision choice. Reduced costs are costs that are decreased or are no longer incurred as a result of the decision choice. Costs that are increased or incurred as a result of the decision choice are additional costs, and reduced returns are defined as income no longer received as a result of the decision choice. When constructing a partial budget, one must decide which items to include. A general guideline is to include any item that may be affected by the decision choice. In some

Box 1. Example template of a partial budget

Additional costs		**Additional returns**	
Item	______	Item	______
Item	______	Item	______
Total additional costs	______	Total additional costs	______
Reduced returns		**Reduced costs**	
Item	______	Item	______
Item	______	Item	______
Total reduced returns	______	Total additional costs	______
Total additional costs + total reduced returns =	______	**Total additional returns + total reduced costs** =	______

Net change in income [a] ______

[a] (Total additional returns + total reduced costs) – (total additional costs + total reduced returns)

instances, these items may not be readily apparent, such as effects on average daily gain, labor inputs, re-treatment rates, and so forth. The net effect is calculated by the summation of additional returns and reduced costs minus the summation of additional costs and reduced returns. This value is an estimate of additional profit realized by adoption of the decision choice.

It must be recognized that decision choices may not be evaluated entirely by net return. Each partial budget user must reach a balance among net return, risk preference, and ability of implementation of decision choice. Partial budgeting, however, provides another evaluation parameter with which to make a sound scientific decision.

Risk assessment modeling (dynamic, stochastic, simulation modeling)

Risk assessment is the process of scientifically evaluating the probability or severity of potential adverse effects attributable to a known risk [10]. Simply defined, risk assessment is the qualitative or quantitative quantifying of the probability and potential impact of risk. Susser [11] described the concept of modeling well, stating the purpose of a model is to take a complex biologic system and reduce it to a model of related variables within the system. This process helps to develop and clarify variables and statements concerning causal relationships.

The first advantage of modeling is the ability to model uncertainty and variability. Uncertainty is defined as the researcher's lack of knowledge about the parameters that characterize the biologic system being modeled, whereas variability is the effect of chance or inherent randomness of the biologic system [12]. Dynamic, stochastic modeling allows each independent variable to have a corresponding probability distribution associated with it. This probability distribution allows for variability in the data or for uncertainty in the biologic system to be modeled by way of many iterations of the model.

Dynamic, stochastic, simulation modeling has the advantage of eliminating much of the guesswork of traditional statistical analysis involving one answer. Traditional statistical analysis provides one answer, an answer that may be the most likely, minimum, or maximum depending on the external validity of the collected data. Simulation modeling relies on many iterations of the model until a static outcome is achieved. In many cases, this means 1000 or more iterations. In essence, the computer has randomly selected a number from the probability distribution for each independent variable, input the number into the model, and allowed for 1000 additional iterations of the model. This technique allows one to determine the median outcome.

After completion of the dynamic, stochastic, simulation model, the researcher has the ability to detect which independent (exposure or study) variables have the most effect on the dependent outcome (morbidity or mortality). Numerous charts, graphs, and tables can be constructed to demonstrate which independent variables are "driving" the model.

Dynamic modeling may include complex feedback loops involving multiple variables, which may have multiple effects on the biologic system at multiple locations or levels. Using modeling allows the feedback mechanism to demonstrate the effect of changing one independent variable.

Dynamic, stochastic, simulation modeling is not without limitations. Perhaps the most severe limitation is human error. Each independent variable may have a probability distribution determined by way of data, literature, or expert opinion. It is plausible for some error to exist due to the use of inappropriate usage of probability distributions. In addition, recognition of which independent variables are driving the model may not lead to the ability to understand the biologic reasons of why certain independent variables are driving the model.

As an example of risk assessment modeling, the authors evaluated several management decisions concerning pregnancy in the feedyard [13]. The model first was developed using a template of a partial budget spreadsheet [14] on an individual-pen basis, with inputs of costs (cattle, preventive medical care, morbidity, mortality, treatments, and performance), inputs of benefits (sales of poorly performing heifers, baby calves, open (nonpregnant) heifers, recently calved heifers, and pregnant heifers), and the output of net return. Three decision choices were evaluated for each lot of heifers: (1) palpate all heifers on arrival at the feedyard and inject with abortifacient only those pregnant (PALABT); (2) inject all heifers with abortifacient on arrival at the feedyard without determining pregnancy status (ABTALL); and (3) do not palpate or administer abortifacient to any of the heifers on arrival at the feedyard (NOTHING). Simulation software (@Risk, Palisade

Corporation, Newfield, New York) was used to incorporate distributions around model inputs and to generate ranges of expected net returns under each scenario. Values derived from the industry, literature, or existing data sets were used as defaults. Distributions were defined to include variability and uncertainty around these inputs when generating values in the simulations.

Results indicated that under the defined input ranges, ignoring heifer pregnancy would not be economically advantageous unless purchased groups were essentially guaranteed to not contain bred animals. Net returns declined rapidly if pregnant animals were retained in a lot. The drop was steeper for rail pricing than live pricing due to trim and carcass penalties. In addition, purchasing groups of heifers likely to have high pregnancy prevalences (≥43%) would be best served by implementing ABTALL. For heifer lots with pregnancy prevalences at or below 36%, PALABT would yield greater net returns. Although net returns increased for ABTALL and decreased for PALABT as pregnancy prevalences rose above 43%, the differences between these strategies in the 36% to 49% pregnancy prevalence range were small, making choice of strategy less critical.

Packing house audits

Many approaches can be taken to monitor the disease status of herds. Inspections at packing houses have long been an important addition to health monitoring in swine and poultry. Before 1980, routine beef cattle inspections were typically limited to monitoring liver abscesses.

Crucial to the success of the inspection is establishing a working relationship with the packing plant management and personnel before trying to conduct a packing plant inspection. The management and personnel should be expecting you on the day of an inspection. They should know what you want to accomplish and what information, data, and samples you are interested in collecting. It is important for the US Department of Agriculture FSIS veterinary medical officer and his or her inspectors to be familiar with your activities. If your activities interfere with the inspection of animals or cause contamination of animals, then not only you will lose your welcome in the plant but you also may be held liable for product loss.

Safety is the most important objective: safety for yourself, safety of the workers, and safety of the product. Remember you are working with food, and cleanliness is the most important mission that packers face everyday. Cross contamination must be prevented, so take three smocks and change as you move from ear tag transfer, offal table, and rail-out area. If you have any questions about how to conduct your activities, do not start until you visit with a supervisor.

Equipment needed to conduct an inspection includes an approved white hard hat (hard hat colors have meaning), hearing protection, safety glasses, clean approved steel-toed boots, multiple layers of clean protective clothing, data collection forms, stopwatch, sample bags, and a permanent marker. Taking knives into the plant is not recommended, but if you do, get approval from the plant and have the appropriate safety equipment.

Standard pre–packing house data you should collect includes description of cattle, number of head, source, background, and health/performance parameters. This pre–packing house examination allows you to formulate a specific approach to gathering the information you need. Standard packing house inspection objectives are found in Box 2 and appear in the order in which observations can be made as calves progress through the packing plant. For each set of cattle inspected, a list of objectives based on the history of the cattle should be established.

Cattle move past an inspection point at approximately five calves per minute, and the typical processing line holds less than 150 calves. When inspecting a group of 150 calves, the first calf processed will be in the cooler before the last animal enters the processing line. At certain inspection points, it will be possible to gather information on only a portion of the animals being processed. Based on your preprocessing examination and evaluation of the cattle, you should be able to prioritize the appropriate objectives. Before you are able to establish the number of observations to collect for each objective, you must estimate the rate of occurrence of each

Box 2. Standard packing house inspection objectives

1. Variation in animal frame size
2. Identification tags
3. Implant retention
4. Implanting technique assessment
5. Hide defects
6. Carcass bruising
7. Carcass contamination from hides
8. Variation in carcass finish
9. Abdominal adhesions
10. Liver abnormalities
11. Lung abnormalities
12. Heart abnormalities
13. Large and small intestinal abnormalities
14. Rumen abnormalities
15. Abomasal abnormalities
16. Reproductive status
17. Kidney abnormalities
18. Carcass trim caused by adhesions
19. Carcass trim caused by injections
20. Carcass retention

defect you expect. Low incidence rates require more observations to be recorded to accurately evaluate the occurrence.

It is important to know exactly where inspection points are located in the plant, exactly how many animals are between inspection points, and exactly how long it will take an animal to get from one location to another. You can accurately determine the rate of cattle processing (chain speed) by using a stopwatch. For example, if the plant is processing an average of 270 calves per hour (4.5/min), but processing 280 calves per hour (4.7/min) during your inspection, then you could miss important data because of a time overestimation between the points of inspection. For example, if 23 calves are on the rail between the lung inspection point and the larynx inspection point, being off by 0.1 animals per minute could cause an important observation to be missed by 6 seconds.

Establish the number of calves you have time to observe at each point by calculating the plant speed, mapping your inspection points, and determining the number of cattle in the harvest group. Start your stopwatch when you begin inspecting, record the number of defects, and calculate the rate of defects based on the observed defects per time. For example, if the chain is moving 5.2 animals per minute past you and you observe 5 implants abscessed in 12 minutes, then the rate would be [5/(5.2 × 12)] or [5/62.4] or 8%. During an inspection, you need to record only the defects per location and the time at the location. If you are organized and have some experience, then there are many objectives on which you can collect data at the same time.

For general quality assurance inspections, it is best to follow the first 30 to 60 calves from beginning to end of processing. This practice allows for an overview of all possible defect areas.

Summary

The progressive feedlot veterinarian must be well versed not only in individual production animal medicine but also in population-based medicine. Feedlot health programs must be goal oriented, and evaluation of these goals is accomplished through diligent use of record systems and analytic evaluation of these record systems. Basic feedlot monitoring parameters include health and economic parameters in addition to the use of benchmarking parameters between and among feedyards. When these parameters have significant changes, steps should be initiated to begin field investigations The major objectives of the investigation are (1) halting the progress of the disease, (2) determining the reasons for the outbreak, (3) beginning corrective measures, and (4) establishing recommendations to reduce the risk of future outbreaks. Successful completion of a field investigation requires a sound, scientifically based, systematic approach to the problem. Feedlot epidemiology has also expanded traditional confines and now uses several novel applications such as partial budgeting, risk assessment, and packing plant audits. Theses applications help to provide scientifically sound and economically feasible solutions for the feeding industry.

References

[1] Edwards AJ, Stokka GL. Feedlot health management. In: Howard J, editor. Current veterinary therapy 2: food animal practice. Philadelphia: WB Saunders; 1986. p. 135–42.
[2] Lechtenberg KF, Smith RA, Stokka GL. Feedlot health and management. Vet Clin North Am Food Anim Pract 1998;14:177–97.
[3] Martin SW, Meek AH, Willeberg P. Veterinary epidemiology principles and methods. Ames (IA): Iowa State University Press; 1987.
[4] Smith RA, Stokka GL, Radostits OM, et al. Health and production management in beef feedlots. In: Radostits OM, editor. Herd health: food animal production medicine. Philadelphia: WB Saunders; 2001. p. 587.
[5] Alexander L, Koshiol J, MacDonald PDM, et al. An overview of outbreak investigations. In: MacDonald PDM, editor. FOCUS on field epidemiology. University of North Carolina School of Public Health, North Carolina Center for Public Health Preparedness. 1.
[6] Dean AG, Arner TG, Sangam S, et al. Epi Info 2000, a database and statistics program for public health professionals for use on Windows 95, 98, NT, and 2000 computers. Atlanta (GA): Georgia Centers for Disease Control and Prevention; 2000.
[7] Jim GK, Guichon DT. Implementation of a feedlot medicine program. Proc Am Assoc Bov Pract 1989;21:38–9.
[8] Boehlje MD, Eidman VR. Farm management. New York: John Wiley and Sons; 1984.
[9] Dalsted NL, Gutierrez PH. Partial budgeting. In: Farm & Ranch Series Economics. Colorado State University Cooperative Extension; 1992. Publication #3.760.
[10] Cassin MH, Paoli GM, Lammerding AM. Simulation modeling for microbial risk assessment. J Food Prot 1998;61(11):1560–6.
[11] Susser M, editor. Causal thinking in the health sciences. 1st edition. New York: Oxford University Press; 1973.
[12] Vose D. Risk analysis: a quantitative guide. Chichester, UK: Wiley & Sons Ltd.; 2000.
[13] Buhman MJ, Hungerford LL, Smith DR. An economic risk assessment of the management of pregnant feedlot heifers in the USA. Prevent Vet Med 2003;59:207–22.
[14] Griffin DD. Economic impact associated with respiratory disease in beef cattle. Vet Clin North Am Food Anim Pract 1997;13:367–77.

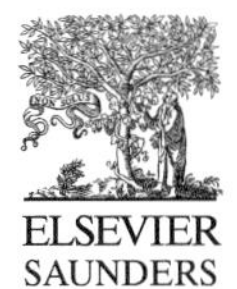

ELSEVIER
SAUNDERS

Vet Clin Food Anim 22 (2006) 53–74

VETERINARY CLINICS
Food Animal Practice

Assessing Performance of Cow-Calf Operations Using Epidemiology

D. Owen Rae, DVM, MPVM

Department of Large Animal Clinical Sciences, College of Veterinary Medicine, University of Florida, P.O. Box 100136, Gainesville, FL 32610-0136, USA

The cow-calf enterprise is a forage- and grass-based cattle production system. The populations of cattle within the enterprise include (1) the productive unit (the cow and her calf); each cow in the population is expected to become pregnant and have and rear her first calf at age 2 years, to repeat this each year thereafter for 8 to 10 years, and to wean a calf that weighs at least 40% of her mature weight; (2) the bull population, which is responsible for breeding these cows; and (3) the heifer population that replaces the cows culled from the herd. Again, the cow is the productive unit within the enterprise; her calf is the product. The greater the proportion of the population that is able to establish a pregnancy, maintain a pregnancy, give birth to a healthy, live calf, and provide the neonate with the nutrition and nurturing (well-being, mothering) requisite for the calf's growth and development, the greater the performance of the herd. Performance becomes a surrogate for health (or a lack of disease). Monitoring the performance of the population using epidemiologic tools provides the practitioner with clues to the subtle (or less subtle) changes that may occur in the population.

Epidemiologic principles are readily applied to the cow-calf population. Cattle, by their nature, are herd animals and best managed as a herd or population. Herd size may be large, including hundreds or thousands of animals, or small, with less than 50 animals, which represents most cattle herds in North America. By establishing methods of monitoring patterns of production, morbidity, and mortality within the population, the veterinarian is able to observe and detect patterns within the monitored events. The selection of monitored events and the use of available detection tools assist in the successful management of the population. Attention to these detection tools assists in identifying the factors or variables associated with impaired performance within the population of cattle. Data are collected and

E-mail address: raeo@mail.vetmed.ufl.edu

doi:10.1016/j.cvfa.2005.11.001 ***vetfood.theclinics.com***

analyzed to determine the strength and importance of epidemiologic associations. The practitioner's intent is to prevent and control conditions that might impede the herd's health or productivity. This article addresses such assessment tools available to the veterinarian.

Assessment protocols

A number of different frameworks or protocols for enterprise/population monitoring have been published and find potential application in the cow-calf enterprise. Three such protocols are the preharvest Hazard Analysis and Critical Control Point process (HACCP) [1], the Standardized Performance Analysis (SPA) cow-calf guidelines [2,3], and the protocol for outbreak investigation and impaired performance [4].

The HACCP concept addresses the total quality management of the enterprise. In addition to the beef quality assurance guidelines [5], it provides for the process verification of the enterprise (Table 1). HACCP is a systematic method used originally in the food industry to identify food safety hazards and to set critical control points to reduce or eliminate the associated risk. These principles can be applied as a preharvest food-source hazard analysis tool and can be incorporated into the SPA guidelines described later.

In the past decade, the US National Cattleman's Association established a format of and guidelines for a standardized performance assessment of the cow-calf herd known as the SPA (Box 1). The SPA guidelines provide a standard for recording and reporting herd production and financial data. This article focuses on the SPA's production application in the context of epidemiologic principles. Before the SPA guidelines were published, there was not a consensus within the beef cattle industry as to how parameters should be measured despite efforts by groups such as the Beef Improvement Federation. The National Cattleman's Association (now the National Cattleman's Beef Association) placed a stamp of approval on the process and has promoted these standardized methods. These standardized descriptors now not only contribute to within-herd monitoring but also to herd-to-herd monitoring and comparison of important production parameters. The

Table 1
Hazard analysis and critical control point process

Quality management	Assessment
Hazard analysis	What is the current status and risks?
Critical control points	How do we measure risks?
Critical limits	When is there a problem?
Monitoring	How is it going?
Corrective action	What change is needed?
Verification	Is the action and monitoring effective?
Record keeping	Record!

Box 1. Standardized Performance Analysis

SPA is

- A tool for beef producers to improve efficiency and lower costs of production
- A select set of specified performance measures
- For any size herd, in any region
- A performance and cost reference point for the beef operation
- Financial and performance data to analyze production
- A measure of reproduction, production, grazing, marketing, finance, and economic measures
- Existing data used to produce standardized information for management decisions
- A cost level and a source of costs determinant for the producer
- An accurate generator of performance information, given that the data are accurate and consistent
- A tool to determine cost and to help identify areas of high production
- A method of performance analysis across a range of herd sizes and localities
- A set of definitions and tables that set a standard by which assessments of the cow-calf enterprise can be made

SPA is the primary tool (in conjunction with the HACCP principles) that is used to monitor cow-calf, bull, and heifer performance in this article. The *Veterinary Clinics of North America: Food Animal Practice* issue on Standardized Performance Analysis in Beef Cattle Operations published in 1995 is a good supplemental resource, especially the articles by Hamilton [3] and Kniffen [6].

A fitting supplement to the previously mentioned approaches is a 10-step strategy to address impaired performance or outbreak investigation [4] (also see article by Waldner elsewhere in this issue).

Population assessment

The beef cattle herd is often a stable and closed population with a minimum of change in its dynamics, which generally permits a minimally rigorous statistical or epidemiologic approach. Populations that are more dynamic (ie, that have movement in and out of the herd or dramatic changes in total herd numbers), however, require more stringent assessments. Individual animal records are often maintained (reviewed in more depth later); however, in most instances, the whole of the cow-calf population is handled or assessed when gathered. All animals may be subject to census, examination (pregnancy, body condition), tests (brucellosis, Johne's), or procedures (immunization, parasite control). The population is thus approached initially as a survey, whereby members of the aggregate population are counted and characteristics of the population are measured. This survey is generally done as a census of the whole population. As the population survey continues over time, a study of the population may ensue, wherein group comparisons are done to investigate cause-and-affect relationships within the population.

The size of the population influences one's ability to do a whole-herd census and assess changes, associations, or risks. A small population may be difficult to evaluate by cross-sectional or even by longitudinal collection and assessments of information. As the size of the assessed population increases, changes within monitored variables are more readily detected as a significant change.

The potential for assessment of the whole target population at risk must be determined. There may be situations in which—due to a large herd size, time, or financial constraints—groups within the herd are "sampled" (ie, for disease detection, screening, and so forth). On these occasions, application of appropriate sampling frames and requisite sample sizes must be defined and applied. The examination of a sampled subunit of the population at risk must be done in such a way as to be able to make some inference of the populations characteristics with an acceptable level of precision (the repeated outcome measure is relatively tight) and accuracy (the repeated outcome measure is close to the true measure of the variable). The subset of the herd that is sampled must be randomly selected and representative of the population. Avoidance of selection bias is essential. The sampling size must be sufficient to detect effect significance within the population. The discussion of sampling, including simple random sampling, systematic random sampling, stratified random sampling, and determination of adequate sample size, is addressed elsewhere.

The assessment of the population, whether as a whole or a subset, begins with taking the herd history and population description (Box 2). What is the profile of the population? A description of the property should include land mass by purpose or use (whether it purchased or leased), a premise identification, and resources available (facilities, water, barns, grasses, forages, and so forth); see also the section on Enterprise Assessment. The animal profile is defined. What is the population of cows, calves, heifers, and bulls? Initial assessment of these populations includes an inventory by population category and basic descriptors such as age, breed, and sex. What are current or presumed mortality, morbidity, and performance measures? What is the temporal pattern of the population cycle? What are the dates of the breeding season (beginning and ending), the herd pregnancy test, the calving season (beginning and ending), and weaning? An example of a profile and assessment form is shown in Box 3. A history of disease conditions that have been seen or are common to the herd should be noted.

Box 2. Herd profile and risk assessment form

Completed by: Date:

General contact information for the herd

Farm name
Premise identification
Owner's name
Key farm contact/management persons (if different from owner)
Address (number, street, route, P.O. Box)
County
City or Town
State
Zip Code
Phone
Fax
E-mail address

General herd information

Type of operation (cow-calf, seed stock, other)
Other animal enterprises
Herd size
Cows
Bred heifers
Heifer calves
Bulls
Total
Herd goals (include future herd size)
Next 2 years
Next 3 to 5 years
Do you plan to be in the beef business in 10 years?
Current and future sources of herd replacements
Current herd performance
Herd performance goals
Herd health concerns you are addressing/plan to address
Management concerns you are addressing/plan to address

Adapted from Rossiter, et al. Johne's disease prevention/control plan for beef herds: manual for veterinarians. *Bovine Pract* 1999;33(2):194-3–4. Available at: http://www.usaha.org/hjwg/njwg.html/ (Florida Johne's Disease Control Program for Beef Cow-Calf Herds); with permission.

Box 3. Sample herd production timeline

Breeding season
Begin: 01Apr05
End: 15Jun05
Length: 75 days

Pregnancy test date
Date: 15Aug05
Gestational age at pregnancy examination
Minimum: 61 days
Maximum: 136 days

Calving season
Begin: 01Jan06
End: 15Mar06
Length: 74 days

Weaning date
Begin: 01Sep06
End: 01Sep06
Length: 0 days
Calf age at weaning
Minimum: 170 days
Maximum: 244 days

Measurements within the population are generally related to reproduction, production, nutrition, and health (morbidity and mortality). Enterprise goals or expectations for reproductive and calf productive performance are established. Example goals are shown in Table 2. The setting of these expectations varies depending on herd and cattle types, environmental and nutritional resources, and management intensity. This process permits identification of the important criteria and objective measures within the monitored herd. For example, What is the expected level of performance (proportion pregnant, calves being weaned, calf weaning weights, and so forth) or maximum expected level of morbidity and mortality (cows, calves)? With these goals and target levels established, a critical intervention point is also set. Intervention points may be based, at least initially, on clinical experience but may later be established based on an accumulation of year-to-year herd or regional expected trends. When the population response exceeds (or falls short) of a critical intervention point, a response is expected from the producer or veterinarian (see Table 2).

As goals and critical interventions are set, outcomes can be monitored by a standardized performance assessment (ie, the measures and standards of assessment are common among those assessing the beef cow populations).

Table 2
Sample herd beef production goals and critical interventional levels in commercial cattle herds

Parameter	Goal	Critical
Pregnancy rate		
Cows (60-d breeding season)	90%–95%	<85%
Heifers (45-d breeding season)	80%–85%	<80%
Abortion rate (pregnancy loss)	<2%	>5%
Calving rate	80%–85%	<80%
Calving interval	12 mo	>13 mo
Still birth rate	<2%	>5%
Dystocia rate		
Cows	<2%–5%	>5%
Heifers	<15%	>15%
C-section rate	<1%	>2%
Weaned calf crop	>75%	<75%
Weaning weights	500 lb or 40% dam wt	<450 lb or <40% dam wt
Weight per day of age	1.6 lb/d	<1.5 lb/d
Female replacement rate	15%	>20%
Mortality rate (annual)		
Calves, birth to 10 d	<5%	>5%
Calves, 11–30 d	<2%	>2%
Calves, 31 d to weaning	<1%	>1%
Calves, postweaning	<1%	>1%
Cows/bulls (breeding stock)	<0.5%	>1%

Values presented in the table are based on the author's observations.
Abbreviation: wt, weight.

To be effective, records must be consistently and meticulously taken, kept, summarized, and used. This practice is not always easy for the producer or the veterinarian but becomes more important as the cattle industry recognizes its role in producing "beef," not just live cattle. The need for product verification and certification is becoming more the responsibility of the producer (and the veterinarian). This information includes verification of animal source, age, and processing or intervention events in the life history of the animal or group of animals. Identification of all animals is becoming more important for production monitoring, total quality management, and rapid disease or event trace back. In the case of a disease outbreak or public health concern, animals must be identified and traceable. Within a few years, this practice will be mandated in the form of premise identification and electronic identification of individual animals entering interstate transport. Producers and veterinarians will increasingly be required to gather and maintain on-farm information that will follow the animal through the production phases. A format of data collection, summarization, and reporting is essential. An important framework for accomplishing this task is the SPA format.

Production and performance records should include readily measurable parameters: animal identification, breed, sex, age, and health (disease/injuries, death). These parameters are the basic animal descriptors or signalment. Evaluation of the cow-calf population should be at the conclusion of the breeding season, at the calving season, and at weaning. In addition, assessment of heifer development and bull development or maintenance is monitored. Each of these topics is discussed later.

Record keeping

Information gathering and summarization is undoubtedly a most critical and often a most difficult task. The practitioner or technician may collect some or much of the desired information, but producer cooperation and assistance is not only desirable but also essential. Information by animal category (cows, calves, heifers, bulls) and production phase is collected as field records. This information is best captured, at present, by use of pocket record books or worksheets that are carried to the field and used where events are occurring. The National Cattleman's Beef Association, in cooperation with other cattle producer groups, prepares an annual pocket record book for this purpose. It follows a format consistent with the SPA standards and guidelines for data acquisition (eg, Box 4). In the future, handheld electronic devices may expedite field data collection, collation, and reporting. Herd records (paper or electronic) should provide timely inputs when cattle are observed, worked, or brought to the processing pens. These field records have limited further use unless they can be collated and maintained in a central data source, usually a personal computer operating in designed data management software. A summary description and independent review of numerous commercially available software programs is available [7]. It should be noted that a simple spreadsheet database program such as Excel (Microsoft Office Excel, Microsoft Corp., Redmond, Washington) or QuatroPro (WordPerfect Office, Corel Corp., Ottawa, Ontario, Canada) meets most recording and monitoring functions. The producer may perform this function, but the veterinarian or his or her staff may perform the role best. It should be noted that the practitioner who has and maintains a current and complete herd record becomes integral and indispensable to a herd operation. The information gathered depends on the operation type and population size, which are discussed in more detail later. Information is summarized and reported in a format conducive to monitoring and the assessment of the herds or the enterprise populations. The important summaries and reports include herd inventory, breeding and pregnancy, calving, weaning and marketing, replacement stock development, and health (morbidity and mortality). A specific description of record keeping and reporting for subpopulations follows.

Assessment of mature cows (and calves)

Description

The cow is the productive unit of the cattle population and the predominant unit of interest. Calf performance is a reflection of cow performance,

Box 4. Definitions and standards for cow-calf population evaluation

- *Calf crop weaned* is determined by the calves weaned during the fiscal year of the analysis. The following definitions are important to this determination.
- *Breeding season*: the dates of the breeding that resulted in the calves weaned during the fiscal year
- *Pregnancy test date*: the dates of the pregnancy test after the breeding season
- *Calving season*: the dates of the calving that resulted in the calves weaned during the fiscal year
- *Weaning season*: the dates of the weaning of calves during the fiscal year of the analysis
- *Beginning breeding inventory*: the total number of females that are exposed for breeding during the breeding season. This number should include replacement heifers exposed for the first time and mature females transferred. This number must be adjusted for any females exposed but not intended to be kept (including females with calves that will be sold when the calves are weaned).
- *Adjustments after breeding* should include all transfers-in after the breeding season that have been exposed and have the potential to calve during the calving season. The only adjustment for transfers-out is for pregnant females transferred out. Animals that are open or have an undetermined pregnancy status should remain in the herd count.
- *Adjustments after the calving season begins* includes all females with nursing calves that are transferred in. Females with nursing calves that are transferred out should be excluded from this total count. Females transferred out without a nursing calf should remain in the inventory count.
- *Births during the calving season* should be recorded in 21-day intervals, if possible. The total number calved is more important.
- *Calf deaths* should be recorded as those that died at birth and those that died during the growth phase.
- *Total calves weaned and weights* is the most important production measurement. Count only calves that are actually weaned and their actual weights at weaning.

Adapted from Hamilton ED. Standardized performance analysis. Vet Clin North Am Food Anim Pract 1995;11:211.

at least until weaning. The cow is defined as a mature female that has delivered at least one offspring. The cow herd is the population "at risk" (ie, the cows that are exposed to the bull for natural service or artificial insemination). It is of importance that the population at risk is well defined because it becomes the denominator in the measurement of many key herd indices. This determination has been approached from a practical inventory standpoint, following rules of inclusion or exclusion defined by the standardized method of SPA (Table 3; see Box 4). Historically, the "coffee shop" estimate of herd performance was based on a liberal censuring of animals at risk. The standard for determining at-risk animals is illustrated in Table 3. The population at risk is that population exposed to a bull at breeding time with the intent to create and rear a marketable calf. Adjustment (or censuring) within this population must accurately reflect departing (or entering) animals, which may influence this denominator. Other methods of determination or estimation of the population biologically at risk may be applicable in other situations [8].

Breeding

Becoming pregnant early in the breeding exposure interval is critical to the operation's success. Measures of importance include the breeding group, sires, and dates of exposure. This information is usually collected by the producer and shared with the practitioner. With conclusion of the defined breeding period, a determination of pregnancy status and gestational age is made. Working from paper or electronic (laptop or handheld computer) herd worksheets, the practitioner, technician, or producer collects/records

Table 3
Sample herd inventory and adjustments worksheet to establish numerators and denominators for calculations through the production phases—the population at risk

Category	Adjusted[a]	Count[b]	Exposed[c]
Female inventory at breeding	—	—	200
Transferred in after breeding	2	—	202
Transferred out after breeding	1	—	201
Total females pregnancy tested	—	176	201
Transferred in after test	3	—	204
Transferred out after test	1	—	203
Total females calving	—	174	203
Total live calves at birth	—	172	203
Transferred out after calving	1	—	202
Transferred in after calving	1	—	203
Calves died at birth	3	171	203
Calves died during growing phase	3	168	203
Total calves weaned	—	168	203

[a] Adjustments to inventory values.
[b] Potential calf count at each point of measurement.
[c] Exposed-female tally through the production cycle.

data in the field. The practitioner and staff best perform summarization of data. The practitioner reports the proportions pregnant by category or strata of interest (ie, age, body condition score, herds/groups) and the gestational age range and distribution. Then, based on the gestational age, an approximation of an expected calving date can be reported. Of course, if reproductive technologies using artificial insemination or embryo transfer are used, then a more certain gestational age and date of calving can be reported.

Evaluation of breeding and pregnancy is measured by several indices (Tables 4 and 5). The pregnancy percentage is the number of females exposed to a breeding opportunity and diagnosed as pregnant divided by the number of females exposed, multiplied by 100. Pregnancy percentage can also be measured by production parameters or strata of interest such as cow age, body condition score (at breeding or at pregnancy examination), or lactation state (cows with and without calves). Time to conception in the breeding season measures the promptness with which animals become pregnant following breeding exposure. This parameter requires the accurate staging of gestation resulting from natural service and concurrence with breeding records if artificial insemination (or other reproductive technologies) is used. The beginning exposure date and days pregnant on the day of examination are used to determine the time to conception, and estimated or projected calving dates for individuals are possible. Gestational age within the breeding season is then categorized according to the units most suited to the pregnancy detector and the needs of the reporting tool.

A distribution histogram can be portrayed as in Fig. 1, using a selected distribution interval (eg, 10-day, 20-day). It is of note that this distribution is generally not a normal (bell-shaped) distribution. An ideal distribution would possess a strong left skew, representing a larger proportion of cows that become pregnant early in a defined breeding season. In other situations, a bimodal distribution or a right-skewed distribution may be observed due to anestrus, inadequate nutrition, or disease events during the breeding

Table 4
Sample herd pregnancy examination summary

	No. of animals	Proportion (%)	TTC[a] (d)	Age[b] (y)	BCS[c]
Female cows exposed	201	NA	NA	3.8	5.1
Pregnant	176	87.6	23	3.8	5.2
Nonpregnant	25	12.4	NA	3.6	4.8
Lactating	128	85.9	26	5.0	5.0
Nonlactating	73	92.0	17	2.5	5.8

Abbreviations: BCS, body condition score; NA, not applicable; TTC, time to conception.

[a] Mean days to conception within the breeding season for each category.

[b] Mean cow age by category.

[c] Mean (or median) body condition score (range, 1–9; where 1 is a thin cow, 9 is an obese cow).

Table 5
Pregnancy distribution

Conception interval	0–20 d	21–40 d	41–60 d	>60 d
Pregnancy by period	70	65	37	4
Cumulative pregnancy	70	135	172	176
Cumulative percentage	39.8	76.7	97.7	100.0

season. A mean time to conception does not represent these distributions well; a median generally serves better as a single term for representation of this population measure.

Strata of interest evaluate the median gestational age. This distribution may suggest nutritional or disease events that may be influencing herd performance. For example, if the proportion of cows pregnant is determined for the range of body condition scores represented within the herd (eg, 3 to 7 on an ordinal scale of 1 to 9), then an upward trend in proportion pregnant is expected when nutrition (predominantly or alone) is influencing pregnancy outcome. If, however, a reproductive disease such as trichomoniasis or campylobacterosis is affecting the herd, then the proportion pregnant by body condition score is more uniformly depressed across body condition scores. This herd may show a delayed relative median time to conception and a distribution of time to conception that has a right-skewed herd conception pattern, suggesting a delay in estrus onset or an early embryonic death loss and subsequent conception. These patterns of change are often subtle and may not be readily observed except by evaluation of distributions.

During the cow breeding period, there is an expectation that cows be in an appropriate nutritional plane to support the potential for pregnancy early in the breeding interval. Thus, regular evaluation of nutritional state is made by measuring body weights (a continuous variable), body condition score (an ordinal categoric variable), or both [9]. As a continuous variable, body weights can be reported as means (and standard deviations) by categories of interest (ie, cow age). Body condition score is an ordinal subjective

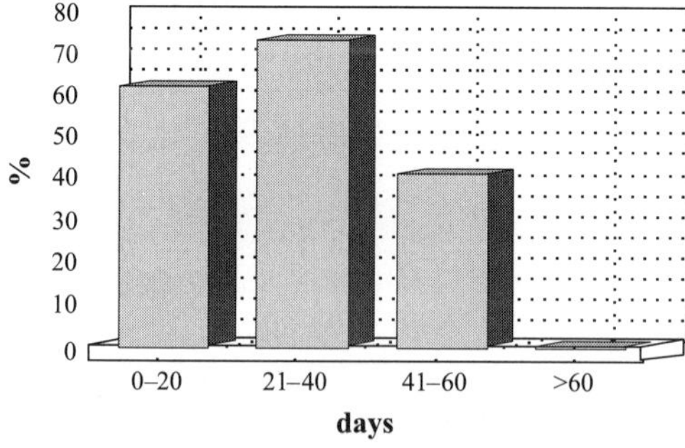

Fig. 1. The pregnancy rate distribution is depicted by time of conception within the breeding season.

measure of fat distribution (or lack thereof) in the animal. It is a categoric score, which is most appropriately reported as a median or a distribution of scores; however, it is also reported as a mean. In most populations, the distribution for body condition score within a herd of adequate size (ie, >50 head) is normally distributed. The normal distribution permits the use of a mean (and variance). It makes a difference whether the distribution is skewed for any reason. The management of categoric data is discussed more in depth by Ruegg elsewhere in this issue.

Calving

The cow reaches the midpoint of the calf production process with the successful delivery of the calf. Maternal information recorded at this time relates to her reproductive health and her maternal or mothering traits. A calf record associated or relationally tied the cow is begun. The pertinent calf information includes calf (and mother's) identification, birth date, birth weight, sex, a measure of calving ease [10], calf vigor [10], health, and mortality. Categoric variables such as calving ease (ordinal) or calf vigor scores (nominal) can be used to compare calves by factors of interest, including cow age (mean), calf sex (cross-tabulation count), birth weight (mean), and calving distribution period (cross-tabulation count).

Evaluation of gestation and calving performance includes calving percentages, pregnancy losses, calving distribution, and calf death losses (Tables 6 and 7). The calving percentage is the number of females calving divided by the number of females exposed, multiplied by 100. Pregnancy loss percentage is the number of cows determined to be pregnant at pregnancy examination minus the number of cows delivering offspring divided by the number of cows determined to be pregnant at pregnancy examination, multiplied by 100. This percentage defines the abortion rate among animals that

Table 6
Sample herd calving season summary

	No. of animals	Rate (%)	TTP[a] (d)	BWt (lb)	CES[b]
Exposed females calving	174	85.7	22	75	1.1
Bull calves	89	—	25	79	1.2
Heifer calves	85	—	19	72	1.1
Pregnancy loss	2	1.0	NA	NA	NA
Calving loss/death	3	1.5	40	82	2.3
Calf death 1–10 d	2	1.0	45	65	1.4
Calf death 11–30 d	1	0.5	25	78	1.0
Calf death >30 d	0	0.0	—	—	1.0
Cow death	1	0.5	—	—	—

Abbreviations: BWt, calf birth weight; CES, calving ease score; NA, not applicable; TTP, time to parturition.

[a] Average number of days to parturition for each category.

[b] Range, 1–5.

Table 7
Calving distribution

Calving interval[a]	0–21 d	22–42 d	43–63 d	>63 d
Calves born by period	66	71	33	4
Cumulative number	66	137	170	174
Cumulative percent	37.9	78.7	97.7	100.0

[a] The starting date for the 21-day periods is 285 days after the bull turn-in date with the mature cows or when the third mature cow calves.

were identified as pregnant. Calving distribution is displayed as the cumulative number of calves born by 21, 42, 63, and greater than 63 days of the calving season divided by the total number of calves born, multiplied by 100. The producer and his or her personnel most appropriately collect calf birth information. The practitioner, his or her staff, or both summarize this information. It should be noted that the calving distribution is expected to mirror the distribution demonstrated at pregnancy examination, as exemplified in Fig. 1. The distribution pattern would ideally be strongly skewed to the left, depicting cows that were reproductively sound and healthy at the initiation of the fixed breeding season and became pregnant promptly. The result is a large proportion of early-born calves relative to the start of calving within the population.

Success of the breeding program and calf survival (or loss) within this neonatal population is the focus of this monitoring strategy. Calf death loss is measured as a proportion of the exposed females or as a proportion of the calves born. Calf death loss based on exposed females is the number of calves that died divided by the number of exposed females, multiplied by 100; calf death loss based on calves born is the number of calves that died divided by the number of calves born, multiplied by 100.

Weaning

At calf weaning time, the focus is the cow's marketable offspring. It is, however, an appropriate time to assess the cow's maternal and reproductive ability in light of her offspring's performance. Age, weight, body condition score, health, and current pregnancy status (the next calf) of the cow are assessed and used at this time as criteria for her continuance in the herd or as reasons for culling her. Culling reasons are assigned to each animal leaving the herd. It is observed that an animal may leave the herd for more than one reason, which may confound assessment due to a recording bias (conscious or unconscious) or clouding of information that may become a source of error or misinterpretation.

Weaning information may be collected by the producer or the veterinarian and his or her staff but is preferentially summarized by the veterinarian (Table 8). Calves are usually weaned at a common date. This date should be recorded for the calf population and for the individuals within the

Table 8
Sample herd weaning summary

	No. of animals	Rate (%)	TTW[a] (d)	WWt (lb)	WDA (lb/d)	W/C (lb)
Weaned[b]	168	82.8	216	502	2.3	415
Bulls/steers	86	—	219	510	2.3	—
Heifers	82	—	218	493	2.3	—
Total weight	—	—	—	84,322	—	415
Market[c]	138	68.0	216	492	2.3	334
Bulls/steers	86	—	219	510	2.3	—
Heifers	52	—	211	462	2.2	—
Total weight	—	—	—	67,879	—	334
Replacement[d]	30	14.8	225	548	2.4	—
Bulls	0	—	—	—	—	—
Heifers	30	14.8	225	548	2.4	—
Total weight	—	—	—	16,443	—	—

Abbreviations: TTW, time to weaning; W/C, weaned pounds of calf per exposed female; WDA, weight per day of age; WWt, mean weaning weight.

[a] Average number of days to weaning for each category.

[b] All calves weaned.

[c] Weaned calves going to market.

[d] Weaned calves being kept as breeding replacement animals.

population not managed as a cohort. This date plus the date of birth provides a measure of age at weaning. The cohort of calves is that year's calf crop. If that crop is derived from a fixed-length breeding season and, therefore, a defined calving period, then the crop will have a relatively narrow range of age from oldest to youngest. Nonetheless, the calf crop can be stratified by cohorts such as calf age (21-day calving intervals), breed composition, or health status. This stratification is demonstrated in Table 9, whereby the distribution of calves by 21-day calving interval categories is used to look at numbers of calves weaned, their mean age and weight at weaning, and the total weaning weight represented within this smaller age cohort. Calf crop or weaning proportion is an important measure of success

Table 9
Weaning distribution

Calving period[a]	0–21 d	22–42 d	43–63 d	>63 d	Total
Calves weaned	66	71	28	3	168
DTW	233	212	191	170	216
WWt	525	500	459	440	502
Total weight	34,650	35,500	12,852	1320	84,322
W/C[b] by interval	171	175	77	8	415
W/C[b] percentage	41.1	42.1	15.2	1.6	100

Abbreviations: DTW, days to weaning; W/C, weaned pounds of calf per exposed female; WWt, weaning weight.

[a] Calving intervals representing birthing distribution in the calving season (ie, the oldest calves are in category 0–21 days).

[b] Contribution by time interval to weight per cow.

in the population. It reports the proportion of exposed females that has successfully traversed breeding, gestation, delivery, and rearing to produce a marketable offspring. Calf crop or weaning percentage is the number of calves weaned divided by the number of females exposed, multiplied by 100. The population at risk continues to be that population of cows initially exposed to a breeding opportunity or a defined adjustment thereto, as previously described (see Table 3). The actual weaning weight reports the cow's nurturing and genetic input to the offspring produced. Note that this measure is very time dependent. Actual weaning weight is the total weight of the weaned calves divided by the total number of calves weaned. This measure is often further evaluated by strata of calf sex (ie, actual weaning weight for all steer calves, bull calves, or heifer calves). This weight may also be evaluated by the 21-day calving interval. Because actual weaning weight is time dependent, individual calf performance can also be calculated as weight per day of age, which is the weaning weight of the calf minus its birth weight divided by the calf's days of age at weaning. Calf weaning weights can be adjusted to a common or standardized age by multiplying the weight per day of age by the adjusted days of age (eg, 205 days) and adding the birth weight to this number. Comparison of strata by standardization methods is possible and occasionally applicable, but from a management standpoint, the time-dependent advantage of early-born calves is desirable and reflective of the maternal fertility.

An important herdwide maternal measure at weaning time is the pounds weaned per exposed female. This measure is the total pounds of calf weaned divided by the total number of females exposed. It reflects a nonspecific but single, overall index of performance for the population of cows, reflecting the combined ability of the population to become pregnant, remain pregnant, deliver a live calf, and nurture that calf to a weaning (marketable) weight. This measure provides a single, year-to-year index of the cow-calf herd performance. It should be noted that year-to-year variation is possible and expected. The cause of variation may or may not be readily determined from the data/information collected and evaluated. The practitioner monitors, measures, and seeks to determine the factors associated with herd performance outcomes.

Finally, calf death loss (mortality) from birth to weaning based on calves born is calculated as the number of calves that died divided by the number of calves born, multiplied by 100. Calf death loss based on the relative time of death (ie, at birth, within the first 10 days of life, between 11 and 30 days of life, and at 30 days to weaning) can be measured as a percentage of calves born (see Table 6).

Analysis and reporting

An annual calf crop summary is prepared as in Table 10, which shows the key performance indices. This summary is the annual report card against

Table 10
Sample herd summary of performance

Measures of reproduction performance	No. of animals	%	lb/head
Exposed females	203	100	—
Pregnancy percentage	176	88.0	—
Pregnancy loss percentage	2	1.0	—
Calving percentage	174	87.0	—
Calf death loss based on exposed females	6	3.0	—
Calf crop or weaning percentage	168	84.0	—
Female replacement rate percentage	30	13.5	—
Calf death loss based on calves born	6	3.4	—
Calving distribution			
Calves born during first 21 d	66	37.9	—
Calves born during first 42 d	137	78.7	—
Calves born during first 63 d	170	97.7	—
Production performance measures			
Weaning weights (mean lb/hd)[a]			
Bulls/steers	86	—	510
Heifers	82	—	493
Mean weaning weight	168	—	502
Pounds weaned per exposed female	168	—	415

[a] Mean age at weaning, 218 days (n = 216 calves).

which goals and critical intervention levels are compared (see Table 2). At this point, goals and critical intervention levels may be adjusted or areas of strength and weakness identified. A more detailed scrutiny of production phases (breeding, see Tables 4 and 5; gestation and calving, see Tables 6 and 7; calf growth, see Tables 8 and 9) may suggest critical factors contributing to outcomes. Strengths can then be reinforced. Weaknesses become the practitioner's focus for medical or managerial intervention strategies. The cross-sectional study of the herd is extended to a longitudinal study (or a sequence of cross-sectional studies). As questions or hypothesizes are generated, other observational (ie, prospective cohort studies, retrospective case-control or cohort studies) or experimental (ie, clinical trials or interventional) studies may be employed.

A final note on the cow-calf herd is that total quality management of the cow herd may include the continued follow-up of marketed calves. This follow-up assesses, by continued observation, whether procedures and practices applied at the ranch level are producing productive, healthy animals in subsequent production phases (ie, stocker, feedlot).

Assessment of heifers

Description

The replacement heifer is usually reared and selected from the source population of cows, and these heifers rejoin that population as a mature cow.

If animals are purchased and added to the herd, then they should have an accompanying record of health and performance. Heifer calves raised on farm have maternal and calf records of performance and health that continue with them.

The planned development of the weaned female is critical to her lifetime success as a cow within the greater cow population. The rearing and development aspect of the enterprise is the foundation for a sound mature cow population. The female replacement rate is measured as the sum of raised replacement heifers exposed and due to calve for the first time plus purchased replacement heifers plus purchased breeding cows exposed, divided by the number of exposed females, multiplied by 100. When the population number remains stable, this measure has greater interpretative value; however, when the population is increasing or decreasing (becoming unstable), it may become a source of error in interpretation. That is, if the mature cow population (the exposed population, denominator of multiple indices) is being retained or culled disproportionately to the number of heifers entering the cow herd, then the perceived replacement rate may give a skewed measure of replacement.

Calf to replacement heifer and cow

Heifer calf records are similar to those previously reported for cows. In addition, as the heifer develops, other data are collected, focusing on growth and condition. The heifer is expected to attain approximately 65% of her mature body weight before she is first exposed to breeding as dictated by good management practice. On a heifer herd basis, there is an expectation that a large proportion of heifers (90%–95%) will attain this target when properly managed. It would be the rare situation that the heifer population is not a relatively uniform genetic population. Thus, the heifers have a similar expected mature weight, and as such, a measure of mean weight and variance may be used as an assessment of development. A birth to mature weight growth chart with an expected mean and 95% confidence interval curve for weight may be developed over time for the breed and management conditions of the operation. Tabular or graphic charts are used to monitor estimates of growth targets for individuals and populations of heifers. Review of these plotted weights should permit the veterinarian to answer whether population targets are being met or whether there are outliers within the population. These weights should be actual as opposed to adjusted weights.

These weights are taken at selected target intervals. Yearling weight is a common measure for the heifer nearing puberty. Because of age differences in the heifer population, this weight reflects a time bias similar to weaning weight. If population standardization is desirable, then the yearling weight is used to produce an estimate of average daily gain within the defined time interval (eg, at a weaning to yearling weight or a weight per day of age). An adjusted yearling weight is then calculated as the mean daily gain multiplied by the adjusted days of age (eg, 365 days) plus the birth weight. Standardization by age is not always desirable because age (time at which conception occurred) is a critical management component.

Two other valuable measures of heifer development are the reproductive tract scores [11] and a pelvic area measurement [10]. The relative merits of these procedures are discussed elsewhere. The reproductive tract score is an objective, categoric measure (range, 1–5) that estimates the relative likelihood that a heifer is cycling reproductively and suggests her probability for pregnancy when exposed to breeding the first time. This measure is an ordinal, categoric measure that may be depicted as a median or as a proportional/count distribution by tract score. The pelvic area measurement, in contrast, is a continuous variable (the height of the pelvic opening multiplied by the width, measured in squared centimeters). This measurement for the individual must be assessed in light of the cohort population mean and standard deviation. The measure is best used to cull heifers that have a relatively small pelvis, as opposed to a criterion for selection. As previously noted, the heifer population is expected to be genetically similar and uniform in age and size. Because the pelvic area measurements within the uniform heifer population are expected to be normally distributed, a mean and standard deviation are fitting measures. Alternately, the veterinarian can produce a graphic distribution. A cutoff point for culling purposes can then be defined by a first or second lower standard deviation.

When heifers are exposed to breeding, they are monitored in a similar way to the mature cow but with a more critical gauge. There is an expectation that heifers will be early maturing and fertile. As a management practice, their breeding season may be shorter than that of mature cows. Nonperforming heifers (due to poor body condition, growth, reproductive tract score, pelvic area, or pregnancy outcome) are not selected. For those heifers that are retained, it must be kept in mind that they are still growing; body weight and condition must continue to be monitored. Heifers preferentially calve at about 85% of their mature body weight. Again, these weights are monitored against the established growth chart for the herd. Continued close monitoring is expected until the heifer is pregnant for the second time and approaching her mature body weight. The heifer's body condition is regularly assessed for reproduction and calf performance as per the mature cow.

Assessment of bulls

Bulls are kept separate from the cow population for much of the year. Their function as breeding animals requires that mature bulls remain healthy and in a maintenance body condition. As the breeding season approaches, bulls should be in a positive energy balance and a good nutritional state and assessed to be fertile by a bull breeding soundness examination and disease-free by selected testing for diseases of concern. These diseases are generally venereal (*Tritrichomonas foetus, Campylobacter fetus* subsp *fetus*) but could also be contagious diseases (bovine virus diarrhea, Johne's disease). Bulls should also be maintained on an immunization and parasite control plan similar to that of the cow population to which they will be exposed.

Bull development focuses on nutritional and health management of the bull. Growth charts on expected growth curves are generated as a result of regular weight (and body condition) monitoring. Bulls should reach puberty by age 12 to 15 months, which means that they will attain 65% to 70% of their mature body weight and demonstrate breeding soundness on examination, including having adequate scrotal circumference. It should be noted that bull growth/development charts could be developed specifically for the bull population, as per the heifers; however because this population size is generally smaller than the heifer population, its creation may be hampered by limited numbers of animals. The bull is capable of limited breeding capacity in the first year. By the following breeding season, the bull should attain full breeding capacity.

Enterprise assessment

Among the important monitoring roles that can be performed by the veterinarian is herd or enterprise surveillance. This assessment establishes a baseline status for the enterprise property or animal populations over time. This assay may relate to nutrient components (excesses or deficiencies), environmental toxins, and disease agents.

Nutrient analysis of major feed components, for example, should be regularly assessed (annually or semiannually). Grasses, forages, and commodity feeds may be analyzed for total digestible nutrients, crude protein, dry matter, and other components. Animals may also be assayed for nutrients or trace minerals of importance (eg, selenium, copper, molybdenum, sulfur, manganese, zinc, cobalt, and iodine). Assessment of micromineral levels provides baseline or normal herd status. These measures should be monitored as population means and standard deviations. The practitioner should be reminded that as the number of tests performed on individual animals increases, so does the likelihood that one or more tests will be abnormal. These individual animal values may be normal but lie outside the population 95% confidence interval or may be temporally deviated from the mean and will regress to a population mean in time. Due to cost and sampling time, representative animal sample collection and selection of adequate sample size become important in the validity of the information collected.

Disease events, diagnostic work-ups, and necropsies within the population should be recorded for an historical perspective. Endemic disease or disease risks are monitored by sampling the population using a suitable testing procedure. Are endemic diseases (eg, infectious bovine rhinotracheitis, parainfluenza 3, bovine virus diarrhea, bovine respiratory syncytial virus, leptospirosis, anaplasmosis, and so forth) a source of risk within the population? What is the baseline parasite burden? What is the parasite burden of the population by age and by season? How and when might strategic or interventional controls be applied? As test procedures are applied, the sensitivity, specificity, positive/negative predictive value, and prevalence of disease principles also become applicable. Test characteristics are discussed in more depth by McKenna elsewhere in this issue. These issues become more pressing as diseases such as Johne's disease (the detection of *Mycobacterium avium* subsp *paratuberculosis*) become more exigent [12,13]. This particular disease complicates communication between the veterinarian and the producer because it is not black or white, positive or negative. Because of moderate-to-poor test sensitivity (15%–85%) for this disease, a test likelihood ratio in which test results provide a probability of disease rather than a positive-negative cutoff point is useful. Population monitoring of Johne's disease is also an appropriate case for application of serial or parallel testing (eg, serum ELISA, fecal culture, polymerase chain reaction) to define disease or disease prevalence within a population. A serial testing strategy considers an animal "positive" if one or more tests are positive. In this case, the condition is less likely to be missed and the animal is asked to prove itself not positive. A parallel testing strategy considers an animal positive if all tests are positive. This strategy minimizes false positives and the animal is asked to prove itself positive. In the process of disease detection, the practitioner potentially determines disease prevalence, quantifies the factors associated with disease and the role of each, and establishes the most fitting intervention strategies.

Other epidemiologic considerations

As the aforementioned information becomes a part of the cow-calf enterprise's norm, other epidemiologic tools are more readily implemented. Some other considerations are enterprise budget, partial budget, benefit-cost analysis, decision tree analysis, and survival analysis. A variety of economic decision-making tools is discussed by Galligan elsewhere in this issue.

Summary

The systematic data collection of population characteristics of interest for the cow-calf herd within the beef cattle enterprise provides a baseline for assessing outcomes of interest, namely, morbidity, mortality, and performance of its populations. The veterinarian and cow-calf producer establish performance goals and critical intervention levels for measurable outcomes of interest. They must then establish a method of data collection that is logistically and economically feasible. They set the groundwork for evaluating the herd performance and detecting evidence of excessive morbidity or mortality. In the cow-calf enterprise, the herd assessment focuses on the cow's establishment and maintenance of pregnancy; the birthing and delivery of live, healthy offspring; the neonate's survival and well-being as a consequence of maternal care and nurturing; and the growth and development of the calf through to weaning. This process is initially a cross-sectional herd survey, which becomes a longitudinal population study over time. As data are analyzed, population studies may be implemented to better characterize the population, interventional strategies may be employed, and ultimately, performance and animal well-being is augmented. The practitioner plays a key role in establishing the groundwork for this process, including data collection, analysis, interpretation, reporting, and overseeing the implemented strategies.

References

[1] van Schothorst M. ILSI Europe concise monograph series. A simple guide to understanding and applying the hazard analysis critical control point concept. 3rd edition. Brussels, Belgium: International Life Sciences Institute; 2004. p. 1–25.

[2] McGrann JM, Hamilton ED, Klinefelter DA. Handbook IRM-SPA. College Station (TX): Texas Agricultural Extension Service; 1993.

[3] Hamilton ED. Standardized performance analysis. Vet Clin North Am Food Anim Pract 1995;11:199–214.

[4] Lessard P. The characterization of disease outbreaks. Vet Clin North Am Food Anim Pract 1988;4:17–32.

[5] National Cattleman's Beef Association. Quality Assurance (BQA) Guidelines. Available at: http://www.geefusa.org/produidelines.aspx. Accessed October 10, 2005.

[6] Kniffen D. Desk record NCA-IRM. Vet Clin North Am Food Anim Pract 1995;11:215–78.

[7] Evans JL, Davies D. Cow-calf production record software. Current report. Stillwater (OK): Oklahoma State University, Division of Agricultural Science and Natural Resources. Publication #WCR 3279.1–3279.8.

[8] Martin SW, Meek AH, Willeberg P. Measurement of disease frequency and production. In: Veterinary epidemiology. Ames (IA): Iowa State University Press; 1987. p. 48–62.

[9] Herd DB, Sprott LR. Body condition, nutrition, and reproduction of beef cows. College Station (TX): Texas Agricultural Extension Service; 1986. Publication #B-1526.

[10] Beef Improvement Federation. BIF guidelines. Available at: http://beefimprovement.org/guidelines.html. Accessed October 10, 2005.

[11] Anderson KJ, LeFever DG, Brink JS, et al. The use of reproductive tract scoring in beef heifers. Agri Pract 1991;12:19–26.

[12] Hansen D, Rossiter CA, Carter M. National Johne's Working Group. Johne's Committee of the US Animal Health Association. Handbook for veterinarians and beef producers. A guide for Johne's disease risk assessments and management plans for beef herds. Richmond (VA): US Animal Health Association; 2003. p. 1–8.

[13] Hansen D, Rossiter CA, Carter M. National Johne's Working Group. Johne's Committee of the US Animal Health Association. How to do risk assessment and management plans for Johne's disease. Richmond (VA): US Animal Health Association; 2003. p. 1–14.

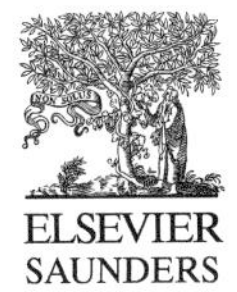

ELSEVIER
SAUNDERS

Vet Clin Food Anim 22 (2006) 75–101

VETERINARY
CLINICS
Food Animal Practice

Disease Outbreak Investigation in Food Animal Practice

Cheryl L. Waldner, DVM, PhD*,
John R. Campbell, DVM, DVSc

Department of Large Animal Clinical Sciences, Western College of Veterinary Medicine, University of Saskatchewan, 52 Campus Drive, Saskatoon, Saskatchewan S7N 5B4, Canada

In addition to excellent observation skills and a good understanding of production medicine, veterinarians require the tools of epidemiology for the successful investigation of disease outbreaks. Food supply veterinary practitioners are often called upon to investigate various types of disease outbreaks. Various investigators have presented general strategies for managing outbreaks [1–6]. Others have developed guidelines for investigating specific disease problems and productivity shortfalls [7–13]. In this article, the authors outline the primary questions a practitioner should address and summarize a systematic approach to determining the causes of an outbreak and minimizing further losses

Initial objectives

The methods for investigating outbreaks of clinical disease are equally applicable to the identification of factors responsible for suboptimal productivity or changes in herd performance. An outbreak is indicated when disease rates are higher than normal or productivity is lower than normal for a particular population [14]. The expected incidence and consequences of different diseases vary considerably, and therefore the threshold of disease that triggers an investigation may vary depending on the disease. An extensive outbreak investigation could be triggered by just one case. For example, the diagnosis of a persistently infected calf in a herd that was thought to be biosecure may require a comprehensive investigation.

* Corresponding author.
E-mail address: cheryl.waldner@usask.ca (C.L. Waldner).

doi:10.1016/j.cvfa.2005.12.001 *vetfood.theclinics.com*

The immediate goal of the practitioner is to take steps to minimize additional herd losses [15]. Actions can often be taken to stop the problem before the specific cause is identified. For example, if a toxic exposure is suspected on pasture, the cattle can be moved to a different field while an investigation takes place to identify the source and type of toxin [16]. After any necessary actions have been taken to address the immediate threat, the next step is to identify the factors that contributed to the development of disease or change in productivity. The practitioner must then determine which of these factors can be controlled by management to reduce the risk of future outbreaks. These objectives can be achieved by addressing the following questions for each outbreak (W5: what, who, when, where, and why) [1]: define the problem—what and how much? identify groups for comparison—who, when, and where? review important risk factors and identify key determinants—why? develop recommendations and follow up to assess the effectiveness of the intervention.

Define and describe the problem—is it worth investigating?

The first and most critical task early in the investigation is to clearly define the problem [5]. An early working definition of the problem provides direction for the investigation. If the veterinarian has an established veterinary-client relationship with the producer, the practitioner should be better able to clearly define the problem. The initial complaint often encompasses a number of different types of health and production issues. The initial complaint can include unexplained mortality, clinical disease [17,18], subclinical disease, impaired performance, and falling trends in productivity [19,20]. Other issues related to a complaint might involve potential public health concerns about food safety [15,21] and environmental issues [22]. The use of herd record systems may allow monitoring trends in herd productivity measures over time or benchmark comparisons by the practitioner. Such systems can identify a problem before an initial complaint is made. The herd veterinarian is also more likely to be aware of any recent changes in management that may have a bearing on the initial complaint.

The development of a case definition is an important step in describing the problem. This case definition is critical when comparing cases with non-cases to determine the importance of potential risk factors for disease. This definition must be reevaluated and refined as more data become available. A simple, easily recognized and applied definition facilitates the consistent reporting of cases by the herd owner, other farm workers, and cooperating veterinarians. A case definition for pneumonia in neonatal calves might include all febrile or depressed animals less than 3 months of age with evidence of increased respiratory effort or coughing. The inclusion of unrelated cases (eg, all calves with an increased respiratory rate) can result in errors in recognizing factors that might have contributed to the outbreak [4]. In some outbreaks, such as in abortion outbreaks, defining the case definition is a relatively simple procedure. However, when morbidity is the primary complaint, a precise case definition helps to avoid differences in treatment thresholds that may exist between various producers or farm workers. For example, using a specific temperature cutoff as part of the case definition for respiratory disease creates a more specific case definition than a case definition that includes just those animals that the treatment crew assesses as "sick."

After developing a working description of the clinical disease or impairment in productivity, the practitioner must determine the extent of the problem that is present in the herd. The answer to this question helps the investigator decide if there really is a problem and then determine the appropriate amount of resources that should be allocated to the investigation.

To determine if the outbreak is real, the productivity and disease frequency in the herd are first measured and then compared with published benchmarks, historical expectations, goals of the farmer, or the performance of neighboring herds. Practitioners that use computerized records may be able to benchmark the performance of their clients from year to year and between herds. The practitioner must have a good understanding of the "normal" production and disease levels for livestock raised under similar management conditions to be able to determine whether or not the observed values are within an expected range [9]. The most appropriate benchmarks against which to compare the production of any herd vary because of economic constraints, physical restrictions, time and management limitations, and individual differences. The targets for performance change over time for a particular herd as these constraints change.

Most outbreaks are identified and reported by the herd owner. The severity of problems presented to the veterinarian varies with the individual owner's threshold of concern [5]. Large-scale disease outbreaks may not be brought to the attention of the local practitioner until significant mortality or production losses have occurred. In these situations, the veterinarian may find it difficult to reconstruct the epidemic because of insufficient client records and the loss of valuable diagnostic material. In some cases, the disease progresses slowly and by the time the veterinarian is asked to investigate, many of the animals have chronic disease. In such cases, determining the original factors that contributed to disease onset may be difficult.

On the other hand, some herd owners are alarmed by disease losses well within expected rates [9]. For example, expectations of acceptable risk of abortion, incidence of calf treatment, and herd average somatic cell count vary wildly among herd owners [5,14]. By confirming the existence and severity of the problem, the investigator decreases time and resources spent on investigating epidemics that do not exist [4].

Identify potential risk factors by comparing groups within the herd

Given that there is sufficient evidence to proceed with an investigation, the immediate goal of the practitioner is to identify risk factors that can be manipulated to resolve the outbreak or improve herd production and profitability. Risk factors are characteristics of the host (ie, animals), agent (ie, causative factor), or environment (ie, actual climatic factors or other management factors) that can increase the occurrence of disease [7]. For example, some of the documented risk factors for increased neonatal mortality in beef cattle include poor cow-body condition at calving, a high degree of crowding and contamination of the calving ground, and a high percentage of heifers in the herd [23]. The risk factors that management can control and alter to affect disease rates or production levels are sometimes referred to as key determinants [9]. Pre-calving nutrition and calving-ground density are examples of important key determinants of neonatal mortality in beef cattle.

The identification of the key determinants that can be most readily manipulated to control the outbreak is called a working diagnosis, an epidemiological diagnosis [9], or a diagnosis of "best fit" [5]. The first steps in identifying these risk factors are to determine which groups of animals are affected (ie, the host characteristics, such as age, sex and breed), when they became affected (ie, time, particularly the date of onset), and where the problem was reported (ie, place or location of affected animals or groups of animals) [24,25]. See the article by Gay elsewhere in this issue for information about determining causal relationship.

Describe who is affected

The amount of information available varies greatly between herds, depending on management, animal identification, and record-keeping practices. The practitioner should collect all relevant and available information on the diseased animals. Sources of this information can include identifying brands, tags (plastic and metal), or tattoos. Types of information can include age, sex, breed, and color of animals; use of animals; origin of animals (ie, purchased or born on farm); an animal's feed and water source; the nature of the animal's housing; stage of reproductive cycle or gestation; lactation status; information about parity; relevant clinical, pathological, or laboratory reports; and processing, vaccination, and treatment histories [4]. A complete and detailed individual animal line listing or inventory is very useful, but often is not readily available.

Where herds are managed in distinct groups, much of this information can be collected and summarized at the group level. Often the herd owner can describe the number of animals in a pen or pasture group and the number affected, while a record of which animals were affected might not be available. In most situations, if individual animal data are available, they should be retained throughout the entire investigation process. This allows the correlation of individual animal laboratory data to individual animal outcomes. If this is not possible, then the collection of data at the next smallest group level is the most appropriate way of proceeding. Simple spreadsheets or databases can be used to enter and sort herd data as they are collected. Other information, including laboratory results, can be added later. Information should be examined for unaffected as well as affected animals and groups within the herd [4]. In some cases, information on neighboring herds can also be useful. Information can be collected by a variety of methods, but personal interviews as part of a herd visit are best.

Determine when the problem occurred

The temporal pattern of disease can provide important clues about the origin of disease in the herd [4]. Is this a new or a long-standing problem in the herd? Are the numbers of new cases increasing, have they stabilized, or have they peaked and started to decrease? The pattern of disease can be described in an epidemic curve by plotting the time of onset of each case (X-axis) in appropriate intervals against the number of cases recognized at each time interval (Y-axis). The distribution of cases in a beef herd abortion storm is provided as an example (Fig. 1). The most appropriate time interval varies with intensity of the outbreak and may be hours, days, weeks, or even months. For example, following the exposure to a potent feed or water toxin, tracking the pattern of disease over a period of hours and days might provide clues to the source of the problem. When examining an outbreak of Johne's disease, cases often need to be tracked over months or years to understand the progression of infection in the herd. Important events and management changes should be indicated on the epidemic curve to help the practitioner visualize the sequence of events.

The epidemic curve can be used to infer whether the problem is endemic in the herd, epidemic in nature, or sporadic. An endemic disease occurs at

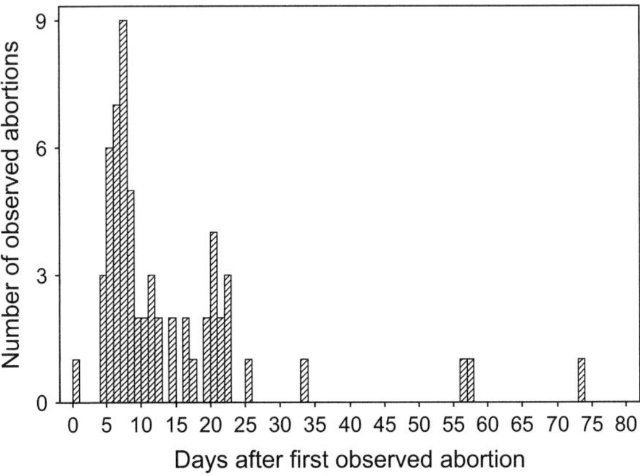

Fig. 1. Epidemic curve demonstrating a *Neospora caninum* abortion outbreak in a beef herd.

a consistent level in the herd with only minor fluctuations over time. For example, subclinical mastitis is endemic in most dairy herds. The percentage of animals affected may be very low or include most of the herd. Epidemic is a relative term used to describe disease within a given time interval that is clearly above its expected rate of occurrence. For example, respiratory disease in feedlot cattle is often epidemic shortly after weaning. A disease is sporadic if it occurs rarely and follows no regular pattern [25]. An example of sporadic disease might be the death of apparently healthy beef calves due to abomasal ulcers.

The distribution of cases can suggest whether the problem resulted from exposure to a single-point source or is caused by an infectious agent moving from one animal to the next. For example, an epidemic curve showing a dramatic upward slope indicates many new cases in a short span of time. Such a curve would be expected when the causative agent is a point source [26]. A dramatic onslaught of cases followed by a rapid decline might be expected following exposure to a toxicant on pasture followed by removal of the cattle at the start of clinical signs. A gradual upward slope followed by a steep down slope with one or more additional peaks can suggest a propagated agent [26]. For example, in an outbreak of calf scours in cow-calf herd, data might show a gradual accumulation of cases to a peak, followed by a downward slope, with additional peaks occurring as the epidemic moves through different management groups. The shape of the curve reflects three factors. One is the incubation pattern, which starts from infection and continues to the time the animal becomes contagious. The second is the timing of transmission. The third is the opportunity of transmission [4,24].

The location and identification of the first case (ie, index case) can be a clue to the source of infection in the group. As an example, several cases of salmonellosis due to *Salmonella typhimurium DT104* were identified in beef cows after visiting a local veterinary clinic. Using clinic records, the index case was identified as a calf that had died in the clinic several weeks earlier. Identification of index cases can be difficult, particularly when the index case is subclinical, such as in the example of a nonsymptomatic animal shedding *Salmonella*, bovine viral diarrhea virus, or Johne's organisms. However, when an exotic or reportable disease is diagnosed, an intensive "trace back" is initiated by the investigating regulatory agency to determine the origin of the first sick animal and potential contacts with other herds. Determining how much time passes from when the animals are first observed sick until they are found dead [6] can also be useful. Where treatment records are limited, however, only the date of death might be available.

Describe where the problem occurred

Differences in where affected animals were housed and pastured in relation to unaffected animals can provide additional clues about origin of the infection outbreak or productivity shortfall [4]. A detailed sketch or map of the farm and surrounding area can be used to record the location of all management groups. For example, dairy heifers can be separated into different facilities based on age and reproductive status. Important risk factors can be identified by investigating the timing of group movement between different housing facilities or pastures and the movement of animals between different management groups. The location of management groups in relation to neighboring herds and the potential frequency of contact with neighboring herds should also be examined. Potential contact information can usually be gathered during producer interviews. The role of contact with other herds may be especially important if the producer uses communal grazing or if there may have been unusual contact with another herd. An unusual contact would be, for example, when a neighbor's bull enters a pasture.

A point map of the farm [27] should include a sketch of housing facilities, corrals, pastures (including details of cross-fencing), feeding facilities, and watering sources. If possible, the location of neighboring herds could also be identified. The location of each management group at the time of the outbreak and the location of individual cases can be overlaid on the map. This map can be used for detecting spatial patterns of disease and developing hypotheses about the location of exposure. A series of maps showing animal movements and patterns of disease over time can also be useful.

Generate hypotheses about key determinants by comparing groups within the herd

The analysis begins with organizing and summarizing the data for the entire herd. A simple spreadsheet is often needed to list animal identifications and other information such as breed, age, laboratory results, pen conditions, and other risk factors. The next step is to quantitatively describe the breed and age structure of the population, the physical examination, and laboratory results. Then the task is to characterize the problem using descriptive statistics. Groups are identified within the herd based on whether or not the animal represents a case. Animals are further sorted by characteristics, locations, and times when they were found sick.

These comparisons form the foundation of information required to determine why the outbreak occurred. Sometimes these comparisons identify one or more key determinants for the disease outbreak. This process may also raise specific questions that can be addressed by obtaining additional information from the herd owner or laboratory testing.

Develop recommendations, provide a written report, and follow up to determine the effectiveness of the intervention

As more information becomes available over the course of an investigation, recommendations for control can be supplemented and modified to reduce losses. The action list evolves as the working diagnosis changes in response to new information. The recommendations for control of the herd problem are developed by addressing the key determinants identified during the investigation [9]. Possible interventions vary depending on the severity of the problem, its potential consequences, and the risks to other producers and public health. Actions available for consideration include changes to the environment, client education, quarantine of affected and suspect animals, test and slaughter, mass vaccination and treatment, and, in extreme circumstances, herd depopulation [1,5]. For example, changes to the environment are often the most effective method of treating an outbreak of calf scours, while mass treatment or metaphylaxis is the most effective response to shipping-fever pneumonia in weaned calves.

Preliminary reports summarizing initial findings should be issued shortly after the first herd visit. A final report can be prepared when all laboratory analyses are completed. The report must be designed for the intended audience. Most reports are prepared for the herd owner, but in some cases the report must be written so that a banker or lawyer can understand it. The report should be well organized, concise, and explain the findings and recommendations of the study without excessive scientific or industry-specific terminology [4,28]. The recommendations should be presented with sufficient detail to avoid confusion. Both short- and long-term recommendations may be necessary. The potential costs and benefits should be explained to the herd owner.

Relatively few complex problems are completely resolved with a single report. Many investigations are done retrospectively with insufficient information to reach definitive conclusions [17]. To address outstanding questions, these cases require protracted herd health and productivity monitoring and, occasionally, planned follow-up studies [19,20]. In outbreaks that were quickly contained through control measures, follow-up field studies may be required to determine if the control measures were effective [18]. In some cases, technical service veterinarians from pharmaceutical companies may be of assistance if a specific vaccine or antibiotic is involved in some fashion in the outbreak. Extension veterinarians and, occasionally, veterinary school investigation teams are also a valuable resource to practitioners in situations where the outbreak is extremely unusual, or when follow-up field studies may be required.

Overview of the process

The basic process of defining the problem; orienting the problem by animal, time, and space; and analyzing the data is common to all outbreak investigations. The steps in this process often overlap and parts of the process may have to be repeated to resolve the problem. The practitioner must be able to adapt these strategies to a wide variety of outbreak situations. The practice of outbreak investigation requires preparation, organization, and communication skills from the initial contact with the herd owner through implementation of the recommendations in the final report. Some suggestions for a structured and consistent approach to field investigations are presented below.

Initial contact and preparation for the herd visit

Veterinarians become involved in outbreak investigations as an extension of routine service to regular clients or, occasionally, as consultants brought in to help trouble-shoot or act on behalf of a third party in the case of more unusual problems. Herd problems can become apparent from a question raised over the counter at the clinic or from an observation while on a visit for a routine procedure. Many herd problems may be initially presented as a complaint about a specific vaccine or treatment recommendation. Problems affecting herd productivity should not be casually diagnosed by phone or "over-the-counter." Although many herd owners can describe the problem very well, incomplete or misleading second-hand information could result in inappropriate recommendations [5] and leave the veterinarian potentially liable for the well-intentioned "free advice." The practitioner should encourage the herd owner to describe the problem as completely as possible. Where the problem appears to warrant immediate further investigation, a herd visit should be scheduled. More subtle changes in productivity may be pursued as a part of the next routine herd health visit.

Communication and preparation before the herd visit can save time on the farm. Background information for all cases must include complete name, address of the herd owner, legal land description of the farm, and contact information. Have the herd owner collect copies of any previous examination or laboratory-testing reports related to the herd. Determine whether or not any other veterinarians are involved in the case. If so, they should be contacted.

Encourage the client to gather all potentially relevant herd records before the planned visit. These may include herd record books, sales receipts, calendars, invoices for purchased feed, and other data, depending on the type of operation. Time can be saved by having the client fill out a short preliminary questionnaire covering basic herd background information [8,12]. Useful information would include a summary of the herd inventory and any recent changes to inventory, breed and age distribution of the herd; an outline of management groupings; and an overview of feeding and vaccination practices. The number of animals to be examined and the number and type of laboratory samples to be collected can be estimated before the herd visit if herd inventory numbers are available.

Whenever possible, arrange to examine the herd in its original location before the herd is disturbed and confined for detailed examination. If the visit is scheduled during feeding, the practitioner can make first-hand observations of both animal behavior and herd management with minimal disturbance to the herd. Close examination of the herd, when possible, could be scheduled during some routine management procedure (eg, pregnancy testing, vaccination, or branding). More than one herd visit might be necessary to make both the necessary herd and individual-level observations. In addition to visiting the herd owner, the practitioner should arrange to visit other family members and farm workers who can provide critical information on the history of the problem and herd management practices. In some cases, these individuals may be more knowledgeable about details of animal management than the actual owner.

A crude working-case definition can be developed from the information provided during the initial contact. The next step, particularly for unusual or complex problems, is to briefly review the current literature on known risk factors. Online access to electronic journals is making access to current information in remote areas easier. Several authors have suggested using a diagram to summarize relationships between known risk factors. This diagram is sometimes called a path model. The purpose of this diagram is to assist in planning for the herd examination and to facilitate discussions with the client. Several good examples have been published, including models related to neonatal mortality in beef herds [9], impaired fertility in beef cattle [7], and factors affecting weaning weights [12].

Taking the time to review the potential risk factors before the herd visit decreases the chance that some area of herd management or the collection of important samples are overlooked. In addition to listing risk factors for the disease, published path models depict the interrelationship among risk factors and their effects [29]. A diagram showing the potential relationships among risk factors can help communicate to the client that herd problems usually have more than one cause, that infectious agents are usually only part of the problem, and that many areas of management should be examined [9].

Preparation for the investigation is important. In many cases, such as in beef cow-calf herds the investigator may only have one opportunity to examine the animals closely and collect samples during routine handling of the animals. While the herd veterinarian may have an advantage over extension personnel in being able to return to the herd, access to extensively managed animals for repeated sampling is often an important limiting factor in outbreak investigations. An animal health technician can help organize sample collection and ensure proper labeling and packaging for transport. Contact the laboratory before the visit to verify the manner of sample collection, quantity of sample, type of container to be used, and packaging and transportation recommendations. Many laboratories have sample collection containers and transportation packages that they provide on request to their clients as part of their service fee or for a small additional charge.

The herd visit

During the herd visit, the investigator collects additional history, examines individual animals from the herd, conducts necropsies, observes herd management, examines the environment, obtains samples for laboratory examination, and examines the herd records. If no clinical cases or mortalities are available, the practitioner may want to make arrangements to have those cases submitted or to be notified when the cases occur. The necessary steps and order of completion vary between problems and often overlap. The objective of data collection during the herd visit is first to determine how the affected or diseased animals differ from those unaffected and then find which of the factors that differ among these groups can be altered by intervention to decrease the risk of disease. The unique characteristics of the nutrition, management, and the environment related to the affected animals become a focus of the examination.

Detailed written notes of all observations are important for constructing a meaningful and accurate report for the herd owner. Few things destroy credibility faster than making a mistake in describing the operation. Digital pictures are inexpensive and useful memory aids as well as great tools for client education and presentations to producer groups. Photos can be particularly useful for recording subjective observations, including body conditions and farm hygiene. Changes over time can be monitored by comparing representative pictures from different dates. When trying to show the size of an object, include a standard reference in the picture, such as a meter stick or a person of a known height. If specific animal identification is important, include the ear tag and brand as applicable in the photo. Alternatively, include a small sign or card in the picture with the necessary information. Video cameras can be used to record behavioral or postural abnormalities and unusual sounds.

All records should be in ink, dated, and signed. Photos and video records can also provide critical information for the visit report. If the case could potentially involve litigation, photos and video should be date- and time-stamped. Record where and when the pictures were taken and include detailed voice narration on the video describing what was seen. If using a digital camera, check on the admissibility of pictures as evidence with a legal expert in the local area.

History

Have the herd owner restate the presenting complaint and encourage him or her to clarify the time sequence of events. Questionnaires prepared for the problem under investigation can help ensure that nothing is overlooked during the interview. Such questionnaires are especially valuable for those inexperienced in this field. Several examples of lists of questions are available for addressing specific herd problems [8,12]. However, while strict adherence to standardized questionnaires is essential for most observational research, this same strict adherence to a prepared questionnaire can hinder the outbreak investigation process. Insistence on following a preformatted series of questions often interferes with the chronological order of the story and no standard questionnaire can fit every situation [5]. Rather than a formal questionnaire, a simple list of required information can be prepared and tailored to the particular problem. This list is used as a check sheet to fill in missing areas not covered in the initial disclosure of information after the herd owner has told his or her story.

Good listening skills and careful questioning can increase the accuracy and reliability of the information collected. Carefully worded open-ended questions allow the possibility of answers not previously considered by the practitioner. Unnecessary industry jargon and scientific terminology should be avoided. Each question should ask for one piece of information at a time and time references in all questions should be unambiguous [30,31]. Unnecessary interruptions or "jumping to conclusions" can disrupt the chronological presentation or lead the herd owner to tell the story that supports the practitioner's assumptions about the cause of the problem.

Emotionally loaded or leading questions can also suggest one answer is better than another and bias the results of the interview. The herd owner can be tempted to give the perceived "correct" or more "socially acceptable" answer and not describe what actually happened. When doubts arise about the completeness of the information provided, alternatives for getting the information should be considered. For example, to evaluate the effectiveness of a particular treatment regime, first-hand observation of the client processing the animals and information on the total amount of drug used often adds important information to that gathered by questions about the dose and frequency of administration. Clues to actual treatment patterns may be discovered through inquiries into the total volume of antibiotic purchased in the previous few months and by investigating remaining inventory.

The completeness of the information can also be improved by using "aids to recall" [32]. By asking the herd owner to refer to relevant records and verify dates and numbers, the practitioner improves the accuracy of information collected during the visit. Where records are not available, simple strategies such as referring to the kitchen calendar can improve recall regarding the chronology of events [5]. A binder filled with examples of labels or parts of the box from common drugs or vaccines can be used when herd owners have difficulty remembering brand names of relevant drugs, vaccines, electrolytes, milk replacers, or mineral mixes.

In addition to basic information about the herd owner, history, and current status of the operation, the practitioner should tactfully ask about other employment and off-farm sources of income. A part-time job as a stockperson in another herd or at an auction market, as examples, could present important biosecurity problems. When there is the potential for zoonotic disease or simultaneous exposures to toxins, the practitioner must also tactfully question the herd owner, employees, and family members about concurrent illnesses [5,18]. While most of the interview should be focused on collecting the owner's observations, The practitioner should also ask the herd owner for his or her opinion about what is causing the problem [5].

Clinical examination of individual animals from the herd

General distant observations should be made of the group and individual animals before the animals are confined and restrained for detailed exams. The distant visual examination of the group could include an assessment of a variety of conditions and characteristics (Box 1) [31].

In outbreak investigations, rarely is it possible to confine and individually examine every animal in the herd. The visual check of different groups in the herd when they are minimally confined or during feeding or grazing is a valuable tool that should not be overlooked. When animals cannot be confined, the body condition can be scored visually from a short distance. Visual appraisal is comparable to palpation, unless the cattle have long hair [7]. Information on diet composition and recent changes or accidental ingestions can also be verified during an examination in the home pen using observations of the amount, consistency, and appearance of fecal material. For example, fecal consistency provides information on the amount of dry hay relative to silage, green grass, or concentrate. Fecal content can reflect recent grain overload or exposure to environmental toxins, such as spilled oil.

Each animal can then be confined and examined individually during the initial visit, if warranted by the severity of the problem, or later, when the examination can be combined with other routine processing activities.

Box 1. Possible factors to assess during distant visual examination of group

- Behavior, mental status, temperament, and exercise tolerance
- Degree of crowding, dominance and aggression problems within the group, and the degree of access and availability of bedding, food, and water
- Respiration rate and character, coughing, and unusual noises or discharges
- Appetite, mastication, and swallowing
- Abdominal shape or contour (eg, bloated, gaunt)
- Defecation characteristics (eg, frequency, consistency, straining) and urination patterns
- Reproductive status, signs of estrus or mounting activity, discharges from the reproductive tract, maternal behavior, udder conformation, and lactation status
- Evidence of libido or successful mounting activity for breeding males
- Posture, gait, lameness and progression of movement
- Body weight and condition score
- Relative frame size and conformation
- Health and cleanliness of the skin and hair coat

The procedure for detailed examination of individual animals has been well documented and will not be reviewed here [25,31,32].

Another way to approach an examination is to confine and examine subsets of severely affected, moderate or mildly affected, and not apparently affected animals from the herd. While no specific guidelines are available for how many animals should be examined, one investigator has suggested a minimum of four severely affected, four mild cases, and four normal animals [31]. Another investigator recommends examining the first few animals that became sick as well as any recent additions to the herd [33]. Identifying and examining early cases that have not yet been treated might also be a valuable diagnostic tool. To minimize the potential for transmitting disease within the herd during the examination, the practitioner should begin where possible by examining the "normal" animals.

The reproductive status and body condition score can also be individually recorded during the detailed examination. For any investigation potentially examining reproductive performance, all animals should be palpated for pregnancy status or evidence of estrus activity and herd bulls should be tested for breeding soundness. This individual animal listing and record of reproductive status are particularly important if the problem requires monitoring over time or there is a potential for ongoing losses.

Necropsy examination of dead or sacrificed animals

Detailed instructions for postmortem examination are not reviewed here as these are available from most diagnostic laboratories and other sources [34,35]. However, some additional factors should be considered when examining losses associated with outbreak investigations.

The results from both gross and histological examination can be critical to refining the case definition where clinical signs are vague and nonspecific [31]. All available cadavers should be examined whenever possible. One or two cases from a major disease outbreak might not be representative of the underlying problem [5]. For example, the authors recently investigated a severe scours outbreak (>70% herd mortality) in calves greater than 4 weeks of age. In this investigation, the first two calves examined were found to have died from causes unrelated to the majority of herd losses. One death was caused by pneumonia. The other was the result of an abscessed umbilical vein. In that example, histopathology on a series of additional calves at different stages of the disease was necessary to define the type of intestinal lesion.

Where the value of individual animals is low, the herd owner might also be willing to sacrifice a small number of affected animals for a complete necropsy examination. If the value of individual animals is high, the herd owner might consent to the euthanasia of one or two chronically diseased animals where the prognosis for recovery is poor [9]. The animals should be submitted for processing at a diagnostic laboratory where possible. The postmortem examination and sample collection can be completed on the carcass within minutes of death. In some cases, very fresh tissue is necessary for specialized testing, such as electron microscopy.

The submission of all samples from one herd to the same laboratory and a single pathologist improves communication, maintains consistency of interpretation, facilitates comparisons between individual cases and identification of trends during the outbreak, and, finally, provides the information to make a herd diagnosis based on quantitative pathology [5]. The practitioner can then determine to what extent the various pathological lesions observed affect overall mortality and mortality within each management group.

By maintaining a consistent protocol for sample collection and a log of all samples collected, the practitioner minimizes the chance of missing important information. Tissues from all important systems should be submitted for histopathology. Reliance on the gross evidence of abnormalities as a basis for sampling can result in a much lower rate of diagnostic success. Call the laboratory in advance for instructions about any nonroutine samples to verify the amount, appropriate sample containers (eg, glass or plastic), storage conditions (eg, frozen, on ice, or at room temperature), preservation, and shipping. Special care improves chances for the survival of the suspected pathogen and reduces the likelihood of overgrowth of contaminants. Samples for toxicological analysis can be contaminated during collection or degrade very rapidly if the wrong container or preservative is used. Small submission errors can result in misleading and inaccurate laboratory results.

Laboratory analysis is expensive and so-called "fishing expeditions," where samples are submitted for a number of tests in the hope something might come up positive, seldom provide useful information. However, because the practitioner has only one opportunity to collect samples from a carcass, it is much better to collect tissue that might not be used than to miss important information. The initial laboratory costs and the potential for important information loss can be minimized by properly storing tissue samples. If the factor to be analyzed is stable for a known period and if the cost of collection and storage are not prohibitive, then the practitioner may find it appropriate to bank tissue samples for future analysis. Small pieces of formalized tissue for histology, for example, do not add much to the cost of the investigation and require little, if any, additional storage space. Frozen tissue samples can be analyzed later for some types of toxins or trace mineral content.

Where herd losses are substantial, the veterinarian should consider asking the owner to transport at least some carcasses to a diagnostic laboratory. Examinations can be conducted by a pathologist under the more controlled conditions of the laboratory. Where this method is not practical or possible, the examinations must be completed in the field using the best possible practices. Use a camera to record gross pathological abnormalities. If litigation is an issue, the identity of the subject animal, the date, a size reference scale marker, and the identity of the pathologist should be included in each photograph [36]. If this is a potential legal case, inform the laboratory before sending the samples. Many laboratories have special chain-of-custody protocol documentation that assist practitioners in ensuring any sample results will be admissible in court [36].

Wobeser [36] summarized from Jaffe [37] common errors made in postmortem examinations that must be avoided in medico-legal examinations. Those are listed in Box 2. Occasionally, tissues from "normal" animals within the herd may be required as controls or for determinations of trace mineral, heavy metal status, or parasite load. Tissue from animals sent to slaughter for the commercial market or for in-home use can be a potential source of reference material.

Observation of herd management

Veterinarians are often reluctant to be perceived as criticizing the management skills of their clients. The practitioner can avoid being judgmental and still collect detailed information on herd management. Most disease outbreaks in herds are the result of some limitation or deficiency in management. Very few of the disease problems important in food animal practice require only the infectious agent to cause substantial herd losses. Almost all outbreaks or suboptimal productivity problems result from a number of factors, including factors related to management. In some cases, the disease outbreak may provide a unique teachable moment for the local practitioner to emphasize the importance of making management changes that may have been suggested in the past but ignored. The objective of the

Box 2. Common errors in postmortem examinations

Incomplete examination (eg, failure to examine the brain)
Inadequate documentation (eg, no written report or photographs)
Too much delay between the examination and preparation of the report
Failure to collect samples for supplementary analysis (eg, microbiology, histology, or toxicology)
Improper collection of samples (eg, inappropriate samples, unsuitable containers, insufficient preservation, inadequate labeling)
Accidental damage to specimens, including contamination with spilled gastrointestinal content, or improper or rough handling of fragile tissues
Confusion of artifacts, including autolysis, or histological damage from freezing with important pathological lesions
Failure to consult with other experts
Bias resulting from too much emphasis placed on the case history

investigation is to identify all factors that can be changed to resolve the current herd problem or minimize the potential for future losses.

A management history obtained with simple questions having yes or no answers provides limited and superficial information on herd management practices. For example, many management questionnaires ask whether or not cattle are vaccinated for bovine viral diarrhea virus and infectious bovine rhinotracheitis. This question seems straightforward. However, if the producer answered yes, the practitioner still has no information on what type of vaccine was used, when it was administered, and if label directions were properly followed.

If management has changed its practices, information about those changes can be important in determining the cause of the outbreak [29]. However, changes that preceded the outbreak need to be carefully differentiated from changes that resulted from the outbreak. The most useful information on herd management comes from seeing how things are done, which can require several visits and extra time. The veterinarian may find it difficult to get paid for this added work. The best management assessments are often collected as part of an ongoing process where the investigating veterinarian works with the livestock owner on a regular herd-health program.

Examination of the environment

Climate, housing, population density, and air quality are all important determinants of disease risk and herd productivity [31]. Historical weather data can usually be obtained from local meteorological stations to confirm observations of herd owners. Weather events should not be taken lightly. For example, snow can dramatically reduce functional pen size. Rain, in combination with poor drainage, can have the same effect [5]. A field that should be of adequate size for a given number of animals can be overcrowded and highly contaminated during certain times of the year because of water accumulation or high snow drifts. Animal density should be calculated based on the usable space at the critical point in time and not total space in the pen. Herd visits should be made as soon as possible, as problematic environmental conditions are often transitory.

Ground conditions (eg, degree of wetness, drainage, type of cover) are also important to livestock health and production. The type and amount of bedding are important to the ground conditions, but bedding management can also affect dust levels in the pen. Air quality is particularly important in dry lots and feedlots where dust levels can potentially affect the occurrence of respiratory disease.

The location and type of shelter within the outdoor pen are important. Sheds, porosity fencing, other types of windbreaks, and wooded areas are all used by various types of operations. Portable calf sheds, if used properly, can help reduce high levels of contamination that often occur in these highly frequented areas. Other potential environmental risks include insect and predator problems on the pasture and the location of carcass disposal sites, garbage dumps, fuel and chemical storage areas, and nearby industrial facilities.

Good ventilation, temperature and humidity control is critical to maintaining health and productivity in housed livestock of all species. The objective evaluation of indoor ventilation may require the assistance of an expert in this area. A number of parameters are typically measured, depending in part on the type of animal being housed. Such parameters include minimum and maximum temperature, the number of air changes per hour, humidity and condensation, the location and size of air inlets and fans, and the presence of drafts. Specialized monitoring equipment can be used to measure levels of a number of suspected problem gases, including ammonia, hydrogen sulfide, and carbon monoxide.

Other factors to be evaluated for indoor environments include the sanitation and hygiene, the type and condition of the flooring, the barn-cleaning and waste-disposal systems, stall or crate design and dimensions, bedding type and adequacy, the ease of movement for both animals and attendants within the unit, and the adequacy of the lighting.

Water quality and availability are important determinants of livestock health and feed intake. Determine the ratio of animals to waterers in each pen. Observe animals using the water source and record any evidence of crowding and dominance problems, stray voltage, or access and footing (eg, mud, manure buildup, or ice). Verify that all automatic waterers are working properly. Is dugout, pothole, or stream water pumped to a trough or do the animals actually enter the water to drink? Is the water clean and free of offensive odors, or are there substantial amounts of mud and manure suspended in the water because of animal movements? Is algae growth an obvious problem?

Collecting samples

Laboratory examination of strategically submitted samples can help rule out or confirm the diagnosis, monitor exposure to potentially important risk factors, determine the necessity for and appropriate level of intervention, and, finally, assess the success of control measures [38]. The only laboratory analyses that should be considered in most investigations are those where the results are likely to directly affect management decisions [38]. Appropriate samples might include blood, milk, feces, urine, nasal and ocular swabs, biopsies or tissue samples from slaughter animals or cadavers, other fluid samples, feed, water, and soil samples. Necropsy sampling has been discussed.

A number of factors determines the success of the laboratory sampling strategy. The appropriate samples must be selected for the question being asked and the number of animals sampled must be sufficient to answer the question with a reasonable degree of certainty. The appropriate technique and collection equipment must be used and the samples must be stored properly and delivered to the laboratory before sample quality is compromised [38]. Laboratories may change their recommendations over time on recommended transport media (eg, those for *Campylobacter fetus* or *Tritrichomonas fetus* cultures) or preferred sample form (eg, serum or whole blood for selenium).

Finally, the laboratory test chosen must have acceptable measurement error, accuracy, and precision standards and be able to discriminate adequately between "normal" and affected individuals. The laboratory should provide the sensitivity and specificity of the test and define how the value for the normal cutoff has been established. Several good additional references are available that discuss the interpretation of diagnostic test results [39,40]. See the article about choosing and using diagnostic tests elsewhere in this issue.

Sample-size determination

Cost considerations often prohibit laboratory testing of every animal in the herd. The most common approach to testing is to submit samples for comparison of laboratory data between cases and a sample of control (ie, unaffected) animals within the herd. All available cases are often needed, depending on herd size and the severity of the problem. The practitioner must select an appropriate comparison or control group. Samples can also be submitted to compare results between animals with acute and chronic disease or among animals from different age cohorts, management groups, or history of exposure to some other risk factor of interest.

Probably the most common question and often the most difficult to address is "How many samples are necessary?" Often, complete herd sampling and testing is too costly. There is no single correct number of samples suitable for every situation. The required number of animals for sampling is based on (1) the acceptable degree of uncertainty in the final estimate; (2) the expected prevalence of the factor of interest, or, for continuous measurements, the variation in the factor within the population, and (3) the size of the population examined [27,41]. The number of samples required also depends on the question being asked. In most cases, the practitioner must take what is available. If few cases are available, there are some statistical advantages to having more controls than cases up to a ratio of about 4:1. Computer programs, such as Win Episcope 2.0, can be used to calculate the required sample size. See the article by Slenning elsewhere in this volume for more about issues related to sample size.

Without a sufficient number of samples across groups, the practitioner often misses differences that are important clues to the underlying cause of the outbreak. As with postmortem examinations, the clinician often has only one opportunity to collect laboratory samples from live animals during the critical time frame. Because of costs, the clinician cannot possibly direct the laboratory to analyze the samples for every potential question that could arise during the investigation. Serum banking should be considered [42].

Feed and water samples

The role of feeding management is central to many investigations. The investigation of nutritional disorders has been thoroughly reviewed by Swecker and Thatcher [43]. Expensive laboratory analysis alone cannot prove that the nutrition program is adequate for the type of animal and environment. While chemical analysis of the feedstuffs is important, this provides only the laboratory report on the components used to formulate the feed. The report does not address what is actually ingested by the average animal and how much variation there is among animals.

Before collecting any feed samples, have the herd owner prepare an inventory of all forages, grains, and purchased supplements. Purchased feeds should be listed by date of purchase, source, type and composition, and amount. Feed tags, which include analysis and instructions for use, or the supplier contact numbers should be collected for all commercially prepared feeds or supplements. Is there any feed left from the time just before the herd problem was noticed? Hancock and colleagues [38] have described the collection of the samples from feed storage and handling equipment, particularly for cases where feed-related toxicity (eg, mycotoxins) is suspected and the practitioner is looking for samples of "old feed."

Good sample-collection technique is important for a meaningful chemical analysis. The samples submitted for analysis must be representative of what is being fed. Use a good quality core sampler for hay, and an auger or probe for grain and concentrates. Silage and haylage are often the most difficult to representatively sample at a single point in time. Collect multiple grab samples from different parts of the open pit or from different times while the conveyor belt is running. There might be substantial differences in quality in different parts of the pit or silo. Sampling of the final or total mixed ration, as compared with the "paper ration," provides a check on the adequacy of the mixing process and the actual composition.

Collect, pool, and mix thoroughly five to ten samples for grain or concentrate and 20 individual samples for hay or silage from each lot of feed before submission to the laboratory. Silage samples should be placed in airtight plastic bags, stored on ice, and shipped to the laboratory as soon as possible. The laboratory should be asked to dry and grind the entire sample before analysis [43,44]. Some laboratories only process a subsample of what was submitted, unless the instructions specify otherwise.

The visual appearance and physical characteristics of the feed observed during sample collection should be recorded [43]. Odor, color, stage of maturity, presence of foreign material (eg, garbage, weeds) and physical form provide information necessary for proper interpretation of the feed analysis. Note the relative stem-to-leaf ratio or the grain-to-forage ratio in the stored feedstuff. Chop length and moisture content should be measured in the field where possible for silage and total mixed rations. Silage pH can also be measured in the field.

Pasture sampling is done relatively infrequently, but may be occasionally necessary in the investigation of metabolic disease or trace-mineral deficiencies [38]. The samples for chemical analysis should not be pulled from the ground but be cut off near the roots with scissors to minimize soil contamination. Toxic plants can be photographed and then collected and dried for identification by an expert in that area.

Before submitting the samples, determine what chemical-analysis packages are available from the laboratory. Because feed analysis can be very expensive, all requested analysis should provide necessary data and the practitioner should understand the limitations of all the tests requested. Commercial feed laboratories also vary greatly in their internal quality-control procedures and the types of analytical, estimation, and calculation procedures used.

Obtain bottles for water sampling directly from the laboratory where possible. Improperly cleaned containers can contaminate the sample. This precaution is particularly important for trace-mineral or organic analysis. Proper sampling technique, special preservatives, and rapid transportation are required for samples being tested for potentially volatile components. Practitioners should call the laboratory in advance if they are planning on requesting tests outside the routine potability parameters.

Water sampling for livestock use should include an assessment of total dissolved solids, sulfates, nitrites, and nitrates. Total dissolved solids in excess of 5000 ppm can reduce water intake and result in diarrhea in all classes of livestock [45]. High sulfate levels (> 1,000 ppm) can interfere with copper status [46] and increase the risk of polioencephalomalacia [31].

Examining the herd records

The quality and completeness of records vary greatly between operations. Some herds have complete records on computer for each animal and others have little or no record of animal health and productivity. Understanding the most commonly used on-farm computerized record systems and third-party data-collection agencies saves time and can increase the amount of retrievable information. For herd managers participating in the National Dairy Herd Improvement Association, computerized herd production records can be obtained for a reasonable fee and imported into common herd-analysis programs. This can save considerable time over what would be required for manual entry and analysis of all important herd data.

A portable photocopier is a valuable tool for on-farm record collection. A laptop computer and printer are also useful where there are questions about invoicing the full value for time at home spent entering records and doing nutritional and performance analyses. Conducting some of this work on-farm with the herd owner can increase the appreciation for the time and effort required.

Too often herd records are scant or nonexistent. Persistence and ingenuity can, however, turn up useful information in unexpected places. Ask the herd owner for any livestock-associated records, including records related to veterinary services, supplies, or drugs; auction mart receipts; old calendars, pocket diaries, and calving books; feed and supplement bills; financial records related to animals bought and sold; and bulk tank receipts showing somatic cell count and bacterial numbers [29].

Individual animal treatment records are often difficult or impossible to obtain in the face of a disease outbreak. During a crisis, however, herd owners might be more likely to record counts of animals treated each day or week than individual animal information. If record compliance is poor, it may be useful to have the herd owner directly identify animals treated with a livestock marker. A different marker color can be used each day. If this method is used, a walk through the herd can provide a quick impression of how many animals have been treated and how long they have been treated.

Definitions of production and health measurements must be clear and used consistently throughout the investigation. Be cautious when comparing findings from other investigations, as there are substantial problems with standardization of terminology and methods of calculation. For example, stillbirth has been defined both as calves dead within the first hour after birth [47] and calves dead within 24 hours of birth [48].

Attack rate tables

The attack rate is the proportion of the group that is affected during a given period. The attack rate can compare those that are and are not exposed with each individual potential risk factor. To easily visualize this comparison across many different risk factors, an attack rate table is used. The table helps identify the exposures most likely to be associated with disease. Alternatively, a table can be constructed to compare the risk of exposure to each potentially important risk factor between case and control animals. Table 1 shows an attack rate table comparing the risk of abortion across various risk factors examined during an investigation.

The application of the appropriate statistical test to this comparison allows the clinician to avoid misinterpreting a chance difference between

Table 1
Partial attack rates for an abortion problem in a cow-calf herd

	Exposed animals				Unexposed animals			
Suspected risk factors	Number affected (not pregnant)	Number not affected (pregnant)	Total number	Attack rate (%)	Number affected (not pregnant)	Number not affected (pregnant)	Total number	Attack rate (%)
Heifers: mature cows	45	39	84	53%	90	180	270	33%
Neospora positive: negative								
All cows	122	160	282	43%	7	58	65	11%
Heifers	38	30	68	56%	2	9	11	18%
Mature cows	84	135	219	39%	5	49	54	9%

groups as a link to a cause [26,29]. To apply statistical methods, the practitioner must assess the probability that the results of the statistical test, or more extreme results, could have been obtained if there really were no association between the risk factor and disease. A chi-square analysis is an example of a simple, commonly used test for significance. This test compares the frequency of observed events to that expected based on chance alone. See the article by Slenning elsewhere in this volume for more information.

The importance of different risk factors can be objectively compared by measuring the magnitude of the association between each exposure and the outcome of interest or disease. The two common indices used to measure the magnitude of effect of a risk factor are the relative risk ratio and the odds ratio. The relative risk is the ratio of the risk (or cumulative incidence or attack rate) of disease in the animals exposed to the factor of interest to the risk (or cumulative incidence or attack rate) of disease in those that were not exposed. If the relative risk is <1, then the exposure is associated with a decreased risk of disease. If the relative risk is equal to 1, then there is no association between exposure and disease status. If the relative risk is >1, then the exposure is associated with an increased risk of disease. See the article by Gay on cause and effect elsewhere in this volume for more discussion about causality.

The odds ratio can be used to measure the association between exposure and disease for any study type. However, the odds ratio is the method of choice for expressing the magnitude of effect in case-control comparisons where the history of exposure to a specific risk factor is compared between case and control animals. The interpretation of the odds ratio is similar to that of relative risk.

Statistical association alone does not prove the identified risk factor is a cause of the outbreak [1,15]. For a risk factor to be considered a potential cause of disease or suboptimal productivity, the risk factor must always precede the outcome. Other potential supporting evidence for a causal association includes a relatively strong association between the risk factor and the outcome, a biologically reasonable link between risk factor and outcome, some suggestion of increasing effect with increasing exposure, evidence that removing or decreasing exposure decreases the risk of disease, and consistency of the association when examined in different studies.

Communicating investigation results and follow-up

The minimum necessary follow-up is a complete written report to the herd owner as described earlier in the article. The report should be direct and concise [49]. To effectively communicate the findings of the investigation, the report must be read by the intended audience. The purpose of the investigation should be stated at the beginning of the report. All investigation results should be summarized using simple tables and graphs where possible. The action list to the herd owner should set clear priorities and include specific details for any recommendations. The report should provide a plan for follow-up and future monitoring. The investigator must consider the potential for future litigation in all statements and recommendations. The report should also clearly discuss any risks associated with the recommendations, describe any risks from the current problem to public health, and promote realistic expectations of the results following any interventions.

This written report may have to be supplemented as the results become available of later laboratory tests or longer-term field studies to identify risk factors. The case definition may need to be revised and the results from the investigation herd compared with other herds in the surrounding area [4]. Practitioners should review their roles and responsibilities, both legal and ethical, to the larger livestock industry as well as their immediate concern with improving health and productivity in a particular herd [5]. If the disease is contagious, consider what risk the herd poses to other livestock producers in the area and consult with the herd owner on minimizing the potential for transmission beyond the herd. If the exposure could potentially result in food residues, contact the appropriate authorities for direction and advise the herd owner of his or her legal and ethical responsibilities. If the disease is potentially reportable, the appropriate regulatory officials should be advised of the results of the field investigation as soon as possible. If the losses are extremely severe, the herd owner should be advised to consider his or her short- and long-term goals and to get advice from a financial councilor before deciding among potential alternatives for control.

For herd problems with significant economic implications, particularly where control or treatment is not well understood, the investigation should not end with the identification of important risk factors and the recommendations for control. Where the effectiveness of proposed control measures cannot be predicted with certainty, one infrequently used, but potentially invaluable, strategy for evaluating the effectiveness of control measures in the herd is the randomized controlled trial [50]. Controlled field trials have been used, for example, to examine the impact of vaccination on treatment rates and weaning weights from a herd with a severe neonatal scours problem [18].

Summary

Because all outbreaks and all livestock operations are different, there is no "recipe for success" that covers all possible situations in the field. The investigating veterinarian must be able to adapt these techniques to each specific situation. The approach outlined here does not have to be followed in the order presented. Often, individual steps are repeated many times before the information necessary to implement a successful control process becomes apparent. The techniques described are sufficient in many investigations. However, situations requiring more complex analysis demand consultation with specialists, including epidemiologists and laboratory diagnosticians.

The role of detective or outbreak investigator can be a refreshing break from the routine of daily practice. The investigation of disease outbreaks provides an opportunity for the herd veterinarian to show clients the advantages of a herd health program and the value of a good record-keeping system. Despite the benefits, the resources required for a thorough herd investigation can seem difficult to justify, particularly when problems are often identified during extremely busy times of year, such as periods of pregnancy testing and calving in beef herds. The decision to conduct an in-depth investigation should depend on the opportunity to control the current problem and minimize the potential for future problems, the severity of the problem and the risk to other producers, the potential risk to public health, and, in some situations, the opportunity for research and training. Some disease investigation units have resources to assist local practitioners in resolving herd problems. These units work out of veterinary colleges and government agencies in both Canada and the United States. A functioning support system for outbreak investigations can assist veterinarians in resolving individual herd problems, while also providing benefits for the livestock industry by enhancing active surveillance for emerging disease problems.

References

[1] Schwabe DW, Riemann HP, Franti CE. Epidemiology in veterinary practice. Philadelphia: Lea & Febiger; 1977.

[2] Kahrs RF. Techniques for investigating outbreaks of livestock disease. J Am Vet Med Assoc 1978;173:101–3.

[3] Blood DC. The clinical examination of cattle. Part II: examination of the herd. Bov Proc 1982;14:14–21.

[4] Lessard P. The characterization of disease outbreaks. Vet Clin North Am Food Anim Prac 1988;4:17–32.

[5] Ribble CS, Janzen ED, Campbell J. Disease outbreak investigation in the beef herd: defining the problem. Bov Proc 1998;31:121–7.

[6] Waldner CL. Investigation of disease outbreaks and suboptimal productivity in herds. In: Radostits OM, editor. Herd health: food animal production medicine. 3rd edition. Philadelphia: WB Saunders Company; 2001. p. 189–210.

[7] Wikse SE. Investigation of impaired fertility in beef cattle herds. Comp Contin Educ 1988; 10:1225–31, 1240.

[8] Mickelsen WD. Investigating the causes of low pregnancy rates in beef cattle herds. Vet Med 1990;85:418–20, 422–7.

[9] Wikse SE, Kinsel ML, Toombs RE, et al. An epidemiologic approach to solving beef herd production and disease problems. Vet Med 1992;87:495–506.

[10] Ruegg PL. Use of basic epidemiologic principles in dairy production medicine. Part II. Investigating herd problems. Comp Contin Educ 1993;15:309–13.

[11] Wikse SE, Kinsel ML, Field RW, et al. Investigating perinatal mortality in beef herds. Vet Clin North Am Food Anim Prac 1994;10:147–66.

[12] Sanderson M, Christmas R. Investigation of depressed weaning weights in beef cow-calf herds. Comp Contin Educ 1997;19:395–9.

[13] Waldner CL. Investigation of reproductive problems in beef herds. Large Anim Vet Rounds 2001;1(5).

[14] Lessard P, Perry BD, editors. Investigation of disease outbreaks and impaired productivity. Vet Clin North Am Food Anim Prac 1988;4(1).
[15] Ruegg PL. Investigating herd problems and production on dairy farms. Bov Proc 1996;29: 96–101.
[16] Waldner CL, Checkley S, Blakley B, et al. Managing lead exposure and toxicity in cow-calf herds exposed to discarded lead batteries. J Vet Diagn Inves 2002;14:481–6.
[17] Waldner CL, Janzen ED, Henderson J, et al. An outbreak of abortion associated with Neospora caninum infection in a beef herd. J Am Vet Med Assoc 1999;215:1485–90.
[18] Gow S, Waldner CL, Ross C. The effect of duration of treatment on weaning weights in a cow-calf herd with a protracted severe neonatal scours outbreak. Can Vet J 2005;16:418–25.
[19] Waldner CL, Henderson J, Wu JT, et al. Continued reproductive losses in a cow-calf herd associated with Neospora caninum following an abortion epidemic. Can Vet J 2001;42: 355–60.
[20] Waldner CL. Precolostral antibodies to Neospora caninum in beef calves following an abortion outbreak and associated fall weaning weights. Bov Pract 2002;36:81–5.
[21] Pritchard GC, Willshaw GA, Biley JR, et al. Verocytotoxin-producing Escherichia coli O157 on a farm open to the public: outbreak investigation and longitudinal bacteriological study. Vet Rec 2000;147:259–64.
[22] Waldner CL, Ribble CS, Janzen ED. Evaluation of the impact of a natural gas leak from a pipeline on productivity of beef cattle. J Am Vet Med Assoc 1998;212:41–8.
[23] Chenoweth PJ, Sanderson MW. Health and production management in beef cattle breeding herds. In: Radostits OM, editor. Herd health: food animal production medicine. 3rd edition. Philadelphia: WB Saunders Company; 2001. p. 189–210.
[24] Radostits OM, Leslie KE, Fetrow J. Herd health: food animal production medicine. 2nd edition. Philadelphia: WB Saunders Company; 1994.
[25] Smith RD. Veterinary clinical epidemiology. A problem-oriented approach. 2nd edition. Boca Raton (FL): CRC Press; 1995.
[26] Gregg MB. Field epidemiology. New York: Oxford University Press; 1996.
[27] Thrusfield M. Veterinary epidemiology. 2nd edition. Oxford (United Kingdom): Blackwell Science Ltd.; 1995.
[28] Gardner I. Techniques for reporting disease outbreak investigations. Vet Clin North Am Food Anim Prac 1988;4:109–26.
[29] Hancock DD, Wikse SE. Investigation planning and data gathering. Vet Clin North Am Food Anim Prac 1988;4:1–16.
[30] Armstrong BK, White E, Sarcci R. Principles of exposure measurement in epidemiology. Oxford (United Kingdom): Oxford University Press; 1994.
[31] Radostits OM, Blood DC, Gay CC. Veterinary Medicine. 9th edition. London: Bailliere Tindall; 2000.
[32] Wilson J, editor. Physical examination. Vet Clin North Am Food Anim Prac 1992;8(2).
[33] Martin SW, Meek AH, Willeberg P. Veterinary epidemiology: principles and methods. Ames (IA): Iowa State University Press; 1987.
[34] Andrews JJ. Necropsy techniques. Vet Clin North Am Food Anim Prac 1986;2(1).
[35] Kirkbride CA. Examination of bovine and ovine fetuses. Vet Clin North Am Food Anim Prac 1986;2:61–84.
[36] Wobeser G. Forensic (medico-legal) necropsy of wildlife. J Wildl Dis 1996;32:240–9.
[37] Jaffe FA. A guide to pathological evidence for lawyers and police officers. 3rd edition. Scarborough (Canada): Thomson Professional Publishing; 1991.
[38] Hancock DD, Blodgett D, Gay CG. The collection and submission of samples for laboratory testing. Vet Clin North Am Food Anim Prac 1988;4:33–60.
[39] Martin SW. The interpretation of laboratory results. Vet Clin North Am Food Anim Prac 1988;4:61–78.
[40] Sackett DL, Haynes RB, Guyatt GH, et al. Clinical epidemiology: a basic science for clinical medicine. 2nd edition. Boston: Little, Brown, and Company; 1991.

[41] Cameron A. Survey toolbox for livestock diseases: a practical manual and software package for active surveillance in developing countries. Canberra (Australia): Australian Centre for International Agricultural Research; 1999.
[42] Moorhouse PD, Hugh-Jones ME. Serum banks. Vet Bull 1981;51:277–90.
[43] Swecker WS, Thatcher CD. The investigation of nutritional disorders. Vet Clin North Am Food Anim Prac 1988;4:127–44.
[44] Holland C, Kezar W. Pioneer forage manual: a nutritional guide. Des Moines (IA): Pioneer Hi-Bred International; 1995.
[45] Jaikaran S. Water analysis interpretation. In: Beef herd management reference binder and study guide. Edmonton (Canada): Alberta Agriculture; 1993.
[46] Larson BL, Arthington J, Corah LR. Recognizing and treating copper imbalances in cattle. Vet Med 1995;90:613–9.
[47] Waldner CL. Serological status for N. caninum, bovine viral diarrhea virus, and infectious bovine rhinotracheitis virus at pregnancy testing and reproductive performance in beef herds. Anim Reprod Sci 2005, in press.
[48] McDermott JJ, Alves DM, Anderson NG, et al. Measures of herd health and productivity in Ontario cow-calf herds. Can Vet J 1991;32:413–20.
[49] Gay JM. Student guidelines for written recommendations. Available at: http://www.vetmed.wsu.edu/courses-jmgay/outbletter.htm. Accessed December 10, 2005.
[50] Perry BD. The design and use of supportive epidemiological studies. Vet Clin North Am Food Anim Prac 1988;4:79–96.

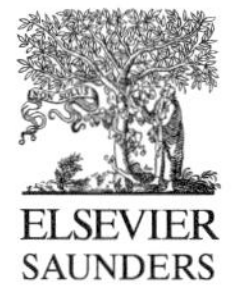

ELSEVIER
SAUNDERS

Vet Clin Food Anim 22 (2006) 103–123

VETERINARY
CLINICS
Food Animal Practice

Designing and Running Clinical Trials on Farms

Michael W. Sanderson, DVM, MS

Department of Clinical Sciences, 111B Mosier Hall, Kansas State University, Manhattan, KS 66506-5706, USA

Clinical trials or field trials are experiments implemented in the real world, such as in a herd setting. As scientific studies, they hold the middle ground between observational studies (cohort, case-control, and cross-sectional studies) and laboratory experiments. In observational studies, the investigator does not exert any control over the study subjects. In laboratory-based experiments, the investigator exerts as complete control as possible over the animals, the environment, and the challenge. In clinical trials, the subjects are left in their normal environment, with the investigator only controlling entry into the trial and allocation to experimental or treatment group. The investigator does not control the environment or exposure to disease or risk (Table 1). Subjects may all be allocated to experimental groups at the beginning of the trial, as in a vaccination or production study, or they may be allocated to an experimental group as the study progresses and as subjects develop disease, as in a therapy trial for mastitis or respiratory disease. Because of this real-world setting, properly done clinical trials are considered the best evidence in clinical questions. Clinical trials are usually done to evaluate therapeutic or preventive products or practices, including vaccines, antibiotics, or management interventions.

Clinical trials, when properly done, are able to assess the relative effect of a practice while controlling for confounding effects. Proper design and statistical analysis of the study isolates the effect of the practice in which the investigators are interested. Well-done field-based clinical trials are the most valuable studies for assisting decision making in production herds. They are useful in the herd or veterinary practice to assist in making rational data-driven decisions for the ranch or farm and for research and pharmaceutic clearance requirements. Pharmaceutic development trials fall into four categories. Phase 1 trials are focused on drug safety/toxicity and include

E-mail address: sandersn@vet.k-state.edu

0749-0720/06/$ - see front matter
doi:10.1016/j.cvfa.2005.11.004

Table 1
Research study types

Research type	Subject and environment control	Statistical control	External validity
Laboratory experiment	High	Low	Low
Clinical trial	Moderate	Moderate	Variable, depending on quality
Observational study	Low	High	High

significant environmental control. Phase 2 trails are small-scale studies usually performed at research farms to identify candidate drugs for further testing. Phase 3 trials are the trials discussed in this article. These trials are generally large scale and done in a field situation with natural environment and management. Phase 4 trials are observational studies done after approval and marketing of a drug to monitor adverse reactions and effectiveness.

Although well-done clinical trials provide the best evidence in clinical questions, a critical evaluation of the scientific literature indicates that not all studies are well done [1,2] and some are little more than uncontrolled informal observations. Clinical trials are prone to confounding and substantial bias if not performed well. This article covers the key concepts in design and implementation of clinical trials for valid, interpretable data. Well-done field trials should include the following factors:

1. a clearly defined research question and assessment of a clinically relevant outcome (morbidity, mortality, performance)
2. an appropriate sample size for the question and study design
3. an appropriate trial design that includes random assignment of animals to treatment and control groups and blinded assessment of clinical outcome (especially important for subjective outcomes such as morbidity)
4. appropriate statistical analysis (correct application of statistical tests and control of herd- or group-clustering effects).

Defining the research question

The interest and direction in answering a specific question generally derives from findings in previous studies or clinical practice experience. General questions must be narrowed and focused into a testable hypothesis. For example, the question, Does deworming calves in the spring before turning out to grass increase weight gain? is a general question that needs to be narrowed based on the type of dewormer, geographic locale, worm burden, pasture management, and numerous other variables. In narrowing the focus of the question, the investigator should become familiar with the published literature on the subject related to what similar questions have been addressed and how well they have been addressed. The literature helps to refine the question to optimize the value of the answer. The final research question should define exactly what the trial is meant to determine. It should be specified in written form before the initiation of the trial and serve to keep the trial focused on the primary objective.

Inherent in the research question is the reference population to which the results will apply. In a refined version of the general question stated earlier, the reference population might be "spring-born beef calves in Missouri that are turned out to grass for the summer." The study population should be selected from the identified reference population (ie, a sample of spring-born grazing Missouri beef calves). If fall-born calves turned out to graze the next spring are used, then they would not be a sample of the reference population from the original question and would not provide useful information in answering the original research question. Even if everything else in the trial is done correctly and quality data are collected, the data would not address the original question.

To further define the question, one needs to decide on the outcome that is to be measured in the study. It should be a clinically relevant outcome such as morbidity, mortality, or performance (Box 1). Surrogate or proxy variables such as antibody titers or egg counts are commonly measured for clinical trials. If such variables are biologically reasonable, then they can be useful supportive data but are not, in and of themselves, clinically relevant outcomes. One does not care that the calves' antibody titers are higher or their egg counts lower unless they also have lower morbidity, mortality, or increased performance (ie, they have increased protection from the negative effects of disease). High antibody titers or low egg counts may be related to disease protection but do not, on their own, assure that. A vaccine may induce high and nonprotective titers or an anthelmintic may decrease egg shedding without improving performance. As such, surrogate variables used as primary outcome variables substantially weaken the study; as supportive variables, they can strengthen the study.

Box 1. Clinical trial outcome measures

Clinically relevant outcomes
- Morbidity rate
- Mortality rate
- Average daily gain
- Milk production
- Pregnancy rate

Surrogate or proxy outcome (not directly clinically relevant)
- Antibody titer
- Fecal egg counts
- Cytokine production
- Lymphoproliferation

The final hypothesis for the trial should be stated in the form of a question that can be answered in the affirmative or negative. It should be constructed in such a way that the results of the trial support or refute it. For example, the general question might be refined into a more specific question such as, Does deworming spring-born beef calves in south central Missouri with product A in May before summer grazing on natural grass pastures increase summer weight gain?

As stated, the trial would be testing for the effect on natural as opposed to irrigated, improved pastures, and summer weight gain as opposed to weaning weight. Therefore, collecting a weight at spring deworming and another at the end of the summer grazing season would be necessary. This research question is then stated in terms of a null and an alternative hypothesis. The null hypothesis is that there is no difference in weight gain between dewormed and not dewormed calves in the trial. The alternative hypothesis is that there is a difference. At the conclusion of a well-designed and implemented trial, the investigators will conclude that one of these hypotheses is correct and accept or reject the null hypothesis (Fig. 1).

This example hypothesis uses a continuous and objective outcome based on weight gain over the summer grazing period. In general, continuous outcomes are preferred to categorical ones, and objective outcomes are preferred to subjective ones. Objective outcomes are based on some measurable trait such as average daily gain or milk production. Mortality is also considered an objective trait for practical purposes in production animal agriculture. Morbidity, however, falls into the subjective category, along with things like change in lameness score. Not everyone agrees on what a morbidity

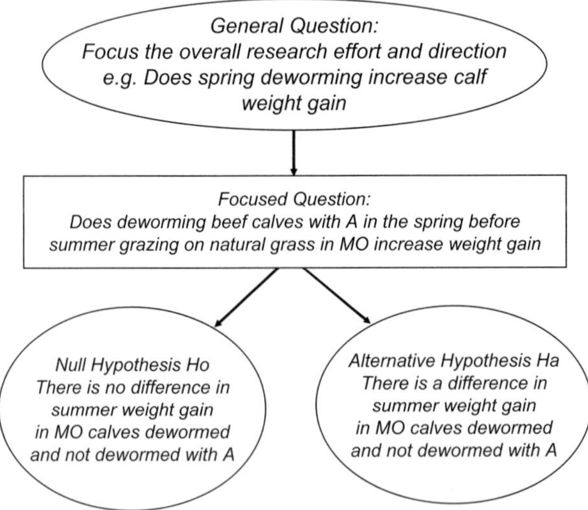

Fig. 1. Question refinement from general to specific.

is (ie, not everyone agrees on which animals are sick). Within a production enterprise, different individuals may not have the same criteria for classifying animals as morbid or well. Even the same individual on an enterprise may not classify animals as morbid or well in the same way every day. When morbidity rates are to be compared between enterprises or sites in the clinical trial, differences in morbidity classification further complicates the issue. If morbidity needs to be classified into syndrome-specific categories or at least to identify a particular disease, then the problem is increased. Investigators need to assign calves correctly to morbid categories, well categories, and to specific morbidity categories and must do so consistently from day to day and from person to person.

A clear definition of what constitutes a morbidity for each syndrome of importance to the trial is necessary for subjective outcomes. For example, a neonatal diarrhea case definition may be set up that involves calf age, depression, dehydration, diarrhea, and temperature. Calves that fulfill the criteria are cases. Not all calves with neonatal diarrhea, however, have diarrhea when they are first recognized as sick, nor do they always have a temperature. The case definition must be carefully thought out and validated if it is to be useful. It can then help to standardize the criteria for a case so that rates are comparable between groups. It may be helpful to think of what other disease entities need to be differentiated and what characteristics would differentiate them from cases of the disease of interest. The assessment of signs that make up a case definition, however, is subjective in nature (eg, there are no objective criteria for what constitutes depression). As such, significant effort should go into validating case definitions. A case definition is validated when it can be shown to identify what it is intended to identify (eg, it correctly identifies neonatal diarrhea cases and is consistently applied over time and between individuals using it). The case definition must agree with reality (identify real cases of the disease of interest and exclude other diseases). Furthermore, all trial participants who have responsibility for identifying cases for inclusion in the study have to agree on what a case is. This agreement is important when multiple individuals within a farm are identifying cases and when studies are performed on multiple farms. Differences in what constitutes a case can introduce significant variation and bias into the study. The case definition must also be stable over time; that is, what is categorized as a case must be the same at the beginning of the trial and at the end (and on Friday afternoon just before quitting time). This consistency is accomplished by training the trial personnel and examining the accuracy with which the case definition criteria identify cases compared with some other established method (perhaps including laboratory support). Some validation and standardization may be achieved by comparing the producer's identification of cases with veterinary identification. In practice, case definitions are rarely rigorously validated, but some level of effort is needed if the resulting data are to be useful.

The idea of a case definition can be extended to that of a clinical scoring system. The intent of a clinical scoring system is to more objectively assess the clinical picture of an animal in assigning it as a case. The most extensive use of scoring systems in beef production has probably been in feedlot respiratory morbidity trials. Scoring systems vary, but typically, each of several signs (nasal discharge, respiratory effort, depression, and so forth) is given a numeric score and the sum of the scores determines the category of the animal. One example of a simple clinical scoring system used in feedlot trials is included in Table 2 [3], and a validated scoring system for coliform mastitis is summarized in Table 3 [4]. Well-designed clinical scoring systems can be useful, but usually some or all of the underlying individual scores are still subjective assessments. The final case assignment is no better than the validity of the underlying subjective assessments, and the outcome variable remains subjective.

This inherent subjectivity in assessing the outcome of the trial provides substantial opportunity for bias. It is easy for those evaluating the trial to let their expectations of the outcome affect their assessment of the outcome. For example, suppose a trial is set up in which calves are vaccinated or not vaccinated for a particular respiratory pathogen on entry to a feedlot. If the feedlot crew that is responsible for checking pens and pulling sick cattle (pen riders) know which pens are vaccinated and which are not, then their biases regarding the effect of vaccination may influence pull rates. If they believe that vaccine is valuable in decreasing morbidity, then they may be influenced to look harder for sick calves in the unvaccinated pen and pull more calves so that they do not let an outbreak get out of hand. If this activity occurs, then it will bias the study toward finding a benefit of vaccination when perhaps no real benefit exists. Similarly, if the producer who is evaluating outcome in the mastitis treatment trial knows the treatment allocation and believes that one treatment is inferior, then he or she may unconsciously evaluate the groups differently. Those who have a vested interest in the outcome may also be tempted to evaluate the groups differently. The most effective way to deal with bias resulting from subjective outcome assessment is blinding of the trial participants to the group assignment. Blinding may be implemented at multiple levels. In single-blind studies, the manager of the trial responsible for follow-up and management of the trial subjects is blind

Table 2
Clinical scores for undifferentiated respiratory disease

Clinical score	Clinical signs
0	Normal, no signs of disease
1	Noticeable signs of depression, weakness usually not apparent
2	Marked depression, moderate signs of weakness but without significantly altered gait
3	Severe depression with signs of weakness such as altered gait or lowered head
4	Moribund, unable to rise

From Perino LJ, Apley MD. Clinical trial design in feedlots. Vet Clin North Am Food Anim Pract 1998;14:356; with permission.

Table 3
Clinical scoring system for coliform mastitis

Clinical variable	Clinical criteria	Clinical score
Rectal temperature (°F)	100–102.7	0
	102.8–103.7	1
	>103.7 or <100	2
Hydration (enopthalmus)	None	0
	Mild	1
	Moderate	2
	Marked	3
Rumen contraction (rate/min)	2 or more	0
	1	1
	0	2
Signs of depression	None	0
	Mild	1
	Marked	2

Clinical scores for each category are summed. A total score of 0–2-mild disease; 3–5-moderate disease; and 6–9-severe disease.

From Wenz JR, Barrington GM, Garry FB, et al. Use of systemic disease signs to assess disease severity in dairy cows with acute coliform mastitis. J Am Vet Med Assoc 2001;218:572; with permission.

to the group assignment. In a double-blind study, the manager and the individuals responsible for assessing the outcome of the trial are blind to the group assignments. To be effective in this instance, blinding may also require blinding of the crew that administers the vaccines so that communication cannot occur with the pen riders. Blinding the vaccination crew means that all calves must get a "vaccine"—a placebo or a real vaccine. Hiding the difference can be difficult but may mean developing a placebo with the same color, consistency, and in the same bottle but without the antigen and adjuvant. Particularly with subjective outcomes such as morbidity, double blinding is crucial to the validity of the trial.

Sample size requirements

Identification of the correct sample size during the planning phase is crucial to the design of a useful clinical trial. Even a perfectly implemented study will fail to answer the research question if the sample size is too small. Conversely, a sample size that is too large will result in needless expense and effort and potentially identify small and meaningless differences. Too large a sample size is usually not the problem. An appropriate sample size is necessary to support or refute the hypothesis with reasonable certainty. A given sample size gives an estimated probability of correctly determining the truth of the research hypothesis and an estimated probability of making an error in the determination (Fig. 2).

These errors are termed type I when a difference is identified that does not truly exist and type II when a difference that truly exists fails to be identified.

Statistical Inference

		Truth: Different	Truth: Not Different
Study Findings	Different	**Power** **1-β**	**Type I error** **α (p)**
	Not Different	**Type II Error** **β**	**1-α**

Errors in Hypothesis Testing
1. Conclude there is a difference when there truly is no difference.
   Type I error – Probability = α (the p-value)
2. Conclude there is no difference when there truly is a difference
   Type II error – Probability = β

Fig. 2. Errors in statistical inference.

The type I error is called α and is the same as the P value. The type II error is called β, and 1-β equals the power of the study. The possibility of an error in the determination can never be completely removed, but attempts should be made to minimize its probability. Increasing sample size is the primary way that the probability of committing an error can be decreased. Increased sample size also increases the power of the study or its ability to detect a difference between the groups if one truly exists. With inadequate sample size, the study has low power and is unlikely to detect real differences. In such a case, the study may find no significant difference but may also fail to provide any credible evidence of a lack of difference. For example, consider a trial of treatment efficacy for disease A that compares two different treatment regimes. Fifty cows were enrolled into each group, and the treatment failure rates observed for the two groups were 20% for treatment 1 and 30% for treatment 2. The calculated P value (the probability that this outcome was due to random variation and not the treatment) was 0.25 and the effect was deemed not significant. A 33% decrease in treatment failure rate (relative risk reduction; see the article by Slenning elsewhere in this issue), however, seems to be potentially important (depending on what it cost to achieve). The power of this study to detect a change in treatment failure from 30% to 20% is calculated to be only about 0.15. Therefore, the probability of failing to detect a real difference from 30% to 20% in this study (a type II error) with only 50 cows in each group is 85%. In this example, the study fails to reject the null hypothesis ($P = 0.25$) but does not have adequate evidence to accept it either (power to find such a difference is only 0.15). So, if the "real" relative risk reduction is 33%, then this study had little chance to detect such a difference. The effect of sample size on precision of estimates is discussed further in Slenning (this issue).

The α and β levels for scientific studies (including clinical trials) have traditionally been set at $\alpha = 0.05$ and $\beta = 0.20$. For studies that are meant to assist in decision making in production enterprises, these levels may not be the ideal values. In a production setting, decisions have to be made and, at times, one may need to accept a decreased level of certainty to make the best possible decision at the time (even though it would not pass muster in a peer-reviewed scientific journal). Where α and β are set should be determined by the relative cost of type I and type II errors. Suppose that a trial is designed to consider implementation of a management change that would require significant economic and labor inputs (ie, the cost of a type I error is high). One might want to be more certain that this costly management change will truly be beneficial before implementing it, so the α level is lowered to 0.01 (the probability of a type I error). If a difference is found, then one is more certain it is real. Conversely, if one wants to increase the probability of detecting a difference in practices or products if such a difference exists—say the cost of making the management or product change is negligible (the cost of a type I error is small) and the potential improvement in cost or production is large (cost of a type II error is large)—then one would decrease β to 0.1 or 0.05 to increase the probability of detecting a difference if a difference exists. For a given sample size, this technique increases the probability of a type I error, which may be acceptable if the cost of that error is small.

For a given sample size, the probability of a type I error (α) is decreased at the expense of increasing the probability of a type II error (β) and the probability of a type II error (β) is decreased at the expense of increasing the probability of a type I error (α).

The first step in calculating the sample size needed for a clinical trial is to decide what effect size is important to detect. This decision should be based on what level of effect would be biologically and or economically important. For example, if the cost of a particular management intervention is such that a breakeven for implementation would require a 50% relative reduction in morbidity, then it may not be justifiable to have a sample size that would detect a smaller difference (even if a 25% relative reduction was found, one would not implement the management change because one could not afford to). Determining economically important levels of risk reduction is discussed further in Slenning (this issue).

The type of outcome variable used also impacts sample size. There are two basic types of outcome variables: categoric and continuous (see the article by Ruegg elsewhere in this article). Generally, sample size is larger for outcome variables that are categorical, such as morbidity, mortality, and pregnancy status, and smaller for continuous variables such as weight gain or days pregnant. This difference in sample size happens because substantial amounts of information are given up in using categoric outcomes. For example, knowing the pregnancy status of individual cows provides substantially less information than knowing how many days pregnant they each are on a certain date.

Categorical variables are those in which the subjects fit into one of two or more categories. Categorical data may be divided into three types (dichotomous or binary, nominal, and ordinal; see Ruegg, this issue) and are commonly tested with the use of a χ^2 test.

In calculating the sample size for categorical outcomes, three values need to be established:

1. α—the probability of concluding that there is a difference between the groups when no real difference exists (the *P* value)
2. β—the probability of concluding that there is no difference between the groups when a real difference exists
3. The magnitude of the difference that one wishes to be able to detect in terms of the proportion with the outcome in each group

To determine the sample size for categorical data with only two groups and when the required sample size is equal among groups, the sample size may be estimated by the following equation:

$$n = \frac{\left[Z_\alpha\sqrt{(2PQ)} - Z_\beta\sqrt{(P_tQ_t + P_cQ_c)}\right]^2}{(P_t - P_c)^2}$$

where *n* is the required number of samples in each group
Z_α is 2.58 for $\alpha = 0.01$, 1.96 for $\alpha = 0.05$, and 1.65 for $\alpha = 0.1$
Z_β is -1.28 for $\beta = 0.1$ and -0.84 for $\beta = 0.20$
P_t is the proportion with the outcome in the treated group
Q_t is $1 - P_t$ and equals the proportion without the outcome in the treated group
P_c is the proportion with the outcome in the control group
Q_c is $1 - P_c$ and equals the proportion without the outcome in the control group
P is $(P_t + P_c)/2$
Q is $1 - P$ and equals $(Q_t + Q_c)/2$

Therefore, the estimated sample size to detect a change in mortality from 10% to 5% between two groups with $\alpha = 0.05$ and $\beta = 0.20$ and with the values of

$Z_\alpha = 1.96$ for $\alpha = 0.05$
$Z_\beta = -0.84$ for $\beta = 0.20$
$P_t = 0.05$
$Q_t = 1 - P_t = 0.95$
$P_c = 0.10$
$Q_c = 1 - P_c = 0.90$
$P = (P_t + P_c)/2 = (0.05 + 0.10)/2 = 0.075$
$Q = 1 - P = 0.925$ is

$$\frac{\left[1.96\sqrt{(2 \times 0.075 \times 0.925)} - -0.84\sqrt{(0.05 \times 0.95 + 0.10 \times 0.90)}\right]^2}{(0.05 - 0.10)^2}$$

$$= 434$$

Continuous variables are those that are measured on a continuous scale and may take on any value. Examples include weight, age, duration of pregnancy, and postpartum interval. Continuous data that are divided into two groups are commonly tested with a *z* test or a *t* test.

In calculating the sample size for continuous variables, four values must be established:

1. α—the probability of concluding that there is a difference between the groups when no real difference exists (the *P* value)
2. β—the probability of concluding that there is no difference between the groups when a real difference exists
3. The magnitude of the difference one wishes to be able to detect
4. The standard deviation (variation) in the groups—this value can come from published data of the variation in the attribute one is interested in or may come from historical production records on the farms one is working on; with production data from the farm, one can calculate the standard deviation in Excel (Microsoft Corp., Redmond, Washington) using the "Stdev" function

For simple studies with two groups and when the sample size and standard deviation in each group are approximately equal, the sample size for each group may be estimated by the following equation:

$$n = 2\left[\frac{(Z_\alpha - Z_\beta)S}{(X_t - X_c)}\right]^2$$

where n is the required number of samples in each group
Z_α is 2.58 for $\alpha = 0.01$, 1.96 for $\alpha = 0.05$, and 1.65 for $\alpha = 0.1$
Z_β is -1.28 for $\beta = 0.1$ and -0.84 for $\beta = 0.20$
X_t is the expected mean outcome in the treated group
X_c is the expected mean outcome in the control group
S is the estimated common standard deviation for the two groups

Therefore, the estimated sample size to detect a change in average daily gain from 3.2 lb/d to 3.5 lb/d between two groups with a common standard deviation of 0.5 lb/d, $\alpha = 0.10$; $\beta = 0.10$

$Z_\alpha = 1.65$ for $\alpha = 0.10$
$Z_\beta = -1.28$ for $\beta = 0.10$
$X_t = 3.5$ lb/d

$X_c = 3.2$ lb/d
$S = 0.5$ lb/d is

$$2\left[\frac{[1.65-(-1.28)]0.5}{(3.5-3.2)}\right]^2 = 48$$

For all sample size calculations, the estimated number is the number of experimental units needed in each group. More complex study designs that involve more than one group, unequal sample sizes, repeated samplings on individuals, or multiple herds with repeated samplings within herds require much more complex calculations and may require substantially increased sample size. Under these circumstances, the assistance of an epidemiologist or biostatistician should be sought. Some issues involved in the analysis of other types of data are discussed in Slenning (this issue).

Trial design and implementation

Inclusion and exclusion criteria

Herd

Standard inclusion criteria can be established for cooperating producers to be included in the trial. These inclusion criteria depend on the trial design and outcome and may include such things as type of operation, physical facilities for handling animals, and ability to collect production and health records. Inclusion criteria essentially define the reference population. For the example, the inclusion criteria for the research question, Does deworming spring-born beef calves in south central Missouri with product A in May before summer grazing on natural grass pastures increase summer weight gain? includes (1) being a south central Missouri cow-calf operator, (2) having a spring calving herd; (3) grazing on natural as opposed to irrigated pastures, and (4) the ability to take weight measurements at spring deworming and at the end of summer.

One could argue that these inclusion criteria limit the application of the results, and indeed, they do. Technically, the results would apply only to herds that meet the criteria for inclusion. Practically, the results may be reasonably applied to other herds for which the management and environment are similar (how similar is arguable and for the practitioner applying the results to decide). The results may not apply to more arid environments, to calves grazed on irrigated pastures, or to herds with a lower level of management. The alternative to this limitation, however, is to have no defined population to which the results apply and no clear results applicable to the original research question. Clinical trials are most useful in answering one or two well-defined questions. A design that attempts to answer too much will be too large and too complex to implement and analyze and will end up answering no question.

Individual subjects

Inclusion and exclusion criteria may also be applied to individual subjects at the time of enrollment to exclude individuals that do not fit the case definition or that have concurrent problems that may confound assessment of the treatment or intervention effect. When not carefully and evenly applied, exclusion criteria can bias the study and damage the generalizability of the results. All exclusion and inclusion criteria should be explicitly written in the trial protocol and applied evenly to all individuals that present for enrollment. This is best implemented in the form of a clear case definition of which animals are appropriate for inclusion and which are not. The previous discussion of case definitions and clinical scores is applicable here.

Cooperator recruitment

After the trial is defined and planned, cooperating producers and their herds are necessary for implementation of the trial protocol. Depending on the defined outcome of the trial, a single herd may provide an adequate number of individuals for allocation to treatment groups or multiple herds may be required to provide individual animals. For some outcomes, it may be most appropriate to allocate whole herds or pens of animals to treatment and control groups. For example, if the management intervention being evaluated is implemented at the whole-farm level, then farms need to be allocated to treatment and control groups. Similarly, in a feedlot vaccine trial, if the vaccination is given to whole pens of cattle, then pens are the units that are allocated to treatment and control groups. This is true even if the cattle were randomly assigned to pens. The intervention is still applied at the pen level, and the pen remains the experimental unit. If the intervention is applied at the individual level and individual response is followed, then the individual is the experimental unit, although farm effects may still need to be accounted for in the analysis of multipen or multifarm trials. The cooperating producers make up the study population and are selected from the reference population as defined in the study protocol. Ideally, the cooperators would be a random sample of the reference population. In practice, this is not realistic and may cause more problems than it prevents. Because producers cannot be compelled to participate, a truly random sample is not possible. Further, some producers who agree to participate may not follow the trial protocols or even finish the trial. Substantial deviation from the trial protocol or loss from the trial due to dropouts can substantially bias the trial and invalidate the trial results. Due to these difficulties, study populations for clinical trials are usually a convenience sample of the reference population. That is, they are the producers to whom investigators have access and who are believed to be able and willing to follow the trial protocol and complete the trial. Ideal cooperators are generally interested in the issues addressed in the trial, willing and able to keep accurate records, and committed to following through with the protocol. They are willing cooperators. If they need to be "talked into" cooperating, then they will be less committed and more likely to deviate from the protocol or drop out completely. This approach improves the likelihood that the trial will be successfully completed in an interpretable form (improves internal validity); however, it narrows the generalizability of the trial results to operations that are similar to the participants' (decreases external validity).

Cooperators included in the study should be clearly informed as to the study protocol, the method of allocation of animals or groups to the treatment and control groups, and the importance of adherence to trial protocol. They should be aware that one of the treatments may be inferior to the other but that its true effect is unknown. As such, one of the treatments may result in poorer response or productivity; however, a true assessment of the effects will require implementation of the trial protocol, including random, unbiased allocation of animals to the groups. (When valid data support that one treatment is better, the better treatment should be implemented and the trial cancelled). These issues should be explicitly communicated in a trial agreement form that the cooperators read and sign. Their signature on this form can serve as an implied informed consent.

Cooperator remuneration should also be discussed and agreed on before the beginning of the trial. For trials run on individual operations with the purpose of generating data to assist in production management decisions, the payment is the expectation that the trial results will provide valuable data to improve decision making and profitability on that operation. For research trials, depending on the trial protocol, producers may be willing to participate out of loyalty to a university program, personal interest, or a desire to further their own knowledge and management. If the trial calls for additional management or labor inputs to collect data, then the cooperators may expect some financial return for their efforts. These agreements should be clearly agreed to in writing and in advance.

Trial implementation

Implementation of the trial involves allocating the subjects to treatment and control groups, collection and management of the data, and monitoring compliance with the trial protocols. Proper allocation of individuals or groups to the treatment and control categories is critical to interpretable data. The experimental unit of the trial is the smallest independent unit that is randomized, whether it is a herd, a pen within a herd, or an individual. The experimental units need to be independent of each other so that even if the randomization takes place at the individual level, the individual is not the experimental unit if the animals are not independent. A common example is calves in a feedlot pen. One might randomly allocate individual calves to pens for a pneumonia vaccination study to assess morbidity, but if the vaccination is applied at the pen level (all calves in a pen vaccinated or not vaccinated), then the individual calves are not independent. These calves are managed as a unit because after one calf in a pen gets pneumonia, the risk of all the other calves changes; their outcomes are correlated and not independent. Therefore, the pen is the experimental unit. This effect is especially prominent for contagious diseases in animals housed in groups and is important to recognize and correctly analyze. The data can be analyzed at the pen level based on the proportion of morbid calves in each pen but cannot be analyzed at the individual calf level without accounting for the pen effect in the analysis.

Numerous methods have been used to allocate subjects, of which some are acceptable and some are not. A formal randomization process is ideal for allocating subjects to groups because it is the most effective way to minimize differences between the groups and distribute confounding factors equally. In a formal randomization process, some random process, such as a random number table (Box 2) or computer-generated random numbers, is used to assign subjects to groups. The process may be simple randomization in which each subject has an equal probability of being assigned to each

Box 2. Random numbers

	1	2	3	4	5	6	7	8	9	10	11	12	13	14	15	16	17	18	19
1	36	09	51	00	21	32	71	51	42	21	07	10	43	24	04	17	19	75	51
2	53	25	11	23	47	10	41	09	52	96	59	89	13	45	41	80	84	20	84
3	07	72	03	43	81	28	10	72	54	66	11	42	75	45	97	02	47	22	41
4	13	01	73	84	83	16	43	14	81	99	75	01	10	33	83	27	76	88	24
5	35	89	44	15	02	72	59	11	52	29	75	30	17	82	18	60	97	10	75
6	23	85	76	71	84	67	26	58	26	41	81	36	64	11	91	99	77	75	70
7	66	91	99	47	77	57	90	66	04	82	16	04	32	80	51	00	48	73	38
8	29	99	04	93	62	05	75	41	38	77	29	25	04	52	85	47	88	47	59
9	90	38	95	62	60	15	20	42	40	47	50	42	54	82	15	23	96	78	07
10	14	60	94	45	30	98	70	86	15	26	82	99	88	16	50	32	95	74	98
11	45	81	70	77	33	91	26	33	59	61	58	59	27	91	25	38	00	53	63
12	11	70	38	00	25	31	68	87	84	02	98	36	07	84	96	36	63	81	07
13	78	83	56	74	83	54	82	70	86	04	61	26	19	90	58	10	90	93	36
14	28	63	84	56	14	37	35	12	41	22	97	31	73	53	33	27	59	01	84
15	21	17	30	79	41	79	42	59	83	81	51	23	35	17	42	57	18	58	20
16	01	53	49	62	66	74	82	72	86	07	15	47	44	23	96	74	95	30	49
17	30	85	27	89	27	57	67	27	42	24	71	38	81	70	97	99	31	81	78
18	71	83	32	28	75	27	05	45	17	83	89	71	37	31	36	29	62	45	30
19	78	04	53	65	80	05	70	01	10	44	72	18	38	82	21	64	52	10	15

Beginning in an arbitrary place in the table, use the numbers to randomly assign groups. For two group assignments, progress through the table and assign units to group 1 if the random number is 0–4 or to group 2 if the random number is 5–9. For example, begin in row 2, column 4 and move horizontally. The random number 2 falls into the 0–4 category, so it is assigned to group 1. Continue assigning groups while moving horizontally:

Random number 2 3 4 7 1 0 4 1 0 9 5 2 9 6 5 9 8 9
Group assignment 1 1 1 2 1 1 1 1 1 2 2 1 2 2 2 2 2 2

group without regard to any other factors. Stratified randomization involves separating the subjects into categories based on potentially important factors such as age, weight, or herd and randomizing them to a group within each category. This process ensures that equal numbers from each category end up in each group (Fig. 3). Simple randomization techniques do not assure an equal number of subjects in each group. For large numbers of subjects, the groups are close to equal, but for small numbers, they can be quite different. One can use block randomization to assure that an equal number of subjects end up in each group. In block randomization, equal numbers of subjects are allocated to each experimental group within each block. For example, when one is allocating to three different groups, the subjects can be blocked into groups of three and allocated to the three groups in random order within the blocks (Table 4). There are six different orders that three units could be assigned to three different groups, so the numbers 0 through 5 from the random number table can be used to determine the allocation order within the block and the numbers 6 through 9 in the random number table can be ignored. At the end of each block, one subject has been allocated to each group and the groups are of equal size (see Table 4).

Clusters of animals, such as herds or pens of cattle, may also be randomized to groups. Randomizing at the herd or pen level is important when the intervention will be given at the herd level or when tracking the response in individual animals is not feasible.

Sometimes a "true" random allocation is difficult to accomplish in a production setting. A realistic alternative is systematic allocation whereby subjects are alternately allocated to groups. When allocating to two groups, the first subject is randomly assigned and each subsequent subject is alternately assigned. This randomization may occur as animals come through the chute for allocation or as they enter the trial as cases. In most instances, this way to allocate subjects is very effective. Systematic allocation, however, is more susceptible to tampering: if the study personnel learn the allocation

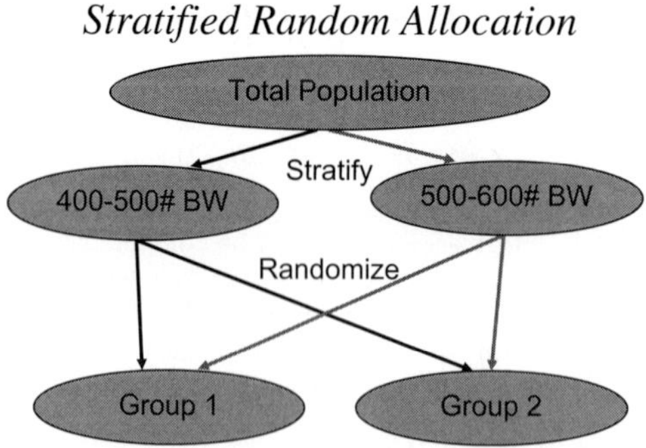

Fig. 3. Stratified random allocation. Population of calves stratified according to weight and randomly assigned to group from each strata. BW, body weight.

Table 4
Block randomization

Random number[a]	Allocation order[b] First experimental unit in the block	Second experimental unit in the block	Third experimental unit in the block
0	A	B	C
1	A	C	B
2	B	A	C
3	B	C	A
4	C	B	A
5	C	A	B

[a] Ignore random numbers 6–9.

[b] Allocate experimental units to groups in blocks of three. Using a random number table (see Box 2), allocate blocks of three units to the three groups in the order indicated.

alternation, they may be able to influence the order in which subjects present and are allocated.

The discussion so far has assumed equal allocation to each group; however, this is not absolutely necessary. Suppose, for example, an intervention is expensive or labor intensive and one wishes to minimize the number of subjects allocated to it. Allocating two control subjects for every treatment subject in the trial will have the effect of modestly decreasing the number of subjects in the treatment group while modestly increasing the total sample size and decreasing the trial cost. One might do the same to decrease the number of placebo controls in a study and offer the supposed beneficial treatment to more animals while still meeting research objectives. Allocating beyond a 2:1 ratio provides little additional benefit.

A final comment on allocation should be made regarding historical controls. When using historical controls, one essentially allocates subjects from the past to the control group and current subjects to the intervention group. Then, the performance or disease rates between the current subjects and the historical subjects are compared. This practice is clearly not random, and historical controls are generally not acceptable. Numerous management, environmental, and exposure variables may be different between current and historical subjects, rendering the comparison between the control and intervention groups invalid. Historical controls may be acceptable in circumstances in which the duration of the trial is very short, such as pre- and post-treatment data, when no other management or environmental factors change, and when the clinical syndrome is stable in the absence of an intervention. The trail duration probably cannot exceed 1 to 2 weeks, depending on the disease or production syndrome. Together, these requirements are very difficult to achieve. Historical controls may be more commonly used in production decision making and, at times, may be the only basis available for decision making. Historical controls, however, provide markedly inferior data for decision making compared with appropriate contemporary controls. The use of disease rates from a previous year to assess the efficacy of a newly introduced vaccine, for example, does not provide good evidence. Numerous factors change from one year to the next that could account for the change in morbidity rates, irrespective of the vaccine efficacy.

Based on the defined research question outcome variables, data collection forms and protocols should be established to ensure that a complete set of the needed data is collected on each subject in the trial. Included should be baseline data on animals allocated to the groups and on those excluded from the study population and the reason for exclusion. Response data on all animals (or groups) enrolled in the trial should also be collected, including reasons for subject dropout. All subjects (treatment and control) enrolled in the study should be followed equally and long enough so that the outcomes of interest are observed should they occur. Finally, the implementation of the trial should be monitored as it progresses to ensure its successful completion. As the data are collected, one should monitor that inclusion and exclusion, allocation to groups, and data collection are progressing in accordance to the protocol. Monitoring is also essential to identify early on problems with the protocol or questions cooperators have and to resolve issues before they endanger the trial. The frequency of monitoring depends on the type and intensity of the trial. For trials in which allocation, treatment, and assessment are ongoing through the study, weekly monitoring may be necessary to keep the trial on track and to avoid drift in the application of the trial protocols. For studies in which allocation occurs at the beginning and assessment is not until the end of the study, such as weight gain trials, less frequent monitoring may be sufficient.

Trial analysis

Analysis of field data is covered in more depth in Slenning (this issue), and the reader is directed there for the details of the tests briefly discussed here. Proper analysis of the trial data is crucial to making good decisions from the data. Selecting the proper analysis is a matter of knowing the design of the trial and the biology of the system and accounting for those factors in the analysis. This process may result in a very simple analysis for two equal-sized groups within one herd that are individually allocated to a treatment group or a control group. Alternately, it may require a very complex analysis that accounts for multiple variables, confounding variables, and clustering at the pen and herd level. The analysis should be based on the level of randomization of experimental units. If the experimental unit in the trial is the herd or pen of animals, then the analysis should not be based on outcomes in individual animals without control for herd- or pen-level clustering effects.

Comparing means

The z test or t test is the simplest method of comparing the mean of two continuous variables, as outlined in Slenning (this issue). For example, suppose there are 50 calves in each group of the summer calf deworming trial to determine whether the average daily gains from deworming to weaning in dewormed calves are different from average daily gains in non–dewormed calves. First, to answer that question fairly, one needs to have randomly divided the calves between the two groups so that the calves of high–milk production cows or greater growth genetics are not more commonly included in one group. If the calf groups are comparable and the same nutritional resources are available to each group, then the groups can be compared by comparing the mean average daily calf gains using a *z* test. The *z* test compares the difference in the two means in relation to the amount of variability in the data (standard error). For the example with 50 calves in each group, suppose that an average daily gain of 2.6 lb/d in the dewormed group and 2.5 lb/d in the non–dewormed group (a difference of 0.10 lb/d) and a standard deviation of 0.5 lb/d in each group are observed. The *z* test would give a *P* value of 0.32, and one would not conclude that there was a difference between the two groups. What the *P* value really means is that if there truly is no difference between the two groups in average daily gain, then one would still expect to observe a difference this big or bigger about 32% of the time. Therefore, the observed difference between the two groups would be fairly common, even if there is no true difference between them. The observed difference between the groups of 0.10 lb/d would equate to a 10-lb difference in weaning weight over a 100-day grazing period. At $1/lb, that would be a $10 return if the difference is real. Economically, if the costs of the dewormer and labor are less than $10, then one would be interested in differences as small as this. So, is there really no difference between the groups or did the study lack sufficient power to detect a difference this size? The power to detect the observed difference in this study with only 50 animals in each group is calculated to be only 17% (17% probability of detecting a difference of 0.10 lb/d). With a power this low, there is no evidence that deworming does not have an effect. The sample size that is needed to have 80% power of detecting a difference of 0.10 lb/d is approximately 393 in each group. Carefully calculating the sample size in the design of the trial would have prevented wasting time and effort with only 50 animals in each group. A *P* value of 0.05 or 0.10 is usually used as the point at which one can conclude there really is a difference. If we had a sufficient sample size, observed the same difference in weight gain, and obtained a *P* value of 0.05, the following interpretation would have been given: if there was no difference between the groups, then this big of a difference would be seen only rarely (5% of the time), and it could be concluded that there probably is an effect of deworming.

Comparing proportions

The χ^2 test is a common way to compare disease counts or proportions between two groups as outlined by Slenning (elsewhere in this issue).

Table 5
Observed outcome for bovine respiratory disease for 50 calves vaccinated prior to weaning and 50 calves not vaccinated

	Pneumonia		
	Yes	No	Totals
Vaccination			
Yes	14	86	100
No	24	76	100
Totals	38	162	200

Suppose, for example, one wants to compare the proportion of weaned calves that get sick in the first 21 days after weaning for calves that were vaccinated 2 weeks before weaning to calves not vaccinated before weaning. The groups need to be comparable except for the attribute of interest (vaccination status). When there are potential confounders between the groups, one can use more sophisticated statistical methods to control for confounding. For the χ^2 test, data are categorized into a 2 × 2 table of the observed distribution of pneumonia and vaccination status (Table 5), and the observed and expected distributions are compared as outlined in Slenning (this issue). The result is a χ^2 statistic that can be compared with a χ^2 table to arrive at a P value. The observed distribution of disease is not different from the expected distribution ($P > 0.1$), so it is concluded that the morbidity is not different between the two groups (differences in morbidity as big as this would not be uncommon if there was really no difference between prevaccinated calves and calves not prevaccinated). Again, there are relatively small numbers in each group, and an assessment of the power to detect differences is in order in light of the nonsignificant result. The observed proportion of vaccinated calves that got sick was 14% and the observed proportion of nonvaccinated calves that got sick was 24%. The calculated power is only about 37%, and the required sample size for 80% power is approximately 260 animals in each group. So again, the inadequate sample size leaves one with no real evidence that vaccination does not decrease morbidity.

For trial designs that involve more complicated analysis, the assistance of an epidemiologist or biostatistician is required. More sophisticated analysis can use analysis of variance and multiple regression techniques to take into account multiple groups, multiple variables, matching of the subjects, and clustering of data from multiple observations within pens or herds.

Summary

Well-designed and -implemented clinical trials provide the most useful evidence regarding clinical questions relevant to food animal practice. The ability to critically identify the factors that make up a well-done (or poorly done) clinical trial in the scientific literature increases one's ability to make quality decisions in production operations. Further, the ability to design and carry out simple clinical trials on producer farms increases one's ability to generate data and make decisions that are most relevant to clients. Consultation with a biostatistician or epidemiologist when necessary makes sure that the planning, implementation, and analysis of the trial are appropriate. Well-done field trials in the scientific literature or performed on client farms should include the following factors:

1. A well thought-out and clearly defined research question that is relevant to clients' operations, including assessment of an outcome that is clinically relevant to the client (morbidity, mortality, performance)
2. Calculation of an appropriate sample size for the question and the study design to assure the question can be answered
3. An appropriate trial design that includes random assignment of animals to treatment and control groups and blinded assessment of clinical outcome (especially important for subjective outcomes such as morbidity)
4. Appropriate statistical analysis (correct application of statistical tests and control of herd or group clustering effects)

Further readings

Dohoo I, Martin S, Stryhn H. Veterinary epidemiologic research. Charlottetown, PEI, Canada: AVC; 2003.

Hulley SB, Cummings SR, Browner WS, et al. Designing clinical research. 2nd edition. Philadelphia: Lippincott Williams & Wilkins; 2001.

Martin SW, Meek AH, Willeburg P. Veterinary epidemiology: principles and methods. Ames (IA): Iowa State University Press; 1987.

Slenning BD. Quantitative tools for production-oriented veterinarians. In: Radostits OM, editor. Herd health: food animal production medicine. Philadelphia: WB Saunders; 2001. p. 356.

Smith RD. Veterinary clinical epidemiology: a problem-oriented approach. 2nd edition. Boca Raton (FL): CRC Press; 1995.

References

[1] Elbers ARW, Schukken YH. Clinical features of veterinary field trials. Vet Rec 1995;136: 187–92.

[2] Perino LJ, Apley MD. Clinical trial design in feedlots. Vet Clin North Am Food Anim Pract 1998;14:343–65.

[3] Perino LJ, Hunsaker BD. A review of bovine respiratory disease vaccine field efficacy. Bovine Pract 1997;31(1):59–66.

[4] Wenz JR, Barrington GM, Garry FB, et al. Use of systemic disease signs to assess disease severity in diary cows with acute coliform mastitis. J Am Vet Med Assoc 2001;218:567–72.

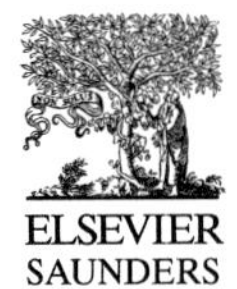

ELSEVIER
SAUNDERS

VETERINARY
CLINICS
Food Animal Practice

Vet Clin Food Anim 22 (2006) 125–147

Determining Cause and Effect in Herds

John M. Gay, DVM, PhD

Department of Veterinary Clinical Sciences, AAHP Field Disease Investigation Unit, College of Veterinary Medicine, Washington State University, P.O. Box 646610, Pullman, WA 99164-6610, USA

Establishing cause and effect is the critical step of many clinical diagnostic work-ups, particularly for herd problems, because understanding cause provides the basis for control and prevention decisions. The confidence required in one's conclusion about cause and effect depends on the situation. Factors include the comparative costs and risks of the problem and potential interventions and the difficulty of implementing interventions, particularly if changes in ingrained human behavior are required. Because of the complexity of biologic systems and processes, the often long lag between cause and effect, biologic variability within the same animal over time and between animals at the same time, and the inevitable continual changes in husbandry conditions (eg, individual animals proceeding through the production cycle, weather changes, feed changes, and personnel changes), defining cause with certainty sufficient for developing control and prevention interventions and with confidence is challenging, even with a definitive clinical diagnosis.

Although the continuing economic loss from a problem usually forces rapid decisions after the problem is recognized, the available information is often incomplete. The cost and delay of acquiring additional information must be balanced against the value of a more timely intervention and the potential cost of error due to incomplete information. To effectively and efficiently determine cause in diverse livestock production environments, considerable background knowledge and creativity are usually required. Although it is important, a definitive clinical diagnosis alone is often not enough to identify the causes of disease problems that are changeable as part of control or prevention interventions. By their nature, most livestock enterprises are complex, dynamic systems with variously lagged positive and negative feedback loops impacted by continual changes in controlled (eg,

E-mail address: jmgay@vetmed.wsu.edu

0749-0720/06/$ - see front matter
doi:10.1016/j.cvfa.2005.12.004 *vetfood.theclinics.com*

change in feed source) and uncontrolled inputs (eg, weather, seasonal climate), changes in location as animals move through the production cycle, and so on. On extensive livestock operations that have low-technology systems, such as grazing beef cow-calf operations in the intermountain West, information is sparse because of infrequent animal observation and the common lack of individual performance records. The coming of mandated individual animal identification from birth may be an opportunity to remedy this lack of information. On intensive livestock operations that have highly technical, tightly interconnected systems, such as large dry-lot confinement dairies, even when sufficient standard operating procedures are in place, uncertainty results from the continual compromises required due to economic and resource limitations, recurring problems due to procedural and technical system drift, and human nature, particularly when poor communication occurrs between personnel.

The purpose of this article is to present the components of the logical process for determining cause and effect and to list common cognitive errors of the medical decision-making process, the thought being if individuals are aware of these errors, then they will be better able to avoid committing them. The first section provides the concepts used in considering cause and effect relationships, the second section provides a logical basis for evaluating cause and effect relationships, and the third section illuminates potential reasoning errors.

Underlying concepts

The following concepts are important for considering cause and effect; the reader is encouraged to consult a dictionary of epidemiology [1] or a veterinary epidemiology text such as Thrusfield [2] for additional details. The **effect** is the outcome of interest, which may be the occurrence of disease, low production, poor performance, or other event or phenomenon. The **case definition** is the set of criteria (eg, death or sickness with certain clinical signs) used to establish which animals experienced the effect. **Risk factors** are individual attributes or exposures that may be involved in the cause of a specific effect, increasing or decreasing the risk of the effect occurring. An **attribute** is a risk factor that is an intrinsic characteristic of an animal, such as genetic susceptibility, immune status, age, sex, breed, or weight. Some attributes can be changed quickly, such as improving host resistance by vaccination, whereas others require a much longer time frame, such as reducing genetic susceptibility by changing the breeding program. An example is reducing the risk of ocular squamous cell carcinoma in future replacement Hereford heifers by using only breeding bulls with dark pigmentation around their eyes. An **exposure** is a risk factor that is in the environment external to the individual, such as nutrition, housing, husbandry practice, or an infectious or toxic agent. A **risk marker** is a noncausal factor associated sufficiently well with a risk factor so that it can be used as a marker, or indicator, of exposure to that specific risk factor when detection of the factor itself is difficult and expensive. For example, serologic titer is often used as a marker for previous exposure to an infectious agent when the agent itself cannot be detected; however, cross-reactions with other antigens and vaccination-induced response can make interpretation difficult.

As defined elsewhere in this issue, a **key determinant**, sometimes called a risk determinant, leverage point, or a critical control point, is a specific risk factor that can be modified or eliminated to control or prevent the effect. In terms of the benefit from changes versus the cost of the changes, some key determinants are more important than others. For example, the risk factors for the transmission of the endemic infectious agents involved in calf scours are more often key determinants than simply the presence of common viral agents because these agents are essentially endemic in almost all livestock operations. The key question is why (if the infectious agents are essentially ubiquitous) some livestock operations have the clinical problem when many others do not. The answer is differences in the key determinants. In such circumstances, rather than limiting interventions to the use of pharmaceuticals for treatment or biologics for prevention, the best interventions often involve long-term changes in facilities and human behavior, which is often expensive and difficult. Carrier cows, however, are certainly a risk factor that could be modified by testing the herd, but for such agents, the cost would likely exceed the short-term benefit.

For diseases with a long latency, such as cancer, the exposure may have occurred much earlier in the host's life. For other diseases such as persistent bovine viral diarrhea virus infection, the exposure must have occurred during a specific period in the animal's life. The **induction** or **incubation period** is the time required from exposure to a specific risk factor until initiation of the disease. These periods are usually distributed in somewhat of a normal or bell-shaped curve that is determined by infectious dose and host susceptibility. Generally, the longer the induction period, the more difficult the assessment of risk factor exposure and disease and, thus, the more difficult the evaluation of cause and effect. The **latent period** is the time between biologic onset of the disease process and disease detection (clinical disease: appearance of clinical signs; subclinical disease: positive diagnostic tests). Potential risk factors that acted on a case in less than the necessary induction and latent periods for their action cannot be components of the cause and effect.

The cause of cause and effect is the presence of a combination of risk factors that alone or in combination and in the correct sequence and timing during the animal's life inevitably result in the effect (such as clinical disease or low production) occurring in that individual. A **necessary cause** [3] is a specific risk factor that must have been or must be present at the appropriate time in the causal model for the effect to occur, such as a specific infectious agent that is the etiologic agent in a particular infectious disease. **Sufficient cause** [3] is that set of risk factors in the causal model whose confluence in an animal's life, with appropriate timing, inevitably results in the effect. Note that if the effect of concern is an infectious clinical disease, many infectious agents are necessary causes but not, by themselves, sufficient causes for the clinical disease for which they are the etiologic agent. **Competing risks** are other sets of risk factors that can cause the condition of concern (such as death or low production) that coexist with the set of factors of interest. These risks are things that cause "red herring" cases at a constant, background rate in the group of animals being worked up for a particular problem.

A **causal model** is the scheme of what happened from the start of the problem to the effect in sufficient detail that potential intervention points are identified as the basis of an effective plan for controlling or preventing the problem. J.P. Box is alleged to have said that all models are wrong; some are just more useful than others. A **causal web**, sometimes called a causal pathway or a path model, contains the specific links that connect each individual risk factor (acting across time or together) and result in the effect in an individual animal or group. The first level of factors are those that act directly on the affected animal, the second level of factors are those that act through one or more first-level factors, the third level of factors act on second-level factors, and so on. The goal is to develop this web in sufficient detail so that risk factors that are the best key determinants are identified. A sketch of the model is often useful in explaining to producers why the problem occurred, how the components are linked, and how to control or prevent it in the future. These models are often unique, with different sets of risk factors for animals in different groups, sometimes even on the same premises. A given disease can be caused by more than one set of sufficient causes and, thus, result from different causal pathways in animals contracting the disease in different management situations. What is effective in one situation is often not effective in another because of farm-specific differences and the basic differences in the component risk factors and their linkages (eg, bronchopneumonia in a barn-housed dairy calf versus a hutch-housed dairy calf versus a feedlot calf; Figs. 1 and 2). Although infectious agents may be necessary causes, for the purposes of prevention, very few cause disease by themselves (ie, are a sufficient cause by themselves) and operate more as opportunists, exploiting weaknesses in livestock management systems. Even for agents that, from a pathology perspective, are a sufficient cause by themselves, the causal web includes the risk factors for introduction into a herd and for continued transmission within the herd after the agent is present.

Evidence is information that tends to support or refute that a cause-and-effect situation exits. Depending on how it was obtained, evidence varies greatly in strength. **Empiric evidence** includes the facts of the situation that are obtained by examining, measuring, or counting rather than by reasoning or from impressions or feelings. The strongest empiric evidence is that obtained from a properly designed and executed experiment, such as a randomized, blinded, controlled clinical trial. The weakest empiric evidence is that obtained from a single case, such as a single necropsy in the

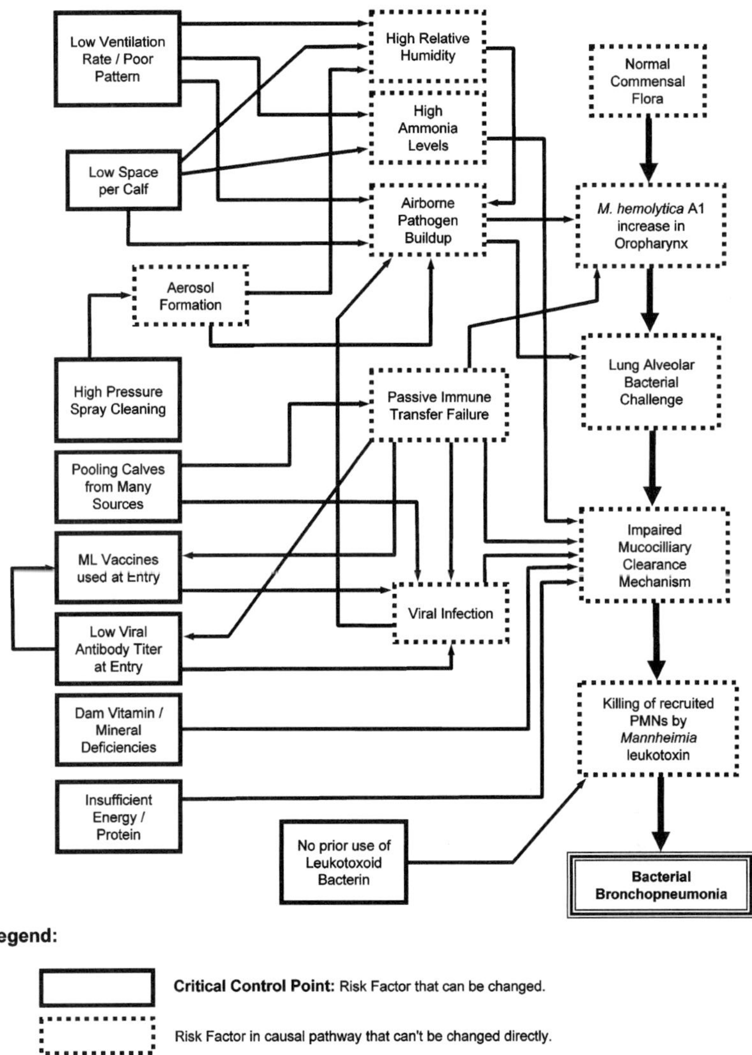

Fig 1. Example of a causal web of risk factors for housed-calf bronchopneumonia.

midst of an outbreak. Empiric evidence for a cause and effect relationship is weakened by the opportunity for other explanations to account for the findings. For example, the necropsied animal may have been one of the sporadic deaths that are at a low but continuous risk of occurrence in groups of animals. For this reason, observational evidence (ie, "an experiment of nature") is inherently weaker than experimental evidence (eg, a randomized, blinded, controlled clinical trial). Stronger observational evidence is obtained from counts, records, or direct observation than from recall, from prospective cohort studies, or from retrospective case-control studies.

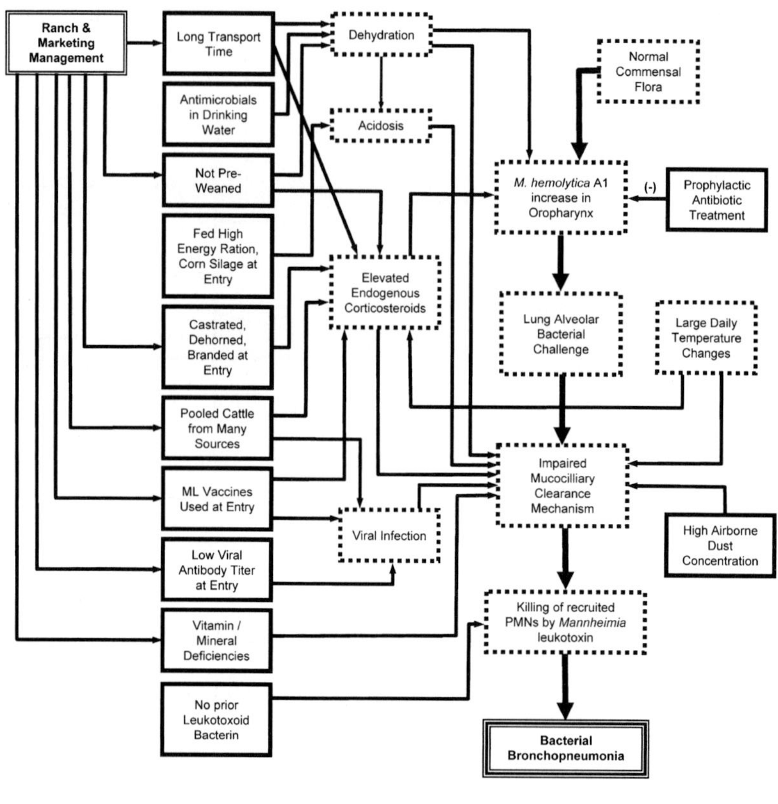

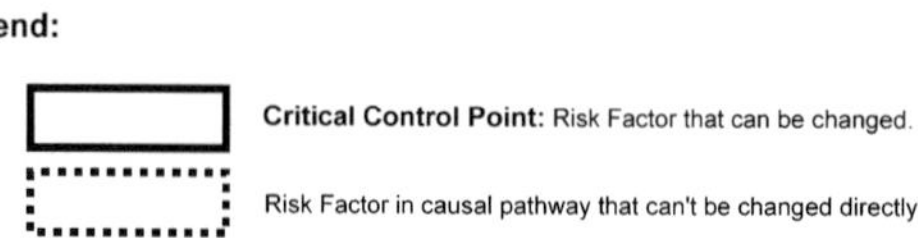

Fig 2. Example of a causal web of risk factors for feedlot-calf bronchopneumonia.

Analogic evidence is the evidence for a cause and effect relationship that is based on reasoning by analogy, which is concluding (from comparing known similarities between two systems) that a relationship shown to exist in one system but unknown in the other system also likely exists in the other. For example, if drug "X" has been shown to be effective against disease "Y" in a species "Z," then perhaps the same relationship exists with a similar drug or a similar disease or a similar species, the other two components of the analogy being identical. Evidence based on analogic reasoning is common in veterinary medicine because it provides a basis for action when the sounder, empiric evidence is lacking. With the broad range of species served by the profession, the many breeds often existing within a species, and the relatively scarce resources for veterinary research, the practice of veterinary medicine is often based on analogic evidence. An example is using a drug in a minor species based on what is known about the pharmacology of that drug in a somewhat similar major species. Analogic evidence is inherently weaker than empiric evidence because of the likelihood that different, unknown factors are operating in the two systems, weakening or invalidating the analogy. Because analogic reasoning yields an inherently weaker form of evidence than empiric evidence, it is likely to be the source of much unexamined dogma and, when possible, better used as a basis for generating hypotheses that can be empirically evaluated.

The weakest form of evidence is **anecdotal evidence**, which is the evidence from a single event such as the medical recovery of a single case or the necropsy of a single animal in an affected group. The probability of apparently unusual events is often considerably higher than is intuitively expected, and other unrecognized factors (confounders) may have invalidated the initial prediction of disease course, thus making the event not that unusual. For example, that a group of only 23 people is required to have a 50% or better chance that two or more of the group have the same birthday is counterintuitive yet easily shown with probability calculations.

Dogma are unexamined beliefs, which can be right or wrong, that are held as established or put forth as an authoritative or expert opinion but that have little or no supportive empiric evidence. An example is the long-held belief that routine intrauterine infusion of antibiotics during prebreeding examinations improved reproductive performance in dairy cows. This practice made biologic sense but was not supported by empiric evidence from subsequent field studies. Medical dogma is usually derived from unevaluated biologic hypotheses and uncritical observation or experience without recognition of the effects of chance, the complexity of biologic systems, natural biologic variation, and observer bias. It is unfortunate that a significant portion of the veterinary medical knowledge base likely falls into this category. Repetition across sources or the number of people (whatever their qualifications and experience) who hold this belief does not change the status of such information until it has been properly examined in light of sufficient strong empiric evidence obtained from sound studies. Because of time and resource limitations, much information conveyed in instructional settings (before and after attaining a doctorate of veterinary medicine degree) is presented in the form of dogma without the associated information necessary to judge its credibility or strength of evidence. The elimination of dogma is the primary goal of the evidence-based medicine paradigm that emerged in human medicine during the last decade.

The **scientific method**, which is a process for obtaining and assessing empiric evidence, provides a sound logical scheme for considering the evidence for a cause and effect relationship. It has evolved as the strongest procedure, given the inescapable limitations of human observation ability and cognitive function, for developing a valid understanding of nature. The basis of the scientific method logic is the **hypotheticodeductive model**. This model comprises (1) the logical deduction of a prediction, (2) the collection of the evidence to examine this prediction by an experiment such as a randomized controlled trial or by observation such as a case-control or cohort study, (3) the analysis of this empiric evidence, and (4) the logical induction that the cause and effect relationship is supported or not supported. **Deduction** is reasoning from the general to the specific situation; **induction** is reasoning from the results of the specific circumstance to conclusions about the general situation. A **hypothesis** is a provisional conjecture that further evidence will support or refute. In this sense, a list of differential diagnoses represents a set of hypotheses that guides the process for determining what additional evidence must be obtained in the diagnostic process and for evaluating that evidence (ruling in or ruling out diagnoses) before a level of certainty sufficient for action is reached. Having a list of specific differentials (hypotheses) guides the clinician in selecting laboratory tests (empiric evidence of varying strength) that will be useful in ruling in or ruling out a differential (further directed investigation). When the risk and cost of treatment is sufficiently low and the differential is sufficiently likely, treatment response is often used as empiric evidence. Similarly, a set of working hypotheses about a herd problem guides the clinician in deciding what herd record data to gather, what animals to examine, what farm procedures to watch, who to interview about management practices and recent events, and so on. A logical problem is that although the facts derived from the test of a hypothesis are correct, the broader underlying theory from which the hypothesis was derived can still be wrong (eg, the laboratory value can be abnormal for reasons other than a problem on the list of differentials).

Hypotheses are most useful if set up as a testable "if…is the cause of…then" statement. The proposed cause and the effect are contained in the "if" component, and the predicted outcome of an evaluation of this hypothesis, such the experimental manipulation of one of those variables or the observation of a natural experiment, is contained in the "then" component. Performing the test (experiment or observation) leads to a logical conclusion that supports or refutes the proposed relationship. For example, if transition pen crowding is the cause of the increased risk of displaced abomasums, then the risk of displaced abomasums should be higher in the weekly calving cohorts with more cows than in the cohorts with fewer cows. This hypothesis could be evaluated visually by creating a graph that contains a smoothed plot of displaced abomasum risk in the weekly calving cohorts and a smoothed plot of number of cows calving by week over a weekly timeline. If the peaks and valleys of the risk plot correlate with the peaks and valleys of the density plot, then it is time to talk to the manager. Establishing these "tests" often involves considerable creativity in identifying on-farm information resources and in execution. The better the "test," the stronger the evidence in supporting or refuting the relationship.

Hypotheses are often confused with theories. In nonscientific contexts, the word "theory" is often used to mean a mere hypothesis or speculation—a much less reliable proposition than is a scientific theory (eg, "I have a theory that it is going to rain today"). A scientific **theory** is the coherent, inter-related structure of scientific propositions and principles derived over time from empiric scientific evidence that explains a class of observed phenomena or facts. Theories enable us to make sense of what we see in nature and to make predictions. For example, a clinician may hypothesize that a down cow has hypocalcemia, but the clinician's treatment of the case and recommendations for prevention in the herd are based on the physiologic theories of calcium regulation in the bovine. A scientific theory must have predictive power (ie, predict phenomena that are observable) and must be testable and falsifiable (ie, the theory is falsified if the predicted phenomena are not observed in the appropriate experiments).

Propositions that are not testable by appropriate scientific research are not theories. Theories are not absolute truth, cannot be verified as such, and are always subject to change due to advancing knowledge and research technology. For example, the physiologic theory about calcium regulation in the bovine has changed over the past several decades as the result of continuing scientific research and, consequently, testing and prevention methods have changed accordingly. Thus, any claim of scientific truth or scientific proof can be immediately disregarded. Any theory that can be tested only by select, unique methods or by certain individuals (usually the promoter of the theory) is highly suspect. A scientific theory must be consistent internally and consistent with broader, more fundamental theories related to other aspects of the phenomenon. For example, a theory of disease physiology cannot be inconsistent with most of the more fundamental and considerably stronger theories of chemistry. It is unfortunate that many of the theories supporting alternative medical practices fail this test. An erroneous underlying theory, however, does not necessarily invalidate a particular treatment because the treatment may represent doing the right thing but for the wrong reason. In these circumstances, empiric evidence derived from the proper application of the scientific method is the only valid basis for evaluating the efficacy of such treatments, and reasoning from the theory should serve only as a source of hypotheses for testing. Depending on relative qualities and amounts of empiric evidence, competing theories explaining the same phenomenon usually differ widely in strength and consistency from more fundamental theories that have broader support. Similar findings replicated by different observers using different but appropriate experimental or observational methods at different locations are regarded as stronger support than is replication by the same investigators or by using identical methods. Although in the end, everything is linked in some way to everything else, the "granularity" or level of detail (eg, atomic, molecular, tissue, organ, body) necessary in a theory depends on the purpose for which it is being used as the basis for prediction.

An **association** exists between two phenomena if a change in one corresponds to a change in the other. An association must be present for a cause and effect relationship to exist, but the presence of an association alone does not prove that the relationship is causal. A positive association or direct relationship exists if the magnitudes of both variables move up or down together. When the correlation coefficient is positive and when the relationship is causal, higher levels of or greater exposure to the risk factor may cause more of the outcome (a dose-response effect). For example, the number of high-string clinical coliform mastitis cases increases when the number of coliforms in the organic bedding is higher. A negative association or inverse relationship exists when the magnitude of one variable moves in the opposite direction of the associated variable. When the correlation coefficient is negative and when the relationship is causal, higher levels of the risk factor are protective. For example, the number of early postpartum metritis cases declines with higher levels of vitamin E in the prepartum ration.

The strength of the association between a risk factor and the outcome in a cause and effect relationship is measured several ways, including the correlation coefficient, relative risk (RR), odds ratio (OR), and logistic regression coefficients. The RR is how much more likely the disease will occur in animals with exposure to the risk factor than in animals without exposure (the risk of disease in the exposed group divided by the risk of disease in the unexposed groups). OR equals the risk of exposure to a risk factor in cases divided by the risk of exposure to a risk factor in controls.

For RR and OR, a value of 1 or close to 1 indicates that a biologically significant cause and effect relationship is not present. The threshold for biologic significance (how close to 1 is important) depends on the relative costs of cases and of prevention. A value larger than 1 is a positive association; a value less than 1 is a negative (protective) association. In scientific studies, the 95% confidence intervals for measures that include 1 are interpreted as meaning that no cause and effect relationship is present for that risk factor in the studies that had sufficient power to detect clinically significant differences. As noted in the statistics article found elsewhere in this issue, in these situations, the χ^2 p-value is larger than 0.05. If, however, a negative study (eg, statistically insignificant findings) had insufficient power to detect the minimum clinically, biologically, or economically significant difference, then the only valid conclusion is that the study should have been larger. In diagnostic work-ups on herds, the width of the 95% confidence intervals is better used to indicate the precision or "stability" of the estimate rather than as a measure of statistical significance. When the estimate is too imprecise (the confidence interval is too wide) for comfort, more sampling and testing is likely in order.

An example of how to calculate an OR from a two-by-two table is provided in the statistics article found elsewhere in this issue. Many on-line calculators are also available for these measures and can be found using Web search engines to search for terms such as "odds ratio calculator." To check that these on-line calculators are programmed and being used correctly, one should enter the numbers from a trusted, worked example and compare the answers. Entering different counts into these calculators, such as doubling the number of controls sampled while keeping the proportion constant, provides an intuitive understanding of how changes in sampling strategies changes the precision of the result.

Although the OR is only an approximation of RR and is a better approximation of RR when the disease is rare than when it is common, as noted in the statistics article found elsewhere in this issue, the OR is often the only valid measure of risk. For example, the OR is the only valid risk measure for a case-control study. A general rule is that the OR overestimates the true underlying RR, being further from 1 than the RR and the OR confidence interval being wider than the RR confidence interval when the RR is valid. When the disease is common, the OR overestimation can be an order of magnitude. Although RR is the preferred measure, it is only valid when all the animals in an exposure group have an equal probability of being included in the calculation (eg, when an entire calving cohort is followed through the risk and disease expression periods with few losses to follow-up, when an entire herd is randomly sampled for testing irrespective of case status, or less commonly, when animals are selected for study on the basis of exposure status). RR estimates are valid only when disease incidence estimates are also valid, such as in cohort studies. In situations in which controls are matched to cases, such as one control for each case, or when cases and controls are selected separately, only the OR is valid. When controls are matched to cases, matching more than three controls per case does not add much additional information on risk relative to the expense. All of these measures are potentially biased by the loss of animals to follow-up when the risk of loss is associated with disease status or exposure status and by misclassification of case or exposure status.

Logical basis for causal reasoning

Ceteris paribus—*holding everything else constant*

The reasoning required for determining cause and effect is often not simple or straightforward. The logical principles for establishing cause and effect relationships have been tempered over the centuries as people struggled to develop sound methods for transforming observations from nature and medicine into reliable, repeatable understandings of cause and effect; namely, to make useful decisions about treatment and prevention. One of the first long-lasting principles to emerge is that of Ockam's Razor (William of Ockam, 1285–1349), which is the principle of parsimony, simplicity, or economy. It states that when two causal models explain a phenomenon equally, the simpler model that requires fewer assumptions and explanatory principles is more likely to be true. Francis Bacon (1561–1626) was the first to develop the methods of inductive reasoning from empiric findings as the basis for developing sound scientific knowledge. His work became the foundation of the modern scientific method.

In the System of Logic, John Stuart Mill (1806–1873) distilled Bacon's methods into several principles of experimental inquiry that provide a logical basis for generating and evaluating hypotheses about cause and effect relationships. The **method of agreement** is that if a risk factor is common to multiple instances of the effect when other factors are dissimilar, then that factor may be a cause. For example, if the same type of feed from the same feed mill is associated with the appearance of the same problem on multiple farms, then that feed is a good candidate to be the cause. The **method of difference** is that if the risk of disease is different when one risk factor is different but other factors are similar, then that risk factor may be a cause. For example, if diarrhea is occurring in pens of horses being fed sweet mix from one bin but not in pens of horses being fed sweet mix from other bins, then the sweet mix in the one bin is a good candidate to be the cause. The **method of concomitant variations**, or simultaneous changes, is that if the risk of disease changes with changes in the level of a risk factor and other factors are more constant, then that risk factor may be a cause. For example, on a dairy where dry cows are kept on a premise separate from the lactating herd, if the risk of displaced abomasum is higher in cows calving a shorter time after being hauled from the dry-cow herd than in cows calving a longer time after being hauled, then hauling is a good candidate to be a cause.

Developed from Mill's methods, the Henle-Koch Postulates (1877) are four sequential criteria for assessing a cause (particular infectious agent) and effect (particular disease) relationship that are familiar to veterinarians. The criteria that must be met before the relationship is accepted as causal are

1. The microorganism must be found in all cases of the disease.
2. It must be isolated from the host and grown in pure culture.
3. It must reproduce the original disease when introduced into a susceptible host.
4. It must be found in the experimental host so infected.

The logical power of these postulates rapidly advanced the germ theory of disease over competing theories of disease cause at the time, such as humors and miasma. Because these criteria focus exclusively on the infectious agent, these postulates are insufficient for identifying the nonagent key determinants involved in infectious or noninfectious diseases or for distinguishing circumstances resulting in subclinical infection from those resulting in clinical disease. Fulfilling the postulates experimentally can be surprisingly difficult, even when the infectious process is well understood and the agent is regarded as a pathogen. Because of these limitations, the Henle-Koch Postulates were superseded by the Hill-Evans Postulates as more generally useful for establishing causality under broader circumstances.

The Hill-Evans Postulates are a set of 9 or 10 criteria, depending on one's interpretation of the original papers, for establishing cause-and-effect relationships. Fulfilling the entire set constitutes very strong evidence for causality but, unlike the Henle-Koch Postulates, the failure to fulfill one or more particular criteria may not significantly weaken evidence for causality. Strong negative evidence for certain criteria, however, logically refutes causality, whereas other criteria provide only weak evidence for cause when fulfilled. Hill [4] proposed the following criteria (Box 1) to evaluate cause and effect relationships for noninfectious diseases, particularly the relationship between smoking and lung cancer.

Based on Hill's [4] criteria, Evan's Postulates [5] provide a direct basis for developing testable hypotheses by constructing comparisons (Box 1).

Creating and evaluating formal hypotheses using these principles provides a powerful basis for establishing cause to the level of certainty needed for action. The unique strength of evaluating cause and effect relationships in herds is that affected animals (clinical and subclinical) can be compared with unaffected animals in a cross-section (at one point in time) and over time to determine the differences and similarities between the animals themselves and the factors affecting them. An expert in systems analysis stated, "Starting with the behavior of the system directs one's thoughts to dynamic, not static analysis—not only to 'what's wrong?' but also to 'how did we get there?' … And finally, starting with history discourages the common and distracting tendency we all have to define a problem not by the system's actual behavior, but by the lack of our favorite solution" [6]. For example, many calf scour agents are ubiquitous and, often, sampling scouring calves only confirms this ubiquity. The critical question is, Why are these individuals on this farm having a problem with this agent when many others are not, even though the infection is most likely present there as well?

Failure to recognize the cause and effect time frame inherent in the type of problem can lead to errors. The three general types of problems are acute, additive or cyclic, and chronic. **Acute problems** are precipitated by a temporally associated management or husbandry error of sufficient magnitude to be the primary cause of the problem. **Additive** or **cyclic problems** are precipitated by a combination of management or husbandry errors over time and the effects of cyclic factors such as season or production cycle stages such that the combination is sufficient to precipitate the problem (eg, the summer coliform mastitis outbreak that is associated with the previous winter change to sawdust bedding). **Chronic problems** are precipitated by the long-term action of management or husbandry errors that require the passage of time before the consequences become of sufficient magnitude to be recognized, such as the slow spread of a contagious mastitis agent or of *Mycobacterium paratuberculosis* (eg, the recognition of a slowly spreading *Staphylococcus aureus* mastitis problem associated with the adoption of a less efficacious teat dipping procedure more than a year previously). For additive, cyclic, or chronic problems, the initial occurrence of the underlying

Box 1. Hill's criteria for causation (1965)

1. Strength of association: the larger the relative effect, the more likely the causal role of the factor. At minimum, a biologically significant association must be present for a cause and effect relationship to be present.
2. Consistency: if similar associations are found in different studies in different populations, then the more likely the causal role of the factor.
3. Specificity: if the effect does not result from other causes, then the more likely the factor is causal.
4. Temporality: risk factor exposure (the cause) must precede the effect. Solid evidence that the effect preceded the exposure to the risk factor indicates, at least, that other risk factors are also causal or, at most, that this factor is not.
5. Dose-response (biologic gradient): if the risk increases with increasing dose of or exposure to the risk factor, then the more likely that a cause and effect relationship exists.
6. Biologic plausibility: given current knowledge, the mechanism is biologically plausible, in that it is consistent with and does not contravene well-established theory.
7. Coherence: associations between the risk factor and the effect are consistent with existing knowledge and do not conflict with the generally known facts of the natural history and biology of the disease.
8. Intervention (experiment): reduction or removal of the risk factor reduces the risk of the effect (the strongest evidence of a cause and effect relationship).
9. Analogy: that a similar but not identical cause and effect relationship has been observed and established elsewhere as causal provides weak evidence for causality.

Evan's Postulates (1976)

1. Prevalence of the disease should be significantly higher in those exposed to the risk factor than in those not exposed.
2. Exposure to the risk factor should be more frequent among those with the disease than among those without.
3. In prospective studies, the incidence of the disease should be higher in those exposed to the risk factor than in those not exposed.
4. The disease should follow exposure to the risk factor with a normal or log-normal distribution of incubation periods.
5. A spectrum of host responses along a logical biologic gradient from mild to severe should follow exposure to the risk factor.

6. A measurable host response should follow exposure to the risk factor in those lacking this response before exposure or should increase in those with this response before exposure. This response should be infrequent in those not exposed to the risk factor.
7. In experiments, the disease should occur more frequently in those exposed to the risk factor than in control subjects not exposed.
8. Reduction or elimination of the risk factor should reduce the risk of the disease.
9. Modifying or preventing the host response should decrease or eliminate the disease.
10. All findings should make biologic and epidemiologic sense.

management or husbandry deficiency is usually not close in time to the recognition of the problem. In many cases, because of the lag between a management change and recognition of the problem, the manager is reluctant to acknowledge that a change precipitated the problem.

Subjective perceptions of employees and managers are valuable sources of hypotheses about risk factors; the clinician's task is to support or refute these and other hypotheses using objective empiric evidence. Unless based on objective evidence (eg, analysis of records), employee and manager perception of the problem may be correct but, more often than not, it is off the mark. The clinician can compare the actual number of cases to the expected number to determine whether the frequency is excessive. The clinician should be very careful of "dangling numerators"; that is, counting the number of cases without considering the number of animals actually at risk of becoming a case during that time period. A large increase or decrease in the number of animals susceptible to a condition causes a corresponding change in the number of cases of that condition, even though the underlying risk remains constant. Because of seasonal effects, few herds maintain a constant number of animals passing through the period of susceptibility year-round. Changes in individual animal performance must be distinguished from changes in total output that are due to changes in the numbers of producing animals.

The strength of herd-focused investigation compared with individual-focused investigation is the opportunity to compare affected animals to unaffected animals. What are the characteristics of affected versus unaffected animals in terms of exposure to potential risk factors, age, production level, stage of production cycle, and source? As noted earlier, because of the spectrum of disease, the clinician must be careful when classifying animals into affected and unaffected groups. Another common error is to overlook the culled or dead animals in the cohort of susceptible animals that entered the risk period because their records were deleted from those of the remaining animals. Where were the affected versus unaffected animals located during the potential exposure period? Because different groups or pens of animals often have different levels of exposures (eg, different amounts of feed ingredients, different water sources, different housing, different pasture, different origins, different stages of the production cycle) and because a dose-response relationship exists for many etiologic agents, this set of clues is important.

Gathering and analyzing objective data on a herd problem is an examination process that is analogous to using laboratory tests or imaging procedures in the diagnosis in an individual animal. These objective data support or refute clinical impressions of the herd problem much like testing or imaging supports or refutes clinical impressions of the clinical case. The clinician should concentrate on the data that will support or refute hypotheses (differential diagnoses). Computer spreadsheets provide a convenient means to enter, validate, and manipulate the relevant individual and group information. If accessing herd data through a production accounting system, the clinician first evaluates the data for quality by verifying that known, relevant events identified by means other than the records system are present and correct in the records. Outliers and logical inconsistencies in the data are detected by sorting variables into numeric order and looking at the minimums and maximums. Plots of production data with variable smoothing over time are easy to create, allowing trends to be discerned amid the noise of random variation. From count data of the numbers of affected and the numbers of susceptible animals, case morbidity and fatality rates by exposure and RRs can be calculated. For endemic problems, risk over time by cohort group can be plotted. The clinician can construct cohorts of at-risk animals passing through a critical point in the production cycle associated with the problem (eg, calving, weaning) over a time interval (eg, day, week, month) that on average, have enough animals (30 or so) to reduce the effects of natural variation but do not obscure trends over time, with wider intervals being needed for smaller herds. The effects of other factors that vary over time (eg, calving pen density, average of weekly high temperature, sources of animals) on risk of occurrence or production can be examined. Detailed weather data from nearby automated weather stations can be downloaded from on-line government sources into a spreadsheet. If the herd does not have a good production accounting system for animal performance information, then the clinician should not overlook clues found in indirect sources of similar information. For example, the delivery dates and weights on feed invoices can provide approximate information on feed batch disappearance and, thus, approximate information on consumption patterns. On this basis, expected disappearance of feeds can be compared with actual disappearance. Invoices from rendering services may provide information on dates of animal deaths if they have not been recorded. Often, events such as calvings and breedings are written on calendars or in pocket books.

Establishing and executing good tests of hypotheses require a large amount of ingenuity. Based on the previous hypotheses, the clinician can predict what should be found in other animals, such as diagnostic test results or production effects, and can evaluate these predictions. As noted earlier, predictions of the form "if this cause is present, then this finding should be present" can be made. Because many causes have multiple effects, finding more of these multiple effects provides stronger support for the presence of the cause than finding only one. Often, a single effect can result from several different causes. Finding what is predicted supports a hypothesis; not finding what is predicted weakens a hypothesis. The key is figuring out what predictions will provide good tests and are "doable." Just as in individual animal work-ups, "scattershot" sampling and testing should be avoided because doing so without an objective in mind is seldom useful and is expensive monetarily for the client and expensive in credibility and time for the clinician. Ockam's Razor should be applied by asking, What is the simplest set of explanations that covers the most findings?

The following are example predictions:

If this infectious agent is being transmitted between animals in this manner, then these other animals are at risk and some will be infected, whereas these others are not at risk and will not be infected.

If overcrowding in the fresh pen (risk factor) is causing displaced abomasums (disease), then the pattern in the associated data that can be expected is a higher proportion of cows experiencing displaced abomasums in the cohorts with more crowding in the fresh pen compared with cohorts with less crowding.

Common causal reasoning errors

When determining cause and effect, veterinarians and their clients are subject to lapses and biases in reasoning and memory recall that can lead the process astray. The following are several important concepts in considering these errors.

Belief is the mental act or state of mind of an individual after he or she accepts and internalizes an external concept or idea, which then becomes part of subsequent thought processes. Internalized deeply, belief becomes part of intuition, particularly for the expert performing conscious and unconscious pattern recognition. Belief can occur after deliberate, systematic, critical thinking or can occur with immediate, nonreasoned, uncritical acceptance. The problem is that after an erroneous belief is established, accepting a more correct belief becomes considerably more difficult than if no previous belief was held. The nature of human thinking is (1) to give more weight to the information that is consistent with the currently held belief and to ignore or discount discordant information, (2) to have better recall of or to give more weight to the unusual or the more recent than the common or the more distant, and (3) to limit the search for additional information to that which has the potential of confirming rather than potentially refuting a belief (eg, selective necropsy to confirm a gross diagnosis). Prior belief biases subjective observation (such as occurs during the diagnostic process or during nonblinded measurement) because it subtly and unconsciously changes perception, particularly of vague or ambiguous characteristics. This bias occurs unbeknownst to the observer despite his or her best intentions and is the reason for many of the aspects of epidemiologic study design and execution such as blinding and randomization. By nature, humans tend to develop explanations from limited, incomplete information, whether in social relationships, from observations of the workings of nature, or when operating in a professional capacity as a veterinarian, often without considering the weaknesses in the information or the assumptions being made.

Bias (systematic error) is any effect at any stage of a process (thinking, observing) or study that produces results or conclusions that differ systematically from the truth. Bias can be reduced by critical thinking and proper study design and execution but not by increasing sample size (which only increases precision by reducing the opportunity for random chance deviation from the truth). The critical question is how likely the results are due to the presence of a large bias rather than the true state of nature, thus making the conclusions invalid. Observational study designs are inherently more susceptible to bias than experimental study designs, but well- designed and executed observational studies can provide more solid evidence than poorly designed and executed experimental studies.

Cognitive bias is the distortion of an individual's perception of his or her world that is due to common observational and reasoning errors. The study of cognitive bias is a relatively young but active area of research in psychology and cognitive science (the study of mind and intelligence). The findings have been applied to behavioral economics and to business and political decision making for 3 decades but only recently to medical decision making. Essentially, the scientific method is a process developed to minimize the effects of cognitive bias on the development of scientific knowledge.

Critical thinking is the disciplined ability and willingness to assess evidence and claims, to seek a breadth of contradicting and confirming information, to make objective judgments on the basis of well-supported reasons as a guide to belief and action, and to monitor one's thinking while doing so (metacognition). The thinking process that is appropriate for critical thinking depends on the knowledge domain (eg, scientific, mathematic, historical, anthropologic, economic, philosophical, moral), but the universal criteria are clarity, accuracy, precision, consistency, relevance, sound empiric evidence, good reasons, depth, breadth, and fairness. One of the more entertaining texts on critical thinking is that of Shick and Vaughn [7].

Some 80 different cognitive biases have been identified, several of which are subtle variations on a theme rather than distinct entities and some of which are opposites. Awareness of these potential errors may reduce their impact. The major cognitive biases that apply to medical diagnostic decision making, selected and modified from Croskerry [8,9], are listed in alphabetical order in Box 2.

The clinician must be careful to detect situations in which the manager has reasoned from a primary problem to what he or she believes is the cause and then presents that conclusion as the primary complaint rather than the original problem. For example, a manager presented a complaint of poor barn ventilation after reasoning that the serious drop in milk production was caused by adult cow pneumonias and further that these pneumonias were caused by poor barn ventilation [10]. In this case, the actual cause of the production loss was the 22% underfeeding of grain due to a miscalibrated scale on a grain auger.

A serious and common error is to jump to generating hypotheses without first developing the quantitative information (the who, when, where counts) beyond vague clinical impressions (eg, these animals seem to be affected more than those) to support or refute a specific hypothesis. This approach is analogous to scattershot ordering of laboratory tests in diagnosing individual animal cases, hoping something will pop up rather than using the laboratory tests to rule in or out specific differentials, and will likely be as unrewarding. After the clinician has communicated a leading hypothesis about cause to a producer, it is difficult for both parties to return later to a more open frame of mind.

The clinician should be careful of "pseudoepidemics" caused by the onset of producer awareness of a more chronic problem or caused by a change in problem definition. For example, changing from detection of fetal loss by visual detection of a conceptus to detection of open cows by repeat palpation post early pregnancy diagnosis will cause a pseudoepidemic of fetal loss in virtually any dairy herd. In one case, a dairy producer invested almost $1,000 in laboratory fees in attempting to establish the etiologic cause of such a pseudoepidemic. The operation had recently switched to a dairy herd records program that classified any cow returning to heat after a positive pregnancy examination as an abortion in addition to those with visible signs of late gestation fetal losses.

The clinician should be aware of what the producer accepts as "normal" (endemic) occurrence. In one high-producing herd, the producer believed that third- or higher parity Holsteins going down with milk fever was a normal occurrence. Thus, he accepted most of his older cows going down with milk fever and did not recognize this situation as abnormal and warranting correction. The producer's veterinarian and nutritionist were not aware of the high incidence of milk fever on the farm. The clinician should be aware of the events that the producer is omitting because of assuming they are not related to the problem of concern. For example, a recent episode of late-term abortions that is not mentioned may be related to the more prevalent metritis problem that is being investigated. One should remember the old

Box 2. Cognitive biases that apply to medical diagnostic decision making

- Aggregate bias (ecologic fallacy, fallacy of composition): the tendency to substitute what is known to be happening in the relationship between group averages of two variables for what is unknown about these two variables at the individual animal level or vice versa. Group aggregate data (eg, bulk tank ship weights, milk composition, pen intakes) is often more readily available than individual data (eg, individual daily milk weights, individual milk composition, individual intakes).
- Anchoring bias ("jumping to conclusions"): the tendency to fixate on limited information too early in the diagnostic process.
- Ascertainment bias: the tendency to allow prior expectations to shape thinking and observation of information, particularly of subtle, vague clues.
- Association as causation fallacy (post hoc, ergo propter hoc fallacy): incorrectly assuming that one event caused another simply because the former was associated with and preceded the latter in a previous occurrence. Many superstitions such as having a lucky token for success in a sporting event are based on this fallacy.
- Availability bias: the tendency to judge things as more likely if they readily come to mind, which tend to be the more recent, the more prevalent, the more striking, or the more readily available.
- Confirmation bias: the strong tendency to look for further confirming evidence to support a weak diagnosis or hypothesis rather than looking for refuting evidence, which is logically more definitive. It is more powerful to ask, What would disprove this hypothesis if found? than to ask, What else would support this hypothesis if found?
- Diagnostic momentum bias: a weak diagnosis may gain momentum without gaining verification, particularly if it is communicated to others without the associated evidence and it induces cognitive bias into their reasoning and recall.
- Framing bias: biased thinking or memory recall that occurs due to being influenced by how the problem is stated, the question is asked, or the information is presented. For example, the question, When did your cow stop eating? is likely to elicit a different response from the 4-H'er than is the question, How is your cow's appetite?

- Fundamental attribution bias: the tendency to take excess credit for one's successes and to deflect responsibility for one's failures while attributing to others insufficient credit for their successes and excess responsibility for their failures.
- Hindsight bias: knowing the outcome profoundly alters interpretation of the events before the outcome, leading to underestimation (illusion of failure) or overestimation (illusion of control) of abilities. In hindsight, events appear to have fit together better and to be explained better than they did at the time.
- Multiple alternatives bias (paralysis by analysis, "wallpaper phenomenon"): multiple options (eg, multiple differential diagnoses) multiply the conflict and uncertainty compared with fewer options, leading to paralysis of action and irrational decision making. Instead of comparing all competing options with each other, one should compare each with a common benchmark such as the status quo, starting with the more relevant or the more likely.
- Null feedback bias: failing to regularly obtain feedback, positive or negative, on the outcomes of previous work-ups and recommendations after the passage of time, and instead, concluding (in the absence of evidence) that the outcomes were successful.
- Order bias: information communicated at the beginning and at the end of an exchange is remembered better than the information communicated in the middle. This bias can be avoided by recording information during the communication process rather than relying on recall later.
- Overconfidence bias: the tendency to spend too little time gathering and synthesizing information before taking action because of placing too much faith in one's opinions and hunches. One should ask whether information been gathered in a logical, thorough, and logical fashion and whether this information supports one's opinion.
- Premature closure bias: the tendency to accept a diagnosis before it has been sufficiently verified by tests for adequacy, coherence, parsimony, and falsification.
- Satisfying bias: the tendency to stop searching for further information after something is found. The questions to ask are, Is there anything else to be found? and Did I look in the right places?
- Support bias: the tendency to judge a hypothesis that has more detailed information as being more likely.

- Sunk cost bias: the greater the investment of funds, time, and mental energy in a diagnosis, the greater the reluctance to let it go and consider other alternatives.
- Vertical thinking bias: the failure to think laterally or "outside of the box," which is reduced by asking the question, What else might explain this?

aphorism, "*More mistakes are made from not looking than from not knowing!*"

The clinician should be careful of a red herring. Often the tendency is to necropsy only a few animals; the necropsies are often incomplete (ie, a wide selection of tissues are not submitted from all major organ systems); and the necropsied animals are often not representative, even when large numbers of animals are dying. The mistaken tendency is to select the worst rather than the representative. When taking samples, the clinician should consider the "regret" factor versus current cost of attainment. For example, when working up a reproductive problem in a grazed beef herd, taking and holding blood samples from palpated animals only to discard them later when they are found not to be needed may be less expensive than finding that such samples are needed when new hypotheses emerge, necessitating rounding up and corralling the herd again.

The clinician should be careful of shortcuts. Failure to perform complete gross necropsies and to submit a full set of properly handled and preserved tissue samples from the major organ systems and instead submitting only those samples that would confirm a leading differential diagnosis is a common error. In a continuing problem in one large dairy herd, the underlying problem was believed to be a severe respiratory condition, but laboratory findings on the lung samples from partial necropsies were inconclusive. Complete necropsies performed on several euthanized cases revealed a severe uterine condition subsequent to improper but widely applied postparturient treatment. The potential regret cost of missing a major gross diagnosis or failure to obtain a laboratory diagnosis must be balanced against the marginal cost of a more complete necropsy compared with a partial.

The clinician should be careful of the overlooked. During an investigation of a large dairy herd, one third of the retained heifer calves were documented to be dying due to salmonellosis. The producer, however, did not recognize the magnitude of these losses because the calves were dying one by one and were being removed by the rendering service during their daily visits. Only by comparing the current young stock inventory on the farm with the calving events recorded on a calendar did the producer recognize the magnitude of this loss. In another large dairy, the manager knew that 10% of the cows calving during a 2-week period were clinically affected by a problem. When the records of all of the cows that had calved during this period were reviewed, however, he was surprised to learn that all had been culled from the herd in the intervening period of 2 months. On larger operations, the discrepancies between what the management intends to happen and what employees do, and what or when major changes in procedures occurred as described by employees versus the management are sometimes amazing.

The clinician should remember the iceberg principle (ie, subclinical cases usually outnumber clinical cases several fold and thus represent the greatest loss) and the spectrum of disease (ie, incubating, clinical, and recovered). Overlooking these concepts in searching for clues can lead to comparing clinically affected animals with subclinically affected and recovered animals instead comparing definitely affected animals with definitely unaffected animals. Doing so may lead to erroneous conclusions about the factors involved in the problem, which defeats the strength of herd investigation (ie, comparison between groups of animals over time). More severely affected animals, however, may have experienced higher levels of a common risk factor than lesser or unaffected animals. Even in general herd problems (eg, low milk production), some individuals are affected more severely than others. For example, in a group of pregnant cattle, approximately 10% of all pregnancies diagnosed before 45 days of gestation are lost and approximately 20% of these losses are observed. The analysis and resolution of the problem will be confused by including cases that are due to other problems.

References

[1] Last J. A dictionary of epidemiology. 4th edition. New York: Oxford University Press; 2000.

[2] Thrusfield M. Veterinary epidemiology. 2nd edition. Malden (MA): Blackwell Science; 1995.

[3] Rothman KJ. Causes. Am J Epidemiol 1976;104:587–92.

[4] Hill AB. The environment and disease: association or causation? Proc R Soc Med 1965;58: 295–300.

[5] Evans AS. Causation and disease: the Henle-Koch postulates revisited. Yale J Biol Med 1976;49:175–95.

[6] Meadows DH. Dancing with systems. Whole Earth 2001;106:58–63.

[7] Schick T, Vaughn L. How to think about weird things: critical thinking for a new age. 3rd edition. McGraw-Hill; 2002.

[8] Croskerry P. The importance of cognitive errors in diagnosis and strategies to minimize them. Acad Med 2003;78:775–80.

[9] Croskerry P. Achieving quality in clinical decision making: cognitive strategies and detection of bias. Acad Emerg Med 2002;9:1184–204.

[10] Bradish SK. A practical approach to the diagnosis of a dairy herd problem: a case report. The Bovine Practitioner 1997;31:111–4.

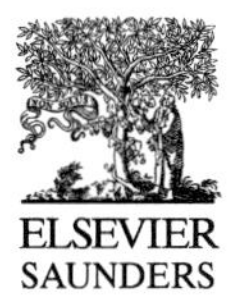

ELSEVIER
SAUNDERS

Vet Clin Food Anim 22 (2006) 149–170

VETERINARY
CLINICS
Food Animal Practice

Hood of the Truck Statistics for Food Animal Practitioners

Barrett D. Slenning, MS, DVM, MPVM

Animal Biosecurity Risk Management Group, Agriculture Disaster Research Institute, Department of Population Health and Pathobiology, College of Veterinary Medicine, Campus Box 8401, North Carolina State University, 4700 Hillsborough Street, Raleigh, NC 27606, USA

Most of us dislike working with numbers. I hate going through my checkbook and bank accounts every month. You probably do, too. If we found some joy in working with arithmetic and columns of numbers, then we probably would have picked careers different from veterinary medicine. In the last few decades, however, our part of the veterinary profession has discovered the power of numbers, which has brought us (sometimes kicking and screaming) to epidemiology and statistics. We often face questions such as

- Is there a true difference in the average weight of grower pigs being fed supplement A versus supplement B?
- A lower percentage of heifers responded to our synchronization program this month. Can we say that this is a real difference on which we should act or a "luck-of-the-draw" thing that we should not get excited about?
- When we purchased this new practice accounting package, we were told we would improve our income per billable hour. Has our income per billable hour gone up?
- Your client thinks that the rate of respiratory disease in her steers is directly related to rainfall. You do not think so, but it is plausible. How do you find out?

Statistics is a discipline whose primary purpose is to help quantify our level of confidence that observed differences are likely due to random events. Business school professors often say "if you can't measure it, you can't manage it." Epidemiology, in general, and statistics, in particular, offer the practitioner a set of tools that allow us to measure, monitor, and make decisions for a variety of events and trends in modern agricultural veterinary practice

E-mail address: barrett_slenning@ncsu.edu

doi:10.1016/j.cvfa.2005.11.002

vetfood.theclinics.com

like those bulleted earlier. This article offers some thoughts and tips on working with statistics and develops four relatively simple procedures to deal with most kinds of data (but not all) with which veterinarians work. The criterion for a procedure to be a "Hood of the Truck Statistics" (HOT Stats) technique is that it must be simple enough to be done with pencil, paper, and a calculator. The goal of HOT Stats is to have the tools available to run quick analyses in only a few minutes so that decisions can be made in a timely fashion. The discipline allows us to move away from the all-too-common guesswork ("that looks about right") about effects and differences we perceive following a change in treatment or management. The techniques allow us to move toward making more defensible, credible, and more quantifiably "risk-aware" real-time recommendations to our clients. Being able to do that is quite a trick.

Basic rules and terminology of all statistical methods

Assumptions of statistical procedures: repeat measures and units of interest

Statistical procedures are basically short-cuts that allow us to distill out important characteristics of a dataset; however, as with any process, they make some assumptions about those datasets and how the data are handled. Much as is the case when we draw blood for a test, the laboratory technician assumes that we did it correctly (correct procedure, correct diluent, correct handling to the laboratory). When we violate the assumption of correct procedure in drawing blood—say, we allow a sample to freeze or get overly hot—we can still get results from the laboratory but will have little confidence in the validity of those results. The same is true for statistics; we must be careful of procedures' underlying assumptions. Overstepping a basic assumption can invalidate a procedure.

In veterinary medicine, we must be especially careful of instances in which repeat measures (ie, using an animal or entity as its own control, which is the case in the third bulleted example question about billable hours) are used or when it is easy to confuse the appropriate unit of interest with another inappropriate factor (ie, whether the cow or the teat is the unit of interest in a mastitis study; whether the steer or the pen is the unit of interest in a feedlot vaccine study).

Repeat measures situations are fairly easy to recognize: if you are measuring the same thing on the same population or group over time, then you are performing repeat measures. Most statistical procedures assume that the sampled observations are independent, but in repeat measures situations, they are not independent (eg, the fastest growing piglets before adding in a new supplement are still likely to be among the faster growing piglets after the supplement is introduced). For that reason, a repeat measures situation will invalidate a number of statistical procedures.

Although it also impacts on independence, the unit of interest is a more complicated thing to figure out. In essence, the unit of interest is the smallest unit to which a treatment could be applied. For instance, in udder health work, environmental conditions act on the entire cow, meaning that it is doubtful you can claim the teat or quarter as the unit of interest (eg, if one teat spends part of the day laying in mud, then it is likely that the other teats also are in mud). In a vaccination study in a feedlot, if two vaccine treatments are allocated by pen over 10 pens of 80 steers each, then the unit of interest is the pen, not the individual steer. That means you will have 10 observations (5 per vaccine treatment), rather than 800 observations (400 per vaccine treatment). An "n" of 10 versus an "n" of 800 makes a huge difference in the resolution and precision of any statistical procedure.

P *values*

We have all seen the term $P \leq 0.05$ used in describing the statistical significance of some finding. But what does that really mean? It indicates that there is a 5% chance that the differences/effects being measured could be due to random variations; that is, there is a 5% probability that the outcome was just a luck-of-the-draw, spurious event. There is no magic about the 0.05 level; it has just become the most typical level of uncertainty with which researchers feel comfortable. As practitioners, however, we must regularly make clinical recommendations and decisions when the uncertainty is well above 5%. Hence, the best level of P is up to you and depends on the situation. A general rule of thumb is if the question at hand is truly life and death (or carries the potential for severe damage) and you already have a good means of working with the situation, a potentially better new procedure should be required to demonstrate very low P values (ie, it is very unlikely that it is better just due to chance) before you consider using it. On the other hand, if the situation is not life or death or your current standard of care is not all that good to begin with, you can probably take a chance on a new procedure, even if the clinical trial's P values that suggest it is the better choice are not very impressive. Do not forget that a P value of 0.2 means you are 80% certain that the effect is real, which is equivalent to 4:1 odds in your favor. Those are pretty good odds in real life.

Confidence intervals

A confidence interval (CI) simply refers to the range of values, at a specified degree of certainty, in which one can expect the underlying true variable to fall. In this view, CIs are really just telling you about the precision of your measurements: the more precise they are, the narrower your CIs will be. We may determine that a 90% CI for average weight gain is 2.1 to 2.5 lb/d. This means we are 90% sure that, given the level of variability in the data, the "true" average lies somewhere within the continuum of the lower limit of 2.1 lb/d and the upper limit of 2.5 lb/d. It is important to realize that no value is more likely than another: 2.4 is just as likely as 2.1, 2.3, 2.5, or any other number in the range. It is human nature to assume that the middle of the range (~2.3 lb/d) is the most likely "true" value, but it is not. Any value within the range is as equally likely as the middle value.

Role of sample size

In general, the larger your sample relative to the overall population, the better precision you will have at any given confidence level and the more likely you will be able to claim that your sample is representative of that population. To take it to extremes, it is intuitive that if you sampled 90 out of 100 milk cows, then you would have more confidence in any statistics generated from that sample than if you had sampled only 9 of the 100. The larger the sample size, in general, the more likely that you will be able to discriminate ever smaller effects of one treatment versus another. The downside, however, is that larger sample sizes are expensive and take time to achieve. Further, if we are looking at historical data or at a report someone else published (Dairy Herd Improvement Association [DHIA] records, Texas Cattle Feeder reports, US Department of Agriculture studies, and so forth), we do not have the option of grabbing larger samples; we must work with what we are given.

Table 1 illustrates the effect that increasing sample size has on the precision of an estimate. The table illustrates how quickly imprecision increases as sample size decreases: the 90% CI for taking 1 animal out of 5 is 20 percentage points wide; the 90% CI for taking 50 animals out of 250 is one half of a percentage point wide. The table also indicates how we quickly strike diminishing returns with larger samples sizes: for many purposes, the precision gained beyond taking 20 samples out of 100 is probably not worth the added effort, time, and cost to get those samples.

Association versus causation

Statistics is an "inferential" discipline: it infers associations or differences, which means that statistical measures, in and of themselves, do not "prove" causality. We may infer causality when we show that bulk tank somatic cell counts rise with daily temperature, but the statistical procedures will only give you information on how likely it is that the association between bulk

Table 1
Effect of sample size on estimation precision

Sample/population	Midpoint estimate (90% CI)
1/5	20% (10.0%–30.0%)
5/25	20% (18.0%–22.0%)
20/100	20% (19.5%–20.5%)
50/250	20% (19.8%–20.3%)
250/1250	20% (20.0%–20.0%)

tank somatic cell counts and daily temperature is due to random chance. It is tempting for us to assume that statistical processes that yield very low P values must be indicative of causality, but that is a false assumption. Remember that P values only measure how likely the difference or relationship being observed is due to chance. Table 2 illustrates how very low P values can have nothing to do with causality. Table 2 shows the biweekly weight of my growing puppy and the price of a gallon of gasoline at my local station over the same period. The Spearman rank correlation test (the fourth statistical method discussed later) suggests that my puppy's body weight explains 94% of the variation in gasoline price and is statistically significant ($P < 0.001$) by anybody's definition of the word "significant."

There is, then, an exceptionally strong and statistically significant association between my puppy's body weight and the price of gasoline over the 5-month period. Nobody would believe, however, that one is causing the other (that if I could get my puppy to lose some weight, the price of gasoline would go down); it just so happens that both values went up over the time period. That consistent movement over time is what gives the two sets of data a strong correlation. This association is what is called a "spurious" association. The article by Gay found elsewhere in this issue addresses issues of causality, so I will not discuss it here. Just remember that statistics only offers us associations; it is up to us and our medical, biologic, economic, and general understanding of the systems in question to determine whether a causal relationship exists.

Statistical versus clinical significance

As stated earlier, statistical significance addresses the likelihood that an effect is due to random chance. Another way to state it is that statistical significance offers us an idea as to how repeatable an outcome might be: the lower the P value, the more repeatable it is; however, it does not say

Table 2
Relationship between a puppy's body weight and the price of gasoline as an example of a statistically significant but spurious association

Wk	Weight (lb)	Gasoline price ($/gal)
0	15	1.77
2	18	1.74
4	19	1.72
6	22	1.81
8	26	1.85
10	32	1.83
12	36	1.83
14	41	1.93
16	46	2.04
18	53	2.13
20	59	2.22

Spearman rank correlation coefficient = 0.94; Student's t value (9 *df*) = 8.34; $P < 0.0001$.

anything about the size of the effect. That is where clinical significance comes into play because it tends to focus on the magnitude of differences or outcomes. Clinical significance, however, says nothing about whether these results are liable to be repeatable.

Hence, each form of significance is near-sighted. For instance, statisticians get excited when they see statements of low *P* values because it suggests that the effects are likely real and repeatable. Clinicians, however, get excited when they see statements such as "twice as likely to return to function" or "three-times the survival rate of controls" because each statement suggests a sizeable magnitude of effect. Both forms of significance are important; however, neither tells us everything we need to know in deciding whether to adopt a new procedure. A method to tie statistically significant results into clinically intuitive measures is described later in the article so that we can get the full story on the different aspects of significance.

Statistical procedures: choice of technique

Type of data determines technique

Which statistical procedure to use and, hence, which outcome to opt for, depends entirely on the type of data with which you are dealing and the kind of question you ask of those data (Table 3). Most (but not all) veterinary data of interest come in the form of means or of counts and frequencies. When the data come to us as means and measures of variation, we usually want to know whether the values for two or more groups differ (Is there a difference in the average weaning weights of two groups of piglets?). When data come to us as counts, frequencies, or percentages, we usually want to know whether the counts that characterize one group differ from

Table 3
Listing of the four Hood of the Truck Statistics techniques by kind of problem and by the type of data required

Kind of problem/question	Data you will need	Hood of the Truck Method
Looking for whether two groups' averages are different	Averages, counts, SDs	*z* test CIs for the difference of two means
Comparing counts, frequencies, and so forth between two groups	Four counts (two groups, two risk factors) based on a risk factor	χ^2 test for contingency tables
Evaluating before/after indices for a group	Number improved, went up, and so forth versus number that did not	Sign test
Looking for whether two variables move together or one is "driving" the other	Two sets of variables to be compared	Spearman rank correlation coefficient

those of another group (Is the proportion of low body condition different between pregnant and nonpregnant animals?) or whether the counts, frequencies, or percentages of a group changed as a result of an intervention (Has the proportion of farm visits achieving a gross income target gone up since instituting our new call sheet?). Finally, whether data come to us as means or counts, we also may ask whether two sets of variables appear to "move" together or whether one variable might "drive" the values of the other variable (For an expanding herd, do the increases in cow numbers appear to explain decreases in average milk production?). Each combination of data and question has its own specialized analytic technique, which is described in the following sections.

When data produce averages and the differences between group averages are of interest

z test confidence interval for the difference between two means

Data in the form of averages are commonly developed in production medicine. In animal agriculture, examples of averages are milk or meat production, growth rates, and days to conception, to name a few. I have observed that most data concerning averages are best evaluated by using a *z* test CI for the difference between two means [1], as shown in Worksheet 1 of Appendix 1.

Worksheet 1 shows two methods to use the technique in generating an answer. The first method determines the level of confidence in which 0.0 would appear in a CI. The second method walks you through creation of the actual CIs. Why show two methods to do the same thing? The first method is a pure HOT Stats procedure: it is quick and simple and offers an answer of known confidence, but it loses out on the information that can be gleaned from calculating the actual confidence intervals, as is done in the second method. Knowing the actual CI width allows you to evaluate the true precision of the method: the wider the CIs for a given level of confidence, the less precise your measures (meaning the more "slop" there is in the underlying data set). That slop may be true, actual biologic variation or it could be due to errors in measurement. Either way, wide CIs warn you that your ability to measure the events might not allow you to find differences that really exist. In short, the first method allows you to say whether you are confident a difference exists. The second method allows you to offer ideas on why you can or cannot claim that a true difference or effect is present.

Note that in the caveats section of Worksheet 1 it claims that normally distributed variables are assumed; however, as indicated in the article by Ruegg found elsewhere in this issue, many of the indices we evaluate (such as somatic cell counts or days open) are not normally distributed. The "normality" assumption, however, applies not to the underlying groups but to whether multiple samples of differences between the means of the two groups (the index being evaluated) are normally distributed. A rough rule of thumb is that the differences between means of multiple samples from even highly skewed data sets tend to be normally distributed, so in the vernacular of statistics, this method is "robust" regarding normality. Put another way, because we are measuring the differences between means of two samples, the odds are that our normality assumption is valid.

One limitation is that you need three aspects of the measures to run the analysis: (1) average values; (2) measures of variation for those averages (SD or variance); and (3) the number of observations that went into forming each average. A frustrating problem with most animal records systems is that they offer us only items (1) and (3); they usually do not report measures of variation and, therefore, limit what we can do with these records. If you have an option of helping clients to choose records software providers, encourage them to seek vendors who will support reporting of measures of variation.

When data produce frequencies or counts

χ^2 test for contingency tables

Another common type of data we encounter comes in the form of counts or frequencies. Examples include gilts versus sows pregnant, proportion of teats dipped, or number of calves with good versus poor plasma protein levels. For this test, when data come to you in the form of frequencies or percentages, you need to convert them to counts (ie, when data come to you as "25% of 80 cows," you can convert to counts: [$0.25 \times 80 = 20$]). Count data are best evaluated using a χ^2 test for contingency tables [2]. The process is demonstrated by using a dairy example in Worksheet 2 of 1.

χ^2 tests can also be used to help understand clinical significance by generating odds ratios or relative risks [3]. The uses of these similar but importantly different epidemiologic measures are explored in articles found elsewhere in this issue, so I will not go into details here about choosing appropriately between relative risks or odds ratio measures or about in-depth interpretations of them. I discuss the computation of odds ratios only because they are applicable (if not optimal) in most situations in which relative risk can also be used, whereas relative risk calculations can be highly misleading in many of the instances in which odds ratios operate well. Again, the primary goal of HOT Stats is to keep things as simple as possible, so we will adopt only odds ratios for this suite of tools. Calculating odds ratios is simple; just multiply the two diagonals in a 2 × 2 table, and divide one by the other; the convention is to do the math as $(a \times d)/(c \times b) =$ odds ratio:

Herd A	a	b
Herd B	c	d

For example, using the statistically ambivalent difference in the proportion of thin beef cows between two ranches ($0.3 < P < 0.4$) from Worksheet

2, an odds ratio of 1.52 indicates the magnitude of the differences seen: we observed cows from herd A to be about 1.5 times more likely to be thin than cows in herd B. Had we calculated the odds ratio backward [(c × b)/(a × d)], the answer would have been 0.66, indicating that the herd B cows were around two-thirds as likely to be thin. In general, odds ratios greater than 2 (or <0.5) usually generate good clinical interest. Results less than 2 are often not seen as sufficiently clinically significant to get our attention. Given that this example yielded a *P* value between 0.4 and 0.3 (not very exciting statistically) and its odds ratio was 1.5 (not very interesting from a clinical point of view), the numbers are telling us to not get too worked up about this apparent difference in condition scores between the two beef herds. It may be worth watching; it may be a good idea to take bigger samples from each herd, if they are available. It is unlikely with the data at hand, however, that we should conclude that a difference exists and, therefore, need to intervene with herd A versus herd B.

When data produce frequencies or counts with repeat measures

Sign test

The sign test is a very simple means of addressing the affects of treatments or programs when you measure the same animals twice (ie, repeat measures). For example, if you follow average daily gain on a group of pastured steers before and after a worming treatment, you have a situation where the measures are dependent and, therefore, appropriate for the sign test [4]. The nice thing about the sign test is that it can be used on any measure that can be categorized in a dichotomous fashion (yes/no, high/low, bigger/smaller, and so forth) that has a "better/worse" meaning to you. Calculation of the sign test is shown in Worksheet 3 of Appendix 1.

Note that in Worksheet 3, I suggested dropping from the evaluation two of the cows whose milk urea nitrogen (MUN) did not change from one month to the other. Because the sign test requires a dichotomous outcome (ie, went up versus went down), we must make decisions on dealing with situations in which the outcomes could reasonably include three or more groups (ie, went up versus stayed the same versus went down). There are actually a couple ways to handle such outcomes. First, just as I did, you can drop them from analysis, so your evaluation compares only those whose values went up versus those whose values went down. The danger here is whether those being dropped signify an important group. In this case, being only 2 of 115, their inclusion or exclusion is unlikely to affect the conclusion. The other way to work with such instances is to recognize that at some unknown level of laboratory resolution, these animals likely did go up or go down. With that assumption, and with no reason to believe there was a bias either way, you could allocate the stayed-the-same group equally between the other two groups. That would have changed our sign test inputs to 48 versus 67, yielding a test statistic value of 1.68, which does not change the decision. Because the calculations are relatively easy and quick, in these kinds of situations, I usually try both solutions (ie, drop the stayed-the-same group observations; divide the stayed-the-same group between the other two groups) to see whether either solution affects the decision.

Whenever something is advertised as "simpler" (as I have done for the sign test), you need to ask what was given up to make it simpler. For the sign test, what was given up is any "awareness" of the magnitude of effect; that is, how much things went up, got bigger, became faster, and so forth, and how much the other things went down, got smaller, became slower, and so forth. For instance, in the Worksheet 3 example, we know that some cows' MUN went up, and some cows' MUN went down, but we are 90% confident that more went down. This finding is good: we were hoping the ration change would lower MUNs. Note, however, that we have no idea how much things changed. What if the MUNs that went up did so only fractionally, and those that went down dropped low enough to suggest that now the ration was too high in rumen-available fermentable carbohydrates? This information is important, but the Sign test cannot tell you about the degree of change—only whether more went up or went down.

When data produce two variables that appear to move together

Correlation (Spearman rank correlation) between two variables

Correlation analysis is a relatively simple way to find out if one index or variable is associated with another; that is, if index X varies in some way that is predictive of how index Y varies. The calculation of correlation is a multistep process; after all, you are now trying to describe variable 1, describe variable 2, and describe whether the two variables appear related. You cannot expect it to be a simple and quick process. In addition, it is complicated by its requiring the user to have several tables of Student's *t*-statistic values because it also introduces the idea of degrees of freedom (*df*), which is a common, if poorly understood concept in statistical theory. In essence, the operational value of including a *df* factor in statistical processes is that you can use the same table of test statistic probabilities for a variety of analyses. Derivation of *df* for each and every problem is beyond this article, however, the general rule is that *df* equals the number of samples or observations minus some number. That number is usually a tally of the number of constraints or estimates that had to be employed in the statistical problem at hand. For this situation, $df = n - 2$ because the process makes assumptions (ie, constraint estimates) for the variations in index X and index Y. Therefore, you can think of *df* as a "penalty" for having to make estimations for some of the inputs. It is fortunate that understanding how *df* values are derived is not required to operate the procedure.

The process of running a rank correlation is illustrated in Worksheet 4 of Appendix 1 [5].

Be aware that correlation analysis is not regression analysis; it does allow you to say that a certain change in X will result in a calculable change in Y. This situation is especially true in the case of Spearman rank correlation work because we are dealing with ranks, not repeatable intervals, and interpreting the importance of an animal moving up or down one ranking is problematic. Correlation analysis, however, lets you know whether X and Y appear to be related.

A previously identified difficulty with the Spearman rank correlation test in a HOT Stats situation is the need for determining *df* and carrying separate tables for Student's *t* values based on those indices. There is a quick and dirty short cut, however, if you are willing to pay close attention to interpretation. If you look at a *t*-statistic table in any standard statistics text, you will see that, relatively speaking, the values for *df* of 10 (ie, n = 12) are within ±10% of the values (for any single confidence level) of *df* of 6 through 18 (ie, n = 8 to n = 20) and within ±5% for *df* of 9 to 13 (ie, n = 11 to n = 15). In general, the *t*-statistic values for *df* below 10 are somewhat larger than those for *df* of 10; those for higher *df* settings have values somewhat lower than those for *df* of 10. I do a rough approximation of the *t* test when I do a correlation by hand: I try to gather 8 to 20 observations and use the *t*-statistic values for *df* of 10. If my calculated test statistic is within 10% or 5% of the published values for any given confidence level (and on the low side for small sample sizes and on the high side for larger sample sizes), then I need to be careful about my conclusions. When that happens, I pull out a *t*-statistic table to get the actual values or I buffer my estimate of the confidence that I can have. After all, if a decimal point or two changes your decision, is it a strong decision to begin with?

Also, remember that a statistically significant correlation does not mean that there is a causal effect going on. Correlations are probably the most "appears-to-be-identifying-causality" seductive technique we perform. For this example, there is a good biologic argument for why higher-producing cows within a herd might have higher days open. Suppose, instead, that rather than days open being the second variable, it was the free-stall lock-up stanchion that the cow was in at time of pregnancy examination. For a given dairy, there might be a plausible causal association between where she locks-up and whether she was pregnant, but I doubt it. Remember puppy weights and gasoline prices: just because it is statistically significant does not mean it has clinical importance or value.

Combining statistical and clinical significance by way of risk reduction techniques

Several times now, we have touched on the differences between statistical significance (eg, the probability that a result is simply due to random chance) and clinical significance (eg, the size of effect due to one treatment versus the other), and how each is important, but how neither gives us the full picture. We looked at one way of quantifying clinical significance in consort with statistical significance for the χ^2 test through developing the odds ratio. That helps, but we need a broader, more general technique to tie the two types of significance together into a single metric that helps us make decisions. An intuitively simple yet equally powerful means to accomplish this is through what is known as risk reduction techniques [6]. These techniques allow us to take statistically significant research results and convert them into intuitive measures that can be prioritized using typical financial methods. In other words, they allow us to convert published outcomes into economically based indices with which we can make decisions.

The process involves identifying "adverse events" (ie, those events we wish to avoid). For instance, we wish to avoid cows relapsing into hypocalcemia after an initial successful treatment. As another example, we desire to prevent abortions. The point of the risk reduction techniques is to help determine the value and ability of different treatments or practices in avoiding adverse events. Risk reduction techniques introduce three new terms:

1. Absolute risk reduction (ARR) shows the absolute disease reduction between treatments, based on the underlying population
2. Relative risk reduction (RRR) sets the magnitude of effect of one treatment relative to another
3. Number needed to treat (NNT) is the number of animals that will need treatment with a new therapy to prevent at least one instance of the adverse effect

The risk reduction process

Suppose a clinical trial (see the article by Sanderson found elsewhere in this issue) appears to have relevant results for clients. It describes a new practice that offers a sizeable and statistically significant reduction in an important adverse event. Its results summarize as:

	Adverse outcome event		
	Yes	No	Total
Reference group	a	b	a + b
Experimental group	c	d	c + d

We can generate five measures for describing risk and risk reduction from this table as shown:

1. Reference event rate (RER) = event risk, reference group = a/(a + b)
2. Experimental event rate (EER) = event risk, experimental group = c/(c + d)
3. ARR = degree of risk reduced = RER − EER

4. RRR = risk drop relative to reference = (RER − EER)/RER
5. NNT = number of new treatments decreasing adverse events by one = 1/(RER − EER)

Let us look at applying risk reduction techniques to a clinical trial [7] in which hypocalcemic dairy cows that had successfully been treated with intravenous calcium were randomly assigned to a reference group (no further treatment) or an experimental group (received oral calcium gel immediately following intravenous calcium). The trial looked at whether the oral calcium treatment decreased relapse rates. Hence, relapsing is the adverse event of interest. The following depiction shows numeric results, statistical outcomes, and the risk reduction values:

	Relapse occurs		
	Yes	No	Total
Reference group	14	25	39
Experimental group	4	2	31

$\chi^2 = 4.78$; $P = 0.03$

Risk reduction calculations are shown as:

1. RER = 14/39 = 0.36
2. EER = 4/31 = 0.13
3. ARR = RER−EER = 0.23
4. RRR = AAR/RER = 0.64
5. NNT = 1/ARR = 4.3

What does any of this mean? First off, we know that a χ^2 test yielded a *P* value of 0.03. Hence, we are 97% confident that the differences shown are real (if you do not believe it, then plug the numbers into Worksheet 2; you will find that it will claim significance between 95% and 99% confidence). Therefore, it is statistically interesting and looks like a repeatable set of outcomes. What about clinical significance? Let us define, in terms relevant to the given study, what the indices indicate. The RER and the EER show how often relapses occurred in the two groups: the reference group suffered 36% relapses; the experimental group suffered 13% relapses. Our clinical significance "ears" just pricked up: this difference looks important. The ARR tells us that using calcium gel reduced the relapse rate by 23 percentage points, and the RRR tells us that this 23-percentage-point decrease represents a 64% lowered risk of relapse following treatment. Now our clinical-significance detectors are going wild; this looks like a good deal.

Clients, however, should always ask us whether "it is better enough" to warrant making a change. For instance, if it bankrupted the dairy to institute this new program, effective though it is, then it would be a bad move. This is where the NNT comes into play. It tells us, based on the clinical trial's own data, how many cows we need to treat with the calcium gel to avoid one adverse event (ie, one case of relapse). Therefore, for every 4.3 cows we treat with the calcium gel, we can prevent one case of relapse. If we do a little bit of financial calculation, we can compare the costs of treating 4.3 cows with calcium gel against the losses suffered by one case of hypocalcemic relapse.

Economic analyses of animal health and performance are covered by Galligan in an article found elsewhere in this issue, so I will not go into details here; however, a simple partial budget analysis using 2004 prices based on the North Carolina State University Teaching Hospital's drug costs and one of my client's records on costs of treating relapses (including probabilities of death/culling but not accounting for future decreases in milk production for survivors, making this a conservative estimate) resulted in the following:

Calcium gel treatment cost = \$12
Relapse median cost = \$67

Therefore, NNT × calcium gel treatment cost = 4.3 × \$12 = \$52

Because \$52 (NNT × treatment cost) is less than the median cost of a case of relapse at \$67, it is economically rational to perform the treatment. The producer will save \$15 (\$67 – \$52) over the cost of the relapse it prevents. Another way to state this result is if the client adopts the calcium gel treatment, the dairy will save 22% (15/67 = 0.22) over the costs of not using the calcium gel.

At this point, the statistician in us (if you have read this far, you know more statistics than most people) has been satisfied with the low *P* value, our "clinician brain" is happy with the sizeable AAR and RRR, and our client (who has to pay for it) is fulfilled because we have shown, through NNT, that he or she can save money by adopting the practice. It does not get any better than that; we got to this "win-win-win" end by using risk reduction techniques to tie together statistical and clinical measures of significance.

Availability of low-cost statistical software applicable to practice

The thrust of this article is to give the reader some statistical methods that need no more resources than a pencil, a piece of paper, and a hand calculator. Two downsides of this thrust, as mentioned several times above, are (1) that these simple methods do not address all of the types of data and questions that food animal veterinarians may face and (2) that the answers we get from these pared-down procedures may miss out on important information and factors that affect a conclusion or decision. Hence, sometimes we need more than a strictly HOT Stats approach. That is, we may need more computational power than what we can do with a pencil, paper, and a calculator. Sometimes we need a computer and statistical software to do the job.

The most ubiquitous source of statistical software is one we already own if our computers came with a "suite" of programs. All the major spreadsheet software packages (Microsoft Office Excel, Microsoft Corp., Redmond, Washington; Corel WordPerfect Office Quattro-Pro, Corel Corp., Ottawa, Ontario, Canada; Lotus SmartSuite Lotus 1-2-3, International Business Machines Corp., Armonk, New York; and so forth) carry statistical functions that largely replicate or explore in more depth the types of questions we have addressed in this article. For instance, these software packages allow you to run tests for differences between means, for performing χ^2 tests (including those larger than a 2 × 2 contingency table), and for different levels of correlation analyses (including the more informative regression techniques and diagnostics). Usually, they will not perform a sign test, choosing instead to offer a paired *t* test procedure that will work in most situations. In some instances, spreadsheets can require a fair amount of work to set up. Specifically, χ^2 procedures are probably easier done by hand than by spreadsheet function. As part of a subtheme in this article, this added complexity carries with it more in-depth analyses and interpretation than what HOT Stats can offer.

In addition to the built-in capabilities of commercial spreadsheets, there are numerous add-in freeware or shareware systems that expand the analytic breadth of these programs. A Google search was performed in November 2005 with the search terms of "excel" and "statistic" being required and requiring at least one of the terms "share," "free," or "add." The first page of the output is depicted as a screen capture in Fig. 1. Over 5 million links were identified as fulfilling the search criteria. No doubt, not all are focused on statistical procedures, but you get the idea that a great deal of support for expansion is out there. Note that this search result is for just one of the spreadsheet packages.

Beyond the statistical resources available through commercial spreadsheet programs, free or shareware statistical packages are available. The most popular of the free packages, EpiInfo, is produced and distributed by the Centers for Disease Control and Prevention, Epidemiology Program Office, Division of Public Health Surveillance and Informatics, Atlanta, Georgia. It is available as a Windows product (version 3.3.2 as of November 2005) and as the older DOS-based product, which runs within a C: window (version 6.04d, no longer under development as of April 2005). Both versions are freely downloadable from the Internet through the URL <http://www.cdc.gov/epiinfo/>.

The EpiInfo DOS version is still very useful for quickly answering simple questions on 2 × 2 tables (such as χ^2 statistics and diagnostics), comparing populations, determining sample sizes, calculating confidence levels (ie, *P* values) for different statistical outcomes, and many other aspects of statistical work. It also has a rudimentary word processor that is useful for developing questionnaires linked to EpiInfo functions. Being DOS based, it is limited in functional, formatting, and output flexibility. Nonetheless, it is fast and relatively small: the whole package occupies between 8 and 9 MB. Its two most useful modules for the veterinarian, STATCALC and EPITABLE, can stand alone and take up only approximately 700 K of disk space.

The EpiInfo Windows version is a large, fully integrated package for gathering, collating, analyzing, and reporting statistical analyses from large datasets. Although not as immediately useful as the DOS version in answering questions for small datasets, it is much more flexible and carries more statistical methodology and procedures than the DOS program. It maintains

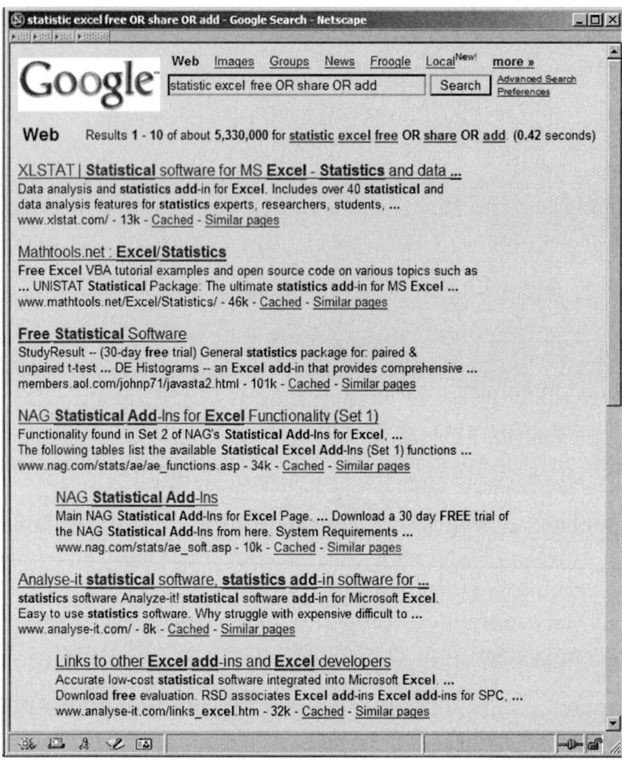

Fig. 1. Results of a Google Internet search run November 2005 in search of spreadsheet freeware, shareware, and other add-ins that enhance Microsoft Excel statistical procedures. Certainly, not all of the nearly 5.3 million links focus on pure statistical procedures, but the results give the user an idea of the wealth of resources that are available. (*From* Google™, with permission from Google Inc.)

the STATCALC module and the questionnaire development ability and brings in a new and in-depth data analysis capacity. The program takes advantage of Windows' ability to visualize data in multiple graphic formats by allowing incorporation of mapping and geographic information system data. Again, for answering basic veterinary questions, this program is likely overkill, but then, so is the depth and breadth of capacity from the spreadsheets discussed earlier. As of April 2005, the version 3.3.2 occupies approximately 130 MB of hard disk space and requires at least 100 to 160 MB of RAM, depending on the Windows version on your computer.

Appendix 1. Worksheets for performing the tests

Worksheet 1. *z* test for the difference between two means based on confidence interval estimation

1. *Setup:* A large farrowing unit is implementing "production pay" for their workers. Two people do most of the breeding at the unit, and the

farm computes weekly conception rates for the breeders, based on ultrasound pregnancy diagnoses. The manager wants your help in deciding whether one breeder has actually done better over the month than the other. The following data are presented to you for consideration:

	Breeder A	Breeder B
Average weekly conception rate	68%	61%
SD	6%	5%
No. of weekly conception rate observations	4	4

2. *Calculation of test statistic:*

$$\begin{aligned}\text{Test statistic} &= \text{Abs}\left[(\text{avgA} - \text{avgB})/\text{SQRT}\left[\left(\text{SDA}^2\right)/\text{countA}\right.\right.\\ &\quad \left.+\left(\text{SDB}^2\right)/\text{countB}\right]\\ &= \text{Abs}\left[(68 - 61)/\text{SQRT}\left[(6^2/4) + (5^2/4)\right]\right.\\ &= \text{Abs}[(7)/(3.91)]\\ &= 1.79\end{aligned}$$

Abs = *absolute value (ie, ignore final negatives)*
SQRT = *take the square root of the expression*

3. *Confidence measures: z* scores for these levels of confidence (from any statistics text or Appendix 2 table):

   95%: 1.96; 90%: 1.64; 80%: 1.28

4. *Decision rule:* Because our test statistic is greater than the 90% confidence level but below the 95% confidence level, we are between 90% and 95% certain that there is a real difference in performance between the two breeders.

To estimate the actual confidence intervals:

2. *Calculation:*

$$\begin{aligned}\text{Interval statistic} &= (\text{meanB} - \text{meanA}) \pm z_{\text{score}}\\ &\quad \times \text{SQRT}\left[\left(\text{SDB}^2/\text{countB}\right) + \left(\text{SDA}^2/\text{countA}\right)\right]\\ &= (61 - 68) \pm z_{\text{score}} \times \text{SQRT}\left[\left(5^2/4\right) + \left(6^2/4\right)\right]\\ &= -7 \pm z_{\text{score}} \times 3.91\end{aligned}$$

3. *Do the math. CI for the difference between means:*

   95%: −14.7 to 0.7; 90%: −13.4 to −0.6; 80%: −12.0 to −2.0

4. *Decision rule:* The decision rule is to reject the conclusion that a difference exists if 0.0 is in the range. Hence, we can be 90% confident that

the weight difference is real (as that CI barely misses having 0.0 included in it) but cannot be 95% confident because 0.0 occurs in that interval.

5. *Caveats:* The z test CI assumes a fairly normally distributed set of data, and the samples were selected at random from the overall population. If these do not apply, it means that you must be more careful in interpreting the results. Note that in the first example, I subtracted the smaller mean from the larger and, in the second example, I subtracted the larger from the smaller—it does not matter.

Worksheet 2. χ^2 contingency tables

1. *Setup:* You evaluated late spring body condition scores (BCS) on beef cattle from two client operations. For the sake of discussion, let us say you believe that cows with BCS less than 5 are too thin and wonder whether the proportion of thin cows differs between the two ranches. The following is what you found:

	Number of cows		Total	
	BCS < 5	BCS ok	Cows	% Thin
Herd A	15	44	59	25
Herd B	9	40	49	18
Total	24	84	108	

2. *Calculation: The equation for calculating the* χ^2*:*

$$[(15 \times 40) - (9 \times 44)]^2 \times 108/59 \times 49 \times 84 \times 24 = 0.77$$

3. *Confidence measures:* χ^2 values for the following levels of confidence (from any statistics text or Appendix 2 table):

95%: 3.84; 90%: 2.70; 80%: 1.64; 70%: 1.07; 60%: 0.71

4. *Decision rule:* Because our test χ^2 is less than the χ^2 statistic for a 70% confidence level but above that for the 60% confidence value, we are only between 60% and 70% confident that there is a difference in the proportions of thin cows between the two herds.
5. *Caveats:* So long as no cell in a 2×2 table has a value less than 5, and so long as the groups are independent and mutually exclusive, the χ^2 CI for contingency tables is a very robust and easy method of determining statistical significance in data sets.
In other words, you cannot use the method for "before-after" comparisons on the same animals (not independent) or in situations in which the classification is not clear (not mutually exclusive).

Worksheet 3. Sign test for proportions with repeat measures

1. *Setup:* Previous clinical work on a client dairy reproductive problem determined that the ration was limited in rumen-available fermentable carbohydrates (RAFC), decreasing protein use, as manifested by increased milk urea nitrogen (MUN). You helped the client increase the RAFC levels in the ration and want to see if it helped. You know that reproductive performance data will take weeks or more to develop, so you focus on changes in MUN—the thinking being if you lowered MUN levels, then your ration was addressing the suspected underlying cause of reproductive inefficiency.
2. *Calculation:* Consecutive monthly DHIA MUN tests for before the ration change and after the ration change were collected. One hundred fifteen cows in the breeding herd string with MUN measures in both tests were evaluated: 47 had higher MUN levels after the ration change; 66 had lower MUN levels over the same period (2 had equal MUN levels and were dropped from evaluation).

   Abs[Total – (2 × lesser of the two counts – 1)/SQRT Total]
   = [113 – (2 × 47) – 1]/SQRT 113
   = 1.69

3. *Confidence measures:* This fits a z test distribution; the appropriate confidence (from any statistics text or Appendix 2 table):

   95%: 1.96; 90%: 1.64; 80%: 1.28

4. *Decision rule:* Because the sign test value is between the z score for 90% and 95% confidence, we can say we are just over 90% confident but not 95% confident that the ration change lowered MUN levels for this herd.
5. *Caveats:* To work well, you should be certain to have at least 25 pairs of measures (ie, 25 cows, evaluated twice).

Worksheet 4. Spearman rank correlation between two variables

1. *Setup:* You have just finished a herd reproduction check and have the impression that the more milk a cow produces, the longer it takes her to get pregnant (ie, number of days open [DA OPN] is related to milk production). Because production is affected by stage of lactation, a transformed index that is based on an entire estimated lactation would remove that confounder. Therefore, you might pick 305-day fat-corrected milk (305 FCM), mature equivalent milk production, or one of a couple other modified production indices. Then, randomly select

a group of just-diagnosed pregnant cows from the current visit, and write down each cow's 305 FCM and DA OPN. The following are the raw data you get for 11 cows:

CowID	305 FCM(1,000's)	DA OPN
A	20.6	103
B	20.1	91
C	19.0	100
D	23.6	109
E	19.2	105
F	22.8	119
G	21.0	113
H	24.8	116
I	19.1	100
J	22.5	99
K	21.7	103

2. *Calculation:* The calculation for running correlations is a bit more complicated than for the others because it requires you to establish rankings for each cow for each index, to take the differences of each cow's rankings (Diff), to square those differences (Diff^2), and to sum the squared differences. And these calculations are just to get started. You then calculate the rank correlation coefficient (which tells you how closely the two variables move together) and, finally, you compute the statistical significance of that correlation coefficient. Each step is detailed in the following:

   2a. Establishing the ranks, the rank differences, the square of the rank differences, and the sum of the squared rank differences (rank 1 = highest, rank 11 = lowest):

			Ranks by cow		Rank difference	
CowID	305 FCM (1,000's)	DA OPN	305FCM	DA OPN	Diff	Diff^2
A	20.6	103	7	6	1	1
B	20.1	91	8	11	−3	9
C	19.0	100	11	8	3	9
D	23.6	109	2	4	−2	4
E	19.2	105	9	5	4	16
F	22.8	119	3	1	2	4
G	21.0	113	6	3	3	9
H	24.8	116	1	2	−1	1
I	19.1	100	10	8	2	4
J	22.5	99	4	10	−6	36
K	21.7	103	5	6	−1	1
					Sum of the Diff^2 =	94

2b. Calculating the Spearman rank correlation coefficient (SRCC). The following formula is filled using the numbers from this problem:

$$\text{SRCC} = 1 - \left[(6 \times \text{sum Diff}^2)/\left(\text{n} \times \left(\text{ n}^2 - 1\right)\right)\right]$$
$$\text{SRCC} = 1 - \left[(6 \times 94)/\left(11 \times \left(11^2 - 1\right)\right)\right]$$
$$= 0.57$$

This result suggests that changes in 305 FCM might account for 57% of the variation in DA OPN.

2c. Calculating the statistical significance of the SRCC.

$$t\text{ statistic} = \text{SRCC/SQRT}\left[\left(1 - \text{SRCC}^2\right)/(\text{n} - 2)\right]$$
$$= 0.57/\text{SQRT}\left[\left(1 - 0.57^2\right)/\left(11 - 2\right)\right]$$
$$= 2.10$$

3. *Confidence measures:* This calculation is more complex that the others because it must use a Student's *t* test. The *t* test confidence values change with the number of observations (calculated as *df*), so it is not a simple "look-up" procedure (from any statistics text):
3a. Calculating the appropriate *df*:

$$df = (\text{n} - 2) = (11 - 2) = 9$$

3b. Establish the *t* statistic value for 9 *df* (from any statistics text or Appendix 2 table):

95%, 9 *df*, 2.26; 90%, 9 *df*, 1.83; 80%, 9 *df*, 1.38

4. *Decision rule:* Because the *t* test value at 9 *df* is between the *t* score for 90% and 95% confidence, we can say we are between 90% and 95% confident that the correlation between 305 FCM and DA OPN is real.
5. *Caveats:* This index works with rankings and, therefore, like the sign test, is oblivious to the magnitude of differences between the raw numbers making those rankings: a cow producing 25,000 lb of milk ranks higher than a cow producing 24,999 lb of milk or a cow producing 14,999 lb of milk. They would rank 1,2,3, respectively, even though most of us would consider there to be no difference between the first two animals and that the third animal is very different. Ranks can change with a move of just a couple of pounds or, in the above example, with a few days' difference in DA OPN (note how close in DA OPN some of the cows in this example are—a couple days difference could really change the rankings). That is just the way it is with rankings versus raw numbers. For ease of calculation, however, we need to use the ranks. Just be aware of and take a look at how the rankings fall out.

Finally, this technique assumes that the animals are chosen randomly from a larger population and are independent of each other (again, no "before-after"–type data can be used here).

Appendix 2. Test values for *z* tests, *t* tests, and χ^2 tests

Confidence	50%	60%	70%	80%	90%	95%	99%
z test	0.68	0.84	1.04	1.28	1.64	1.96	2.57
t test							
(6 *df*)	0.72	0.91	1.13	1.44	1.94	2.45	3.71
(10 *df*)	0.70	0.88	1.09	1.37	1.81	2.23	3.17
(14 *df*)	0.69	0.87	1.08	1.35	1.76	2.15	2.98
χ^2 test	0.45	0.71	1.07	1.64	2.71	3.84	6.63

Examples:

A *z* **test** value of 1.17 is calculated. This yields a confidence of between 70% and 80% (ie, *P* is between 0.2 and 0.3) that the observed difference is real.

A ***t*** **test** value from a sample of 12 ($df = n - 2 = 10$) of 0.83 is calculated, which corresponds to a confidence between 50% and 60% (ie, *P* is between 0.5 and 0.4) that the correlation is real.

A χ^2 **test** value of 4.46 yields a confidence between 95% and 99% (ie, *P* is between 0.01 and 0.05) that the observed difference is real.

References

[1] Hamburg M. Confidence interval estimation (large samples). In: Statistical analysis for decision making. 3rd edition. New York: Harcourt Brace Jovanovich; 1983. p. 228–30.

[2] Fleiss JL. Sampling method I: naturalistic or cross-sectional studies. In: Statistical methods for rates and proportions. 2nd edition. New York: John Wiley & Sons; 1981. p. 60.

[3] Martin SW, Meek AH, Willeberg P. Disease causation. In: Veterinary epidemiology—principles and methods. Ames (IA): Iowa State University Press; 1987. p. 130.

[4] Snedecor GW, Cochran WG. Shortcut and nonparametric methods. In: Statistical methods. 8th edition. Ames (IA): Iowa State University Press; 1989. p. 138–40.

[5] Mansfield E. Regression and correlation techniques. In: Statistics for business and economics. New York: WW Norton & Co.; 1980. p. 401–3.

[6] Sackett DL, Haynes RB, Guyatt GH, et al. Deciding on the best therapy. In: Clinical epidemiology—a basic science for clinical medicine. 2nd edition. Boston: Little, Brown and Co.; 1991. p. 187–210.

[7] Oetzel GR, Vagnoni DB, Nordlund KV. Effect of an oral calcium chloride gel on prevention of hypocalcemic relapses in dairy cattle [abstract]. Presented at the 30th Annual Conference of the American Association of Bovine Practitioners, Montreal, Quebec, Canada, 1997.

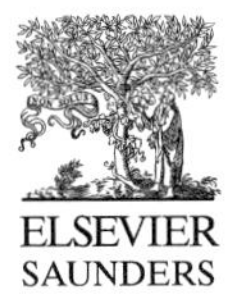

ELSEVIER
SAUNDERS

Vet Clin Food Anim 22 (2006) 171–193

VETERINARY
CLINICS
Food Animal Practice

Using Statistical Process Control Methods to Improve Herd Performance

Jeffrey K. Reneau, DVM, MS*, Joanna Lukas, MS

Department of Animal Science, University of Minnesota, Haecker Hall, 1364 Eckles Avenue, St. Paul, MN 55108, USA

How consistently are livestock farms managed? How consistently and compliantly do employees carry out the management protocols? It is common knowledge that livestock thrive well when herd management is consistently excellent. Dairy cows, for example, perform best when they are healthy, milked exactly the same every day, and fed palatable diets that consistently provide all nutrient requirements day after day.

Variation is the opposite of consistency and considered the enemy of process performance. Excessive variation interferes with the evaluation of performance. It is true that high variability makes performance outcome unpredictable and difficult to interpret; however, understanding variation is the diagnostic key to improving process performance. Statistical process control (SPC) is an analytic approach using the theory of variation as a means of explaining with statistical certainty when process performance is improving, staying the same, or getting worse.

Livestock farm managers and their consultants have, in the past, restricted their analysis to limited comparisons of performance means without full consideration of variation (eg, comparing last month's average of some herd performance variable with this month's average). Such an analysis may not only be misleading but is also usually out of context with the daily management activity. Ironically, although consistency in herd management is intuitively sought, analysis of variation in process output has been neglected. Consequently, consultants or employees may be blamed or rewarded for random variation in performance but not on the basis of "real" change. This confusion leads to management decision errors and frustration for everyone: the consultants, the managers, and their employees [1]. The need for fact-based management decisions as understood

* Corresponding author.
E-mail address: renea001@umn.edu (J.K. Reneau).

0749-0720/06/$ - see front matter
doi:10.1016/j.cvfa.2005.11.006 *vetfood.theclinics.com*

by Ishikawa [2] is apparent. Applying statistical methods to analyze data already available on the farm has the potential of improving process and personnel performance monitoring, thus providing more effective management tools for livestock farm managers and their consultants. Moreover, it can assure more timely performance feedback to those directly responsible for the process (ie, milkers, feeders, breeders) compared with the retrospective monitoring garnered from once-per-month record analysis that is often out of time-order context with daily management.

The livestock production system

Every livestock production system comprises many interconnected processes that eventually result in the production of milk or meat. Every process has inputs that result in some output variable (Fig. 1) that can often be routinely and accurately measured. Monitoring of these key process output variables by SPC techniques characterizes the data, providing, with statistical certainty, a "voice of the process" prediction of future performance.

What is statistical process control?

SPC is more than another analytic methodology. It is a philosophy, a strategy, and a set of analytic methods for the improvement of systems, processes, and outcomes [3]: "SPC builds an environment in which all individuals in an organization seek continuous improvement in quality and

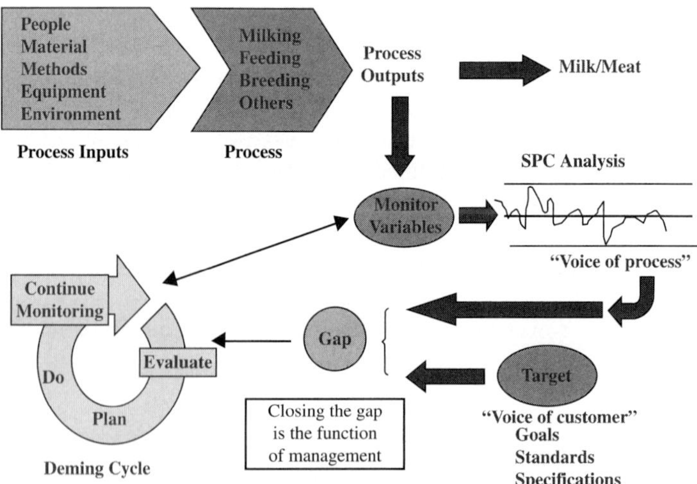

Fig. 1. Process flow diagram.

productivity" [4]. Making quality a responsibility of every employee starts with the management and its commitment to creating the right working environment [1]. Continuous improvement is achieved by implementing the following SPC family of problem-solving tools that have the aim of process improvement by reducing variability [4]:

1. Histogram
2. Check sheet (used to record process performance data: who? what? when?)
3. Pareto chart (used to identify the most common problems)
4. Cause-effect diagram (used to search for root cause of errors/defects/ process performance changes)
5. Defect concentration (used to identify defect location)
6. Scatter diagram (used to identify relationships between process variables)
7. Control charts

Although this article focuses almost entirely on the use of control charts, the authors recommend that readers familiarize themselves with the other six SPC tools.

Control charts were developed in 1920 by Walter A. Shewhart for the purpose of identifying and distinguishing between normal (common cause) and abnormal (special cause) variability. The output of every process is characterized by a certain level of variation that is due to a cumulative effect of many factors that are out of our control. This is called common cause variation. The level of common cause variation can be reduced by finding a way to control these contributing factors. For example, if a bulk tank somatic cell count (BTSCC) is considered to be too high, then the herd manager might try to find a way to improve (1) milking personnel skill by training them in standard operating procedures or (2) the cows' environment by more frequent changing of bedding.

Some level of variation is unavoidable: one may not know all of the possible factors that affect process output or it may not be economically justifiable to control some of the factors that are known. For example, a certain drop in milk production or an increase in somatic cell count (SCC) in hot weather may be tolerable because building a barn with a fully controlled environment would be too expensive.

When only common cause variation is present in process output, the process is said to be operating under the state of statistical control. The process enters an out of control state when some aspect of the process that is usually under control changes and impacts process performance. The resulting variation is usually caused by machine/equipment problems, operator/personnel errors, or defective raw materials. This variation is called special cause variation because its source can usually be traced and eliminated, returning the process back to the state of statistical control. Table 1 summarizes the differences between the two types of variation.

Table 1
Source of process variation

	Sources of variation	
	Common cause	Special cause
Synonyms	Normal, unassignable cause, random, noise	Abnormal, assignable cause
Definition	Predictable variation inherent in the process itself resulting from factors that we may not control	Unpredictable variation resulting from factors that we usually have under control
Cause of variation examples	1. Variable milking prep time per cow 2. Effect of atmospheric humidity on dry matter content in feed 3. Biweekly fluctuations in milk yield in cows supplemented with bovine somatotropin	1. Increased incidence of pneumonia among calves 2. Decrease in BTSCC after milkers' training
Solution	Work on improving the process by 1. Changing the procedures 2. Investing in equipment or other measures that enable better control of factors we previously were not able to control 3. Identifying factors influencing the output and learn how to control them (experiments)	Identify the reason for this variation and 1. Remove it if it is undesirable 2. Try to repeat it if it is desirable
Solution examples	1. Adopting a milking procedure that minimizes the variation in milking prep time 2. Routine measurement of forage dry matter and adjusting diets to correct for moisture changes 3. Administering bovine somatotropin to half the herd each week to level out milk yield	1. Check for wet bedding in calf hutches 2. Establish mandatory yearly retraining for all employees

After the underlying principles of the control charts are understood, application to a livestock operation can begin. Developing SPC charts involves four steps: deciding what to chart, determining how the samples will be collected, developing the charts, and plotting the process output data.

Deciding what to chart

The data should

- Be sensitive to changes (in method, people, the environment, machines, materials, and so forth) so that they can be used to monitor their performance
- Be easily, inexpensively, routinely, and frequently collected (to provide timely feedback)

- Have an economic value attached
- Have a measure that is possible to standardize/specify
- Be familiar to or easily understood by process operators
- Be collected at an appropriate process level (ideally, low enough to tie process performance with possible sources of variation but high enough to avoid plotting too many charts that may eventually be ignored)

Determining how samples will be collected

Rational subgrouping determines the sampling scheme. Rational subgrouping basically means grouping data in a way that makes logical sense so that only random effects are responsible for observed variation within a sample. Decisions about when to sample, how frequently to sample, and how big (single or multiple) the individual samples should be are critical to achieving meaningful analysis. The subgrouping should be designed to help detect possible sources of special cause variation between samples. In summary, the key to creating rational subgrouping is to sample as much the same as possible yet assure that the samples are representative of the process characteristic that is to be monitored.

Developing the charts

This step involves choosing the appropriate charts. A wide range of charts has been developed for measurement (continuous) data (I, X-bar, S, moving range charts) and attribute (count or proportional) data (NP, P, C, U charts) (Fig. 2). With measurement data, both variations can be monitored for change by separate charts.

X-bar and S charts

X-bar and S charts are used to monitor the mean and variation, respectively, in situations in which rational groups of multiple measurements can be collected (eg, collecting all the individual cow milk weights to calculate the mean and standard deviation of all the milk weights in a group of cows each day). In a production setting, however, the variation between animals (common cause, within sample) could be greater than day-to-day variation (special cause, between samples). Therefore, in a biologic system, plotting an X-bar chart may not be a recommended approach unless relatively homogeneous groups can be sampled.

I and moving range charts

I and moving range charts are generally used when rational grouping requires a single measurement (eg, the simple daily milk production average for a pen of cows expressed in pounds per cow per day, or a daily BTSCC or milk component test result).

When using attribute data, due to the relationship between mean and variance, it is sufficient to monitor only the mean.

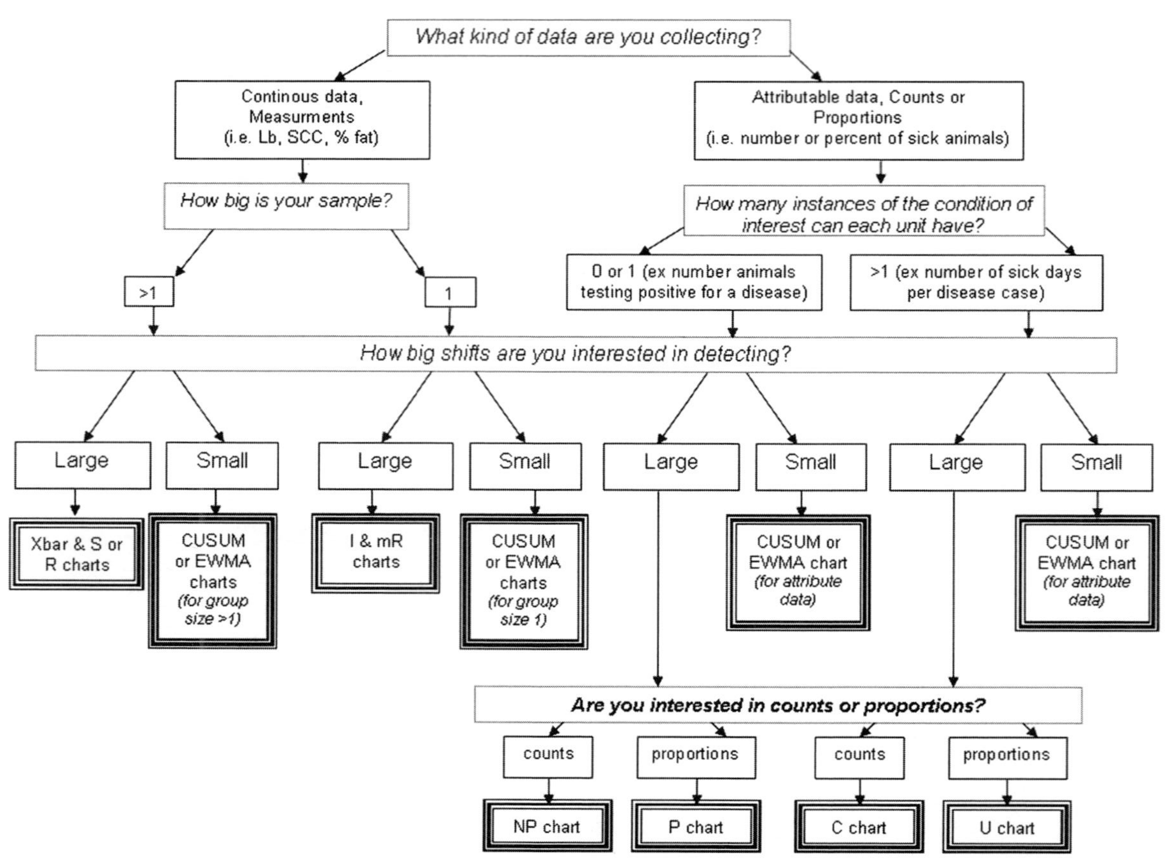
What kind of data are you collecting?
Continous data, Measurments (i.e. Lb, SCC, % fat)
Attributable data, Counts or Proportions (i.e. number or percent of sick animals)
How big is your sample?
How many instances of the condition of interest can each unit have?
>1
1
0 or 1 (ex number animals testing positive for a disease)
>1 (ex number of sick days per disease case)
How big shifts are you interested in detecting?
Large
Small
Large
Small
Large
Small
Large
Small
Xbar & S or R charts
CUSUM or EWMA charts (for group size >1)
I & mR charts
CUSUM or EWMA charts (for group size 1)
CUSUM or EWMA chart (for attribute data)
CUSUM or EWMA chart (for attribute data)
Are you interested in counts or proportions?
counts
proportions
counts
proportions
NP chart
P chart
C chart
U chart

NP chart

The NP chart requires a constant sample size. It is used for monitoring the number of times a condition occurs when each unit can have this condition or not have this condition (eg, the number of dystocias or retained placentas per 20 consecutive calvings).

P chart

The P chart does not require a constant sample size. It is used for monitoring the proportion of samples having the condition when each sample can have the condition or not have the condition (eg, the percentage of animals with some disease or condition during a defined period of time).

C chart

The C chart requires a constant sample size. It is used for monitoring the number of times a condition occurs when each sample can have more than one instance of the condition (eg, the number of recurrent cases of clinical mastitis per a set number [20 or more] lactating cows over a specific period of time).

U chart

The U chart does not require a constant sample size. It is used for monitoring the percentage of samples having the condition when each sample can have more than one instance of the condition (eg, the number of cow days in the sick pen per week).

More detailed information about choice, design, and application of SPC charts can be found at the following Web site: www.qualityamerica.com/knowledgecente/index.htm.

In general, control charts for measurement data are more powerful for detecting special cause change than charts for attribute data; X-bar and S charts are more powerful than I charts; and the C chart or the U chart is more powerful than the P chart [3]. Control chart choice also depends on what degree of anticipated change is expected. Classic Shewhart charts (I charts and X-bar charts) are designed to detect large shifts in process performance; however, run rules like the following Western Electric rules have been developed to make possible the detection of more subtle changes on I and X-bar charts:

1. A single point more than 3 σ away from the mean
2. At least nine successive points on the same side of the mean
3. At least two of three successive points 2 σ away and on the same side of the mean
4. At least four of five successive points 1 σ away and on the same side of the mean

Fig. 2. Chart choice diagram. CUSUM, cumulative sum; EWMA, exponentially weight moving average; MR, moving range.

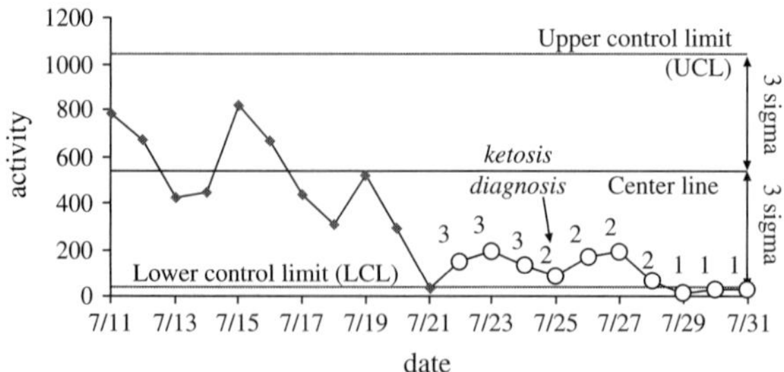

Fig. 3. Anatomy of an I chart. Upper control limits (UCL) and lower control limits (LCL) are marked as lines 3 σ away from the center line. The data points labeled by white circles indicate points out of control. The numbers above data points indicate which Western Electric rule identified the point to be out of control. The arrow indicates when the diagnosis of ketosis was made.

Whenever any of these conditions is met, one can be sure that real change has occurred. When using all of the Western Electric rules, there will be a false alarm approximately 2% of the time, which means that for most management circumstances, there is a 98% probability of being right about whether a change is "real."

Monitoring dairy cow activity with pedometers has been shown to help detect developing metabolic disorders [5]. Fig. 3 is an example of a Shewhart I chart of daily single-cow activity (Richard Wallace, DVM, MS, University of Illinois, personal communication, May 2005). To develop the chart, an arithmetic mean was calculated and a sigma estimated from the average moving range (average moving range of size 2). A center was plotted at the mean, along with upper and lower control limits 3 σ above and below the center line. Applying the Western Electric rules 2 and 3 identified a significant drop in activity as a result of developing ketosis as early as 7/22. The 3-σ rule [1] did not signal until 7/29, 4 days after diagnosis of ketosis was made. This example shows how additional run rules increased the sensitivity of the control charts, as opposed to using only the 3-σ rule.

More recently, however, more sensitive and specific charts have been developed to detect smaller sustained shifts in process performance. These more sophisticated techniques include exponentially weight moving average (EWMA) and cumulative sum (CUSUM) charts [4], which can be designed for optimal performance in detecting shifts from 0.5 to 2 σ. Classic Shewhart charts are easy to develop and interpret. Supported with Western Electric rules, they are usually the first step in monitoring process for change and gaining familiarity with SPC tools. The currently recommended technique, however, is to plot classic Shewhart and CUSUM or EWMA charts simultaneously. In this way, large and small sustained shifts can be detected.

Plotting the process output data

This step involves plotting the process output data and applying the control limits to observe for special cause variation. After a data point is observed to be "out of control" (outside the control limits or meets run rule criteria), one searches for the root cause, eliminates it, and restores the process to its state of statistical control.

Why use statistical process control in livestock management?

SPC has proved to be an effective quality management tool in manufacturing businesses for over 80 years, improving product quality and reducing process waste. The first attempts to implement the principles of SPC in the livestock industry were in 1977, when Wrathall [6] studied the applicability of individual-measurement SPC chart application. Since then, the use of SPC charts has been researched in all four major livestock species: swine [7–9], beef [10], poultry [11,12] and, more recently, dairy [13–15]. Wrathall and Hebert [16] first identified the need for SPC application in livestock because of growing herd size and increasing remoteness between managers and livestock. More current studies underline the applicability of SPC methods in continuous improvement effort at the farm [17,18]. Although the research in SPC application in livestock production has at least a 28-year history, the idea has become practical only recently, largely due to advances in computer capability. News of SPC has been reaching livestock producers' through professional magazines (*Progressive Dairyman*, *Midwest Dairy Business*, *International Pigletter*, and others) and through practical application by way of Web sites that chart process output variables on SPC charts (ie, MilkLab at www.dairyperformance.com, Ag Information Management, Ellenburg, Washington) and include SPC in software packages that analyze farm performance data (ie, 100-Day Contract Manager, Pfizer Animal Health, New York, NY). In addition, increased use of on-farm technology (computerized milking, feeding, and estrous detection systems, to name a few) provides resources by creating enormous amounts of data available on a daily or hourly basis. Analyzed properly, these data can be helpful in monitoring the performance of critical processes and the employees who carry them out.

Below is a summary table of the SPC charts' application to variables across the four main species (Table 2). The table includes only variables that have been considered by previous research. As mentioned earlier, the automation of many processes on the farm, including data collection, creates the opportunity for SPC charting of many other performance measures. For example, in dairy production, these performance measures could include feed efficiency, activity monitoring, electric conductivity of milk, parlor throughput, milk bactoscan test results, water and dry matter intake, and others.

The goal of a commercial dairy farm is to consistently produce high-quality and safe milk in a manner that enhances animal health and productivity [19]. This goal is consistent among all food-producing livestock enterprises. Controlled basic research studies provide cause and effect knowledge of the effectiveness of a management or product intervention. Although such

Table 2
Application of statistical process control charts to monitor livestock production variables

Species	Variable	Chart type	Reference
Dairy	Bulk tank MUN	I	www.dairyperformance.com
	Bulk tank protein percentage	I	www.dairyperformance.com
	Bulk tank milk fat percentage	I	www.dairyperformance.com
	Milk/cow/day	I	www.dairyperformance.com
	Dry matter/cow/day	I	www.dairyperformance.com
	BTSCC	I	[14,28]
	Percentage pregnant	P	[13]
	Estrous detection ratios	P, CUSUM	[15]
Swine	Percentage return to service	I, CUSUM	[6,7]
	Number of pigs per litter	X-bar	[6]
	Percentage fetuses born dead/alive	I	[6,8]
	Snout-deformity score	CUSUM	[10]
	Farrowing rate	I	[8]
	Number of piglets weaned	I	[8]
	Number of services	I	[8]
	Feed conversion rate	I	[8]
	Nonproductive sow days	I	[8]
	Water usage	I	[8]
	Shots administered	I	[8]
	Weight out (nursery)	I	[8]
	Number of sows and gilled culled	I	[8]
	Number of females mated	I	[8,9]
Beef	Weight gain	X-bar	[10]
Poultry	Weight	X-bar	[11]
	Survival rate	I	[12]

studies are possible, they are not practical under day-to-day conditions on commercial livestock facilities. There is no control group and only a single stream of data on commercial livestock facilities. Yet, it is important to determine with some degree of certainty whether a management intervention or product introduction is working and whether the processes are improving or getting worse. It is in this circumstance that SPC analysis is not only appropriate but also superior to other statistical or monitoring techniques. This argument alone provides a compelling reason for the application of the SPC tools in commercial livestock production systems. Because before and after comparisons are being made from a single stream of data, however, it is important to emphasize a need for the process to be stable (in a state of statistical control) before the new protocol or product is introduced to be sure that any observed process change is valid. It should be further noted that the smaller the process variation before introducing a known intervention, the greater the sensitivity for detecting small changes before and after comparisons.

The authors conclude that SPC can be successfully applied in livestock production systems. The time is right. The availability of large amounts of automatically collected data, the advances in computer capability, and the obvious need for more timely fact-based information for day-to-day management make SPC application the next step forward in improving herd management quality.

Examples of control chart use

Monitoring swine water intake by a time series plot and an I chart

Recent studies [20] show that monitoring water intake can help detect potential health problems in growing pigs. Individual readings plotted on a time series plot can provide insight into a developing crisis (Fig. 4) and offer a quick and easy way to monitor water intake on growing pigs in the barn; however, two difficulties arise in using time series plots. Reading a time series plot is subjective and leads to differences in interpretation depending on the person examining the plot. Was there a "real" change in water intake between days 15 and 27? How sure could one be by looking at this time series chart? When did the change begin and end? Using SPC charts to present the same data (Fig. 5) standardizes the interpretation so that every person reading the chart draws the same conclusion and can implement an appropriate standard intervention procedure without hesitation. As with any intake monitor for growing animals, however, readings have a tendency to increase with time. Plotting the raw values on an SPC chart will eventually cause signals to occur due to a natural increase of water intake in growing pigs rather than due to any special cause. Different methods have been developed to deal with this lack of independency between subsequent data points (autocorrelation). One of the methods is to model the dependency (in this case against time) and plot the residuals on an SPC chart. Fig. 5 is an example of an I chart in which the time effect has been modeled and the residuals are plotted to monitor for special cause variation. As mentioned previously, control limits on an SPC chart make the interpretation independent of who is looking at the plot and, therefore, help in making

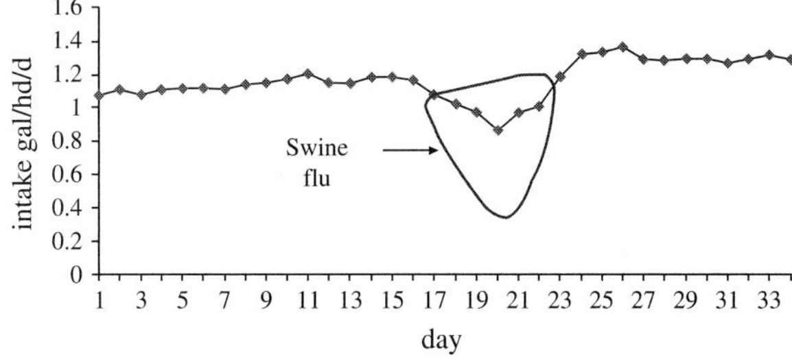

Fig. 4. Time series plot monitoring water intake (gallons/head/day) for growing swine. The circled period indicates time when swine flu occurred. (*Data from* http://porkcentral.unl.edu. Accessed June 29, 2005.)

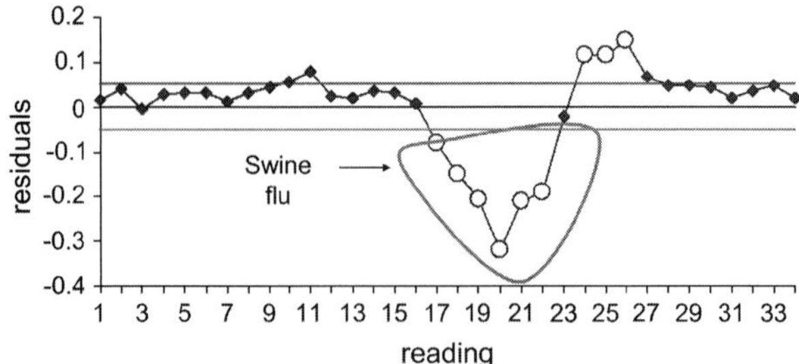

Fig. 5. I chart monitoring water intake for swine by plotting residuals of the fitted model. The data points labeled by white circles indicate points out of control according to the 3-σ rule. The circled period indicates time when swine flu occurred.

timely, fact-based decisions (in this case, concerning potential health problems among growing pigs).

I and EWMA chart comparison used to monitor bulk tank somatic cell counts

BTSCCs are a reflection of many on-farm processes that contribute to milk quality (milking routine, milking system, bedding routine, dry/fresh cow management, and so forth). They are therefore a good monitor of people, equipment, and animal performance. The following shows an example of BTSCC being monitored by an I chart (Fig. 6) and an EWMA chart (Fig. 7). A change in milking routine was implemented on 3/22. A significant drop in BTSCC was identified by the I chart 2 days later, whereas the EWMA took another 5 days to signal. This difference illustrates an important characteristic of EWMA (and CUSUM) charts. They can be designed for optimal performance for a specific change in mean/variation and perform well when the magnitude of occurring change is reasonably close to the anticipated design value. Generally, however, the I or X-bar chart signals a large shift sooner than an EWMA or CUSUM chart. Therefore,

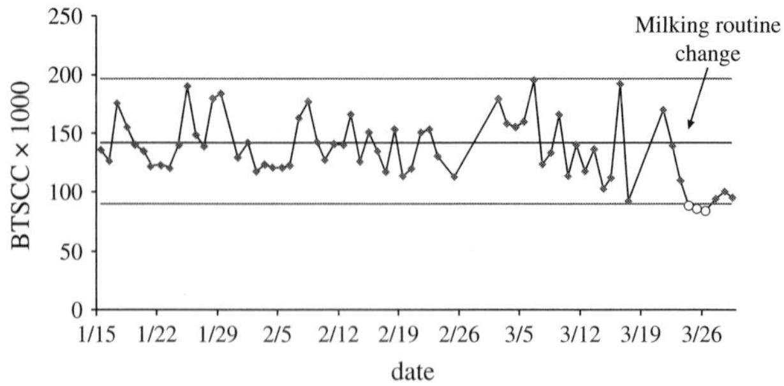

Fig. 6. I chart for BTSCCs. The arrow indicates the time when a change in milking routine was implemented. The data points labeled by white circles indicate points out of control according to the 3-σ rule.

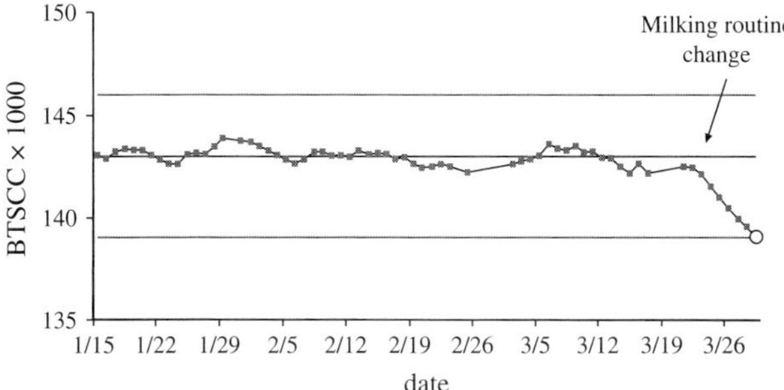

Fig. 7. EWMA chart for BTSCCs. The arrow indicates the time a change in milking routine was implemented. The data point labeled by the white circle indicates a point out of control according to the 3-σ rule.

when large and small shifts are to be detected, the recommended approach, as mentioned previously, is to plot both charts alongside each other.

Percentage of fresh cows in the first week post calving with fever monitored by a P chart

The number of fresh cows with fevers during the first 10 days after calving is indicative of dry, close up, and fresh cow management (Mark Kinsel, Ag Information Management, personal communication, June 2005). On a 2000-cow dairy, the proportion of cows with fever was monitored daily and compiled on a weekly basis, giving a sample size of around 40 (Fig. 8). For simplicity, it is assumed that the sample size (number of cows calving per week) is fairly constant throughout the year. Three "out of control" points on the lower side of the mean following a manager change indicate a significant decrease in the percentage of cows calving with fever and provide excellent feedback to the owner on his hiring decision (assuming the old and new managers recorded all the fever incidences among fresh cows).

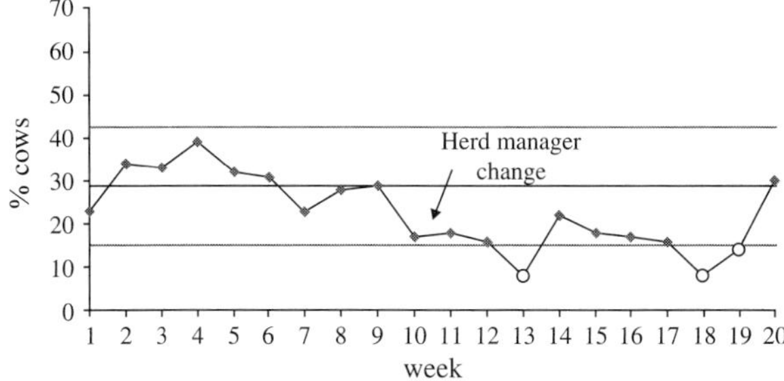

Fig. 8. P chart for monitoring percentage fresh cows with fever. The data points labeled by the white circles indicate points out of control according to the 3-σ rule. The arrow indicates the time a new herd manager was hired.

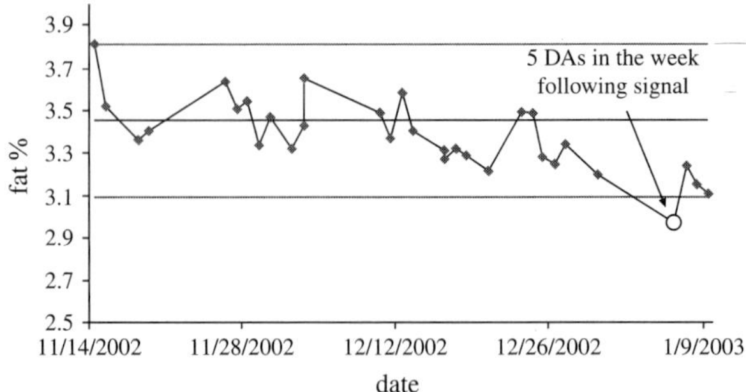

Fig. 9. I chart for monitoring daily milk fat percentage in the first lactation heifer group sampled with a line sampler. The data points labeled by the white circles indicate points out of control according to the 3-σ rule. The arrow indicates the time of signal.

As mentioned previously, many variables that can potentially be plotted on SPC charts to monitor process performance are already being collected on farms. The following are examples of two such variables and their possible role in monitoring herd nutrition.

Milk fat depression in a group of first lactation cows

Fig. 9 is an I chart of milk fat depression in a group of first lactation Holstein cows preceding an episode of displaced abomasums. An investigation into the root cause of the increased occurrence of displaced abomasums revealed a problem with the feeding process. A newly hired feeder had been routinely overmixing the total mixed ration (TMR) prepared for the heifer group, causing the feed to be deficient in effective fiber, resulting in milk fat depression and an increased occurrence of displaced abomasums in the group. There were five displaced abomasums in that group during the week following the control chart "signal."

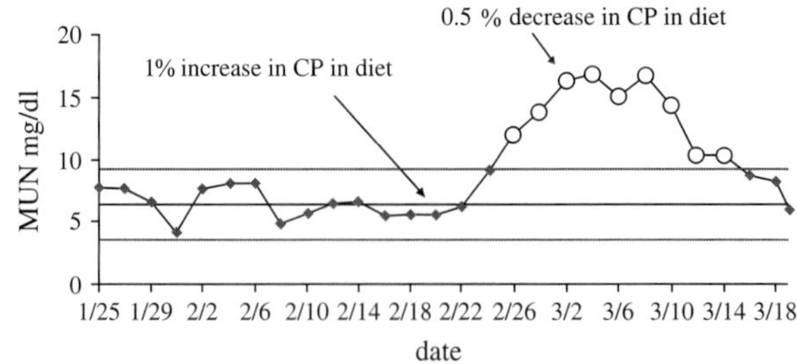

Fig. 10. I chart monitoring the MUN response to dietary crude protein (CP) change. The data points labeled by white circles indicate points out of control according to the 3-σ rule. Arrows indicate the time of change in CP concentration change in diet.

Milk urea nitrogen response to changes in dietary protein

It has been well documented that milk urea nitrogen (MUN) responds quickly to dietary changes [21]. Fig.10 shows a response of the bulk tank MUN to known changes in crude protein concentration in the diet of a group of late lactation cows at the University of Minnesota research herd in Morris, Minnesota.

Benchmarking variation

Benchmarking variation is not traditionally recognized as an SPC technique; however, benchmarking is a recognized quality management tool for determining the strengths and weaknesses of a business and an excellent method of motivating improvement. Because many livestock databases are standardized, benchmarking between farms is possible. Because each Shewhart control chart provides calculation of the process variable means and a sigma value, comparisons of process variation between farms is possible. The following dairy experience provides an example of how benchmarking variation can give insight into process quality or protocol consistency.

Variation as a tool in managing milk quality

Deming [1] summarized his theory of management in this often-quoted sentence: "If I had to reduce my message to management to just a few words, I'd say it all has to do with reducing variation." Although the authors have found this idea intuitive among dairy managers, study of herd data indicates that there is a great amount of process variation found on dairy farms today. Perhaps this process variation can best be demonstrated in exploring day-to-day variability in BTSCCs. It has been widely documented that the SCC level is inversely correlated to the quality of herd management [22]. The incidence of intramammary infection is correlated to the quantity of bacteria on teat surfaces [23–25]. Bodoh and colleagues [26] concluded that daily management and cow hygiene has more influence on BTSCC than dry cow therapy. Dairies with management styles described as "clean and accurate" had lower BTSCC compared with those described as "quick and dirty" [27].

Determining how consistently clients manage their livestock operations is important in assessing the quality of herd management. Understanding process variation is helpful in differentiating whether it is the process or the personnel (or both) that needs improvement.

In a study of 1500 Upper Midwest dairies for which SPC control charts [28] were completed for each milk pickup during 2003, the authors found a positive correlation between mean BTSCC level and day-to-day variation (sigma values). Herds with low BTSCC also had low day-to-day variation, and vice versa. The R^2 value was 0.4997 (Fig. 11), indicating that although

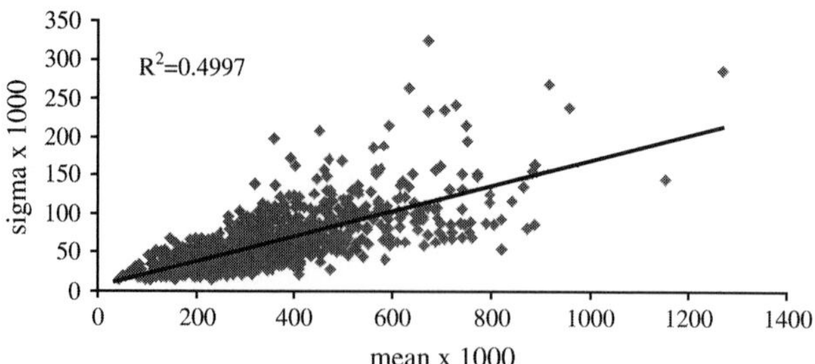

Fig. 11. Scatter plot of BTSCC sigma versus mean. Solid line plotted on the figure marks the regression line. R^2 value indicates the strength of the relationship between BTSCC mean and sigma.

50% of the variation can be explained by the change in SCC level alone, 50% of the variation can be attributed to the quality of the processes that result in the BTSCC. In a related study of 275 Minnesota Dairy Herd Improvement (DHI) herds for which SPC control chart techniques were used to evaluate SCC and milk components, it was found that the herds with the highest milk production also had the lowest mean BTSCC and the lowest BTSCC variation (Figs. 12 and 13). This finding confirms Deming's hypothesis that variation can be used to assess process quality.

There are two factors needing consideration in assessing process quality. The first is the process itself as measured by a variable mean. For example, in the case of BTSCC, a low mean BTSCC indicates that the management procedures (protocols) are appropriate and effective for achieving a low BTSCC. The second factor to consider is the process variation. Low day-to-day sigma values (variation) are a strong indication that personnel are applying protocols consistently every day. High sigma values (variation), on the other hand, indicate a need to improve the consistency in applying process protocols. Benchmarking of process means and sigma values can serve as a method of determining answers to common management questions such as Is this a process problem? or Is this a personnel problem?

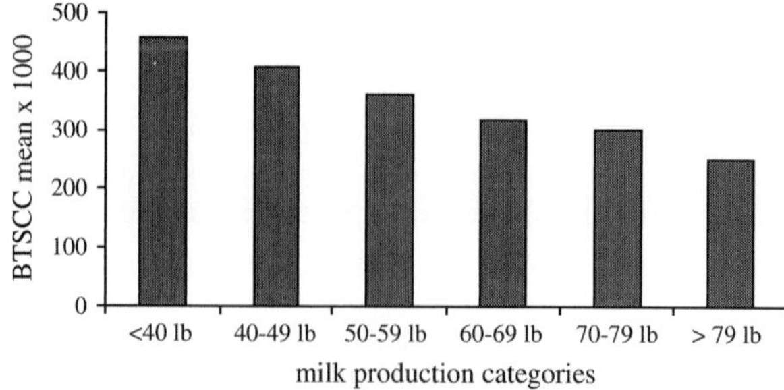

Fig. 12. BTSCC mean by production category for 275 Minnesota DHI dairies. The herds were divided into six production categories based on the average pounds of milk per cow.

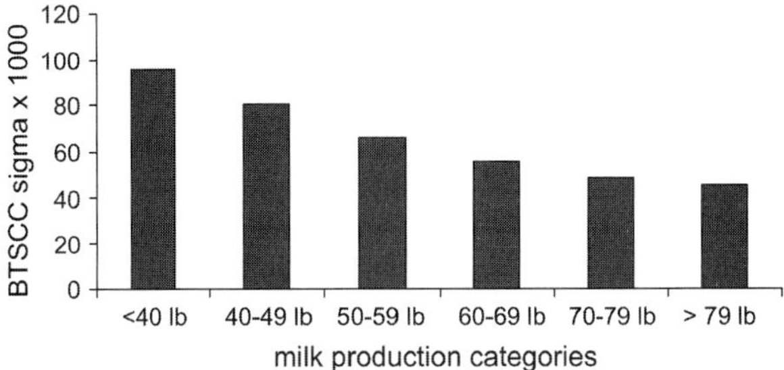

Fig. 13. BTSCC variation by production category for 275 Minnesota DHI dairies. The herds were divided into six production categories based on the average pounds of milk per cow.

Fig. 14 indicates the relationship between BTSCC level and the expected day-to-day variation based on analysis of daily BTSCC control charts for 1500 Upper Midwest dairies over 2 years. Because herd size has an effect on the degree of expected BTSCC variation, the 1500 herds were categorized into herds greater than 100 cows and herds less than 100 cows.

When a herd's average BTSCC and the day-to-day variation (sigma) are known, it is possible to determine the process quality relative to the level of herd management and the consistency with which protocols are being applied at the farm.

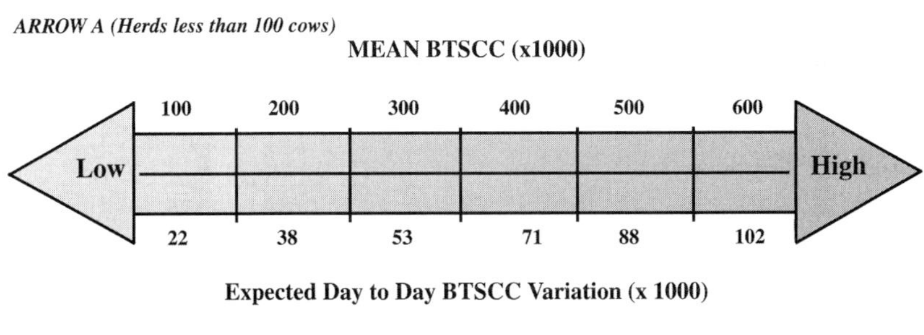

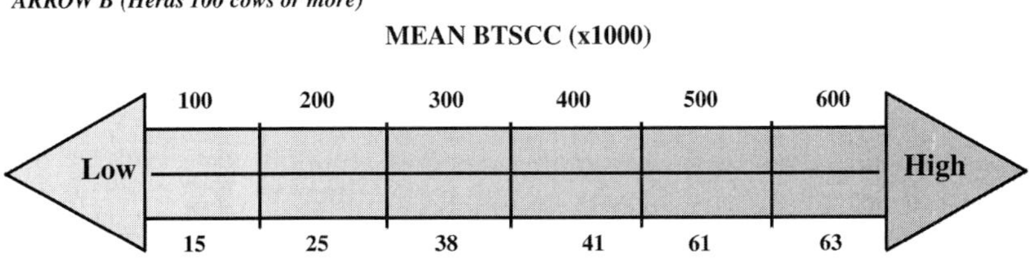

Fig. 14. Diagram for benchmarking BTSCC mean and variation. The data is based on milk tests of 1500 dairies for one year.

What if variation is low?

When the variation is low, the good news is that personnel are being consistent in their work. The bad news is that if the dairy is still not producing milk of desired quality, some things are being done consistently wrong. The consultant should take a closer look at how all tasks are performed, take measurements, and make observations. Some examples of the measurements to take when attempting to lower the SCC are cow density, bedding cultures, cow hygiene score, bulk tank cultures, and a number of other indicators that might help identify the root cause of the problem.

What if variation is high?

When the variation is higher than expected, it suggests a need to improve process compliance and consistency. Evaluation of employee compliance to protocols or the consistency with which protocols are followed is needed. On farms where standard operating procedures are not in place, encouragement should be given to write them. Routine employee training should be implemented to be sure that each employee understands his or her duties and is committed to following all standard operating procedures. Training is effective in reducing variation. Recent University of Wisconsin studies [29] indicate that herds with more frequent training of milkers had lower BTSCCs.

What if variation is average?

If the variation for BTSCC is somewhere in the middle of the indicated range and there is a desire by the dairy to lower BTSCC, then improvement in consistency of personnel performance and the processes themselves is needed. Experience has shown that it is best to start by improving consistency and protocol compliance because it makes it easier to identify true improvement in performance. By reducing the variation in performance first, it is easier to determine whether the implemented changes actually result in any improvement in milk quality after changes are made in the processes.

A 200-cow dairy with a BTSCC mean of 300,000 cells/mL and a day-to-day variation of 22,000 (sigma value of 22) can be used as an example. Assuming the herd's goal is to qualify for the quality premium for a BTSCC under 200,000, what should be done? Should personnel be hassled about the consistency of milking and bedding management routines or should methods of improving the total process be explored? The answer is obvious. Because day-to-day variation is lower than expected for a BTSCC of 300,000, the current BTSCC level is not likely to be the result of inconsistent application of protocols by milking personnel. It is more likely that the personnel are consistent in applying the protocols but the protocols themselves are not capable of delivering a BTSCC of less than 300,000. What is the solution? Work should be done to improve the process protocols.

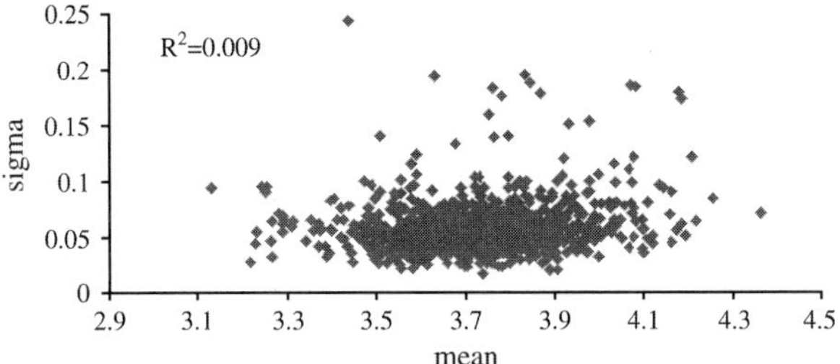

Fig. 15. Scatter plot of bulk tank (BT) milk fat percentage sigma versus mean in 1500 upper Midwest dairies. R^2 value indicates the strength of the relationship.

Benchmarking variation as a tool in managing feeding consistency

Can analysis of day-to-day variation of milk fat, protein, MUN, dry matter, dry matter intake, pounds of milk per cow per day, or feed efficiency give insight into feeding management? Although the jury is still out, evidence is building that SPC use could be useful for managing dairy herd nutrition. Regardless of how well a diet is formulated, it needs to be fed consistently to achieve its desired results. Variation between the formulated diet and the diet consumed by the cow is common. This variability can be caused by variability in the feeds, the feeder, or the cow [30,31].

Figs. 15, 16, and 17 show the correlation between day-to-day variation in and levels of milk fat percentage, protein percentage, and MUN, respectively. These plots are interesting because they indicate that there is no relationship between the degree of variation and the level of milk fat percentage, protein percentage, or MUN. In contrast to BTSCCs, whereby only half of the variation can be attributed to the processes involved in producing a BTSCC, all the variation at any milk fat, protein, or MUN level may be due to the management or biologic processes that effect these variables. In addition, there are no great differences in the degree of variation because of herd size. This news may be good for nutritionists because interpretation of variation is simplified.

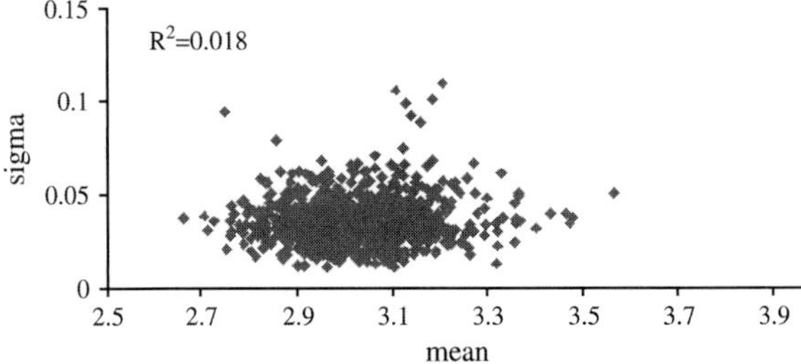

Fig. 16. Scatter plot of bulk tank (BT) milk protein percentage sigma versus mean in 1500 upper Midwest dairies. R^2 value indicates the strength of the relationship.

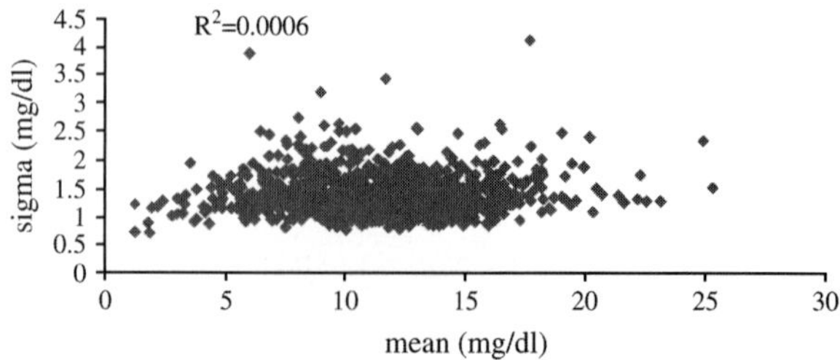

Fig. 17. Scatter plot of bulk tank (BT) MUN sigma versus mean in 1300 upper Midwest dairies. R^2 value indicates the strength of the relationship.

Fig. 18A and B shows the spectrum of day-to-day variation in bulk tank milk fat percentage and protein percentage for 1500 Upper Midwest dairies monitored at each milk pickup in 2003. The MUN variation (see Fig. 18C) was from 1300 dairies of the same data set monitored at each milk pickup for 6 months and, therefore, may not fully represent seasonal variation in MUN. It should also be pointed out that these milk component data represent whole-herd bulk tank samples and not individual feeding groups.

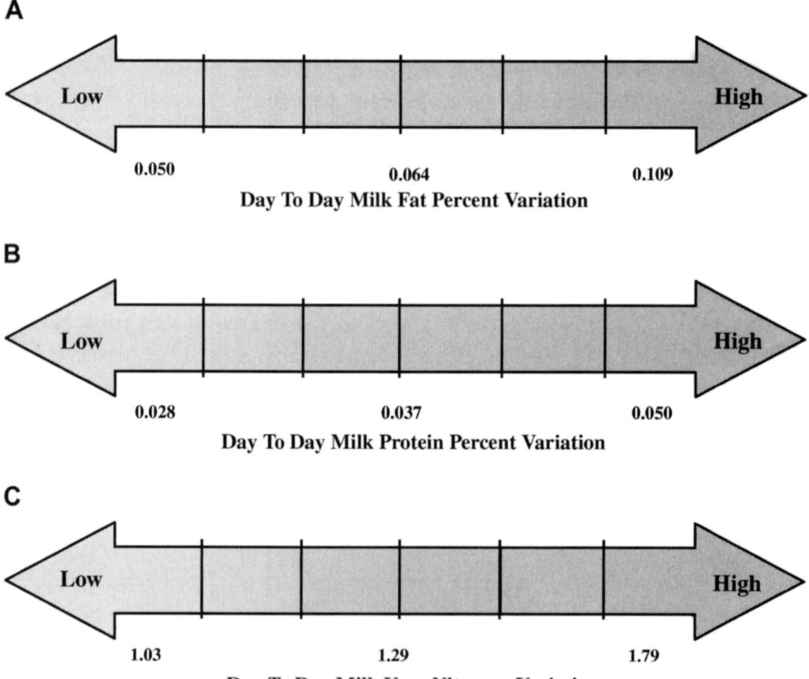

Fig. 18. (*A*) Diagram used for benchmarking variation in bulk tank milk fat percentage. (*B*) Diagram used for benchmarking variation in bulk tank milk protein percentage. (*C*) Diagram used for benchmarking variation in bulk tank MUN.

It is currently thought that benchmarking day-to-day variation of milk components can be useful in giving insight to dairy farm feeding management of lactating cows. Generally speaking, low day-to-day variation in milk fat, protein, and MUN implies that a very consistent feeding program is being implemented on the farm. High variation implies the opposite is true. Because most larger dairies have several feeding groups, greater sensitivity in assessing the feeding process variation can be achieved by collecting line samples from each feeding group [32]. This sampling is consistent with the previous discussion about rational subgrouping design. Each feeding group could have control charts completed simultaneously for lactating group inputs (ie, dry matter intake) and process outputs (ie, milk components and average pounds per cow per day), providing well-rounded real-time feedback to facilitate more timely day-to-day nutritional management decisions.

High variation suggests a need to improve process compliance and consistency. When the variation is low, the good news is that the feeds, the employees, and the cows are consistent. The bad news is that if the cows are still not performing up to expectation, then perhaps some things are being done consistently wrong (eg, consistently feeding poor-quality forages or routinely overmixing the TMR). What should be done? A closer look should be taken at how all tasks are performed, measurements should be taken, and observations should be made. The evaluation should include bunk space, feed dry matter change, TMR mixing time, manure score, particle size of feed that is fed to the cows, and refusals, to name a few. As was previously mentioned but well worth repeating, experience has shown that it is best to start by improving consistency and protocol compliance. This practice makes it easier to identify true improvement in performance. After changes are made to the processes, it will be easier to determine whether the implemented changes resulted in any real improvement in process quality if the variation in performance is first reduced.

Available statistical process control tools

Personal computer–based software

There are numerous SPC software products available for personal computer application, ranging from Microsoft Excel (Microsoft Corp., Redmond, Washington) add-ons to very sophisticated stand-alone SPC software products. The price range for these products is $129 to $600. The advantage of personal computer–based software is more independence and flexibility. The disadvantage is that the user not only must be more knowledgeable in SPC software use but also the custodian of the data, which usually includes the time-consuming effort of data entry and report generation. The following are recommended Web sites where product information can be found:

http://www.qualityamerica.com/QAProducts/softwareproducts.htm
http://www.statistix.com/home.html

http://www.excel-spc-software.com/excel-spc-software.html
http://www.ozgrid.com/Services/statistical-Quality-Control.htm

Web-based statistical process control tools

The advantages of Web-based SPC tools are numerous. The Web-based system allows freedom from data storage and software updates. Consultants and their clients do not need to worry about software compatibility, and SPC results can be accessed from any Internet computer terminal anywhere, at any time. Because much of the data is automatically uploaded to the web server, manual data entry is minimized or entirely eliminated. Automated electronic mail alert systems can provide the consultant and the client with a "24/7" vigilance over critical farm processes without having to be physically at the farm. The disadvantages of a Web-based system are that only a few variables are tracked and there may be less flexibility in tracking the variable of interest. At the time of this writing, there is only one Web-based SPC product that is limited to dairy use: MilkLab at www.dairyperformance.com, offered by Ag Information Management.

Summary

SPC techniques have been used successfully for 80 years in manufacturing as a quality management tool to improve the timeliness and accuracy of management decisions and to improve personnel performance. It is apparent that these techniques can be applied equally well to livestock production systems and can improve herd management and profitability.

References

[1] Deming WE. Out of the crisis. London: MIT Press; 1986.
[2] Ishikawa K. What is total quality control? The Japanese way. Englewood Cliffs (NJ): Prentice-Hall; 1984.
[3] Carey RG. Improving healthcare with control charts. Milwaukee (WI): ASQ Quality Press; 2003.
[4] Montgomery DC. Introduction to statistical quality control. New York: John Wiley & Sons; 2005.
[5] Edwards JL, Tozer PR. Using activity and milk yield as predictors of fresh cow disorders. J Dairy Sci 2004;87(2):524–31.
[6] Wrathall AE. Reproductive failure in the pig: diagnosis and control. Vet Rec 1977;100: 230–7.
[7] Wilson MR, McMillan I, Swaminathan SS. Computerized health monitoring in swine health management. Pig Vet Soc Proc 1980;6:64–71.
[8] Kniffen T. Potential uses of SPC in a pork production system. In: Veterinary Outreach Program. Statistical process control. Proceedings of the Allen D. Leman Swine Conference. St. Paul (MN): University of Minnesota; 1998. p. 1–12.

[9] Koketsu Y, Duangkaew C, Dial GD, et al. Within-farm variability in number of females mated per week during a one-year period and breeding herd productivity on swine farms. J Am Vet Med Assoc 1999;214:520–4.
[10] Sard DM. Dealing with data: the practical use of numerical information—(14) monitoring changes. Vet Rec 1979;105:323–8.
[11] Ravindranthan N, Unni AKK. A study on consistency in body weights of chicks using Shewhart control charts. Cheiron 1990;19:156–8.
[12] Cowen P, Fernanadez D, Barnes HJ. Surveillance strategies for monitoring variation in animal health and productivity: the use of statistical process control in turkey industry. Kenya Vet 1994;18:202–4.
[13] Marsh WE, de Vries A, Reneau JK, et al. Monitoring performance: statistical process control in dairy herd management. In: Proceedings of the Annual Northeast Dairy Production Medicine Symposium. 6th edition. Syracuse (NY): 1997. p. 34–46.
[14] Reneau JK, Kinsel ML. Record systems and herd monitoring in production-oriented health and management programs in food producing animals. In: Radostits OM, editor. Herd health: food animal production medicine. Philadelphia: WB Saunders; 2001.
[15] de Vries A, Conlin BJ. Design and performance of statistical process control charts applied to estrous detection efficiency. J Dairy Sci 2003;86:1970–84.
[16] Wrathall AE, Hebert CN. Monitoring reproductive performance in the pig herd. Pig Vet Soc Proc 1982;9:136–48.
[17] Cowen P, Fernandez D, Barnes HJ. Surveillance strategies for monitoring variation in animal health and productivity: the use of statistical process control in turkey industry. Kenya Vet 1994;18:202–4.
[18] Polson D. SPC = statistical pig control. Int Pigletter 1998;18:43–6.
[19] Natzke D. 'Statistics' key piece of process analysis. Midwest Dairy Business 2005;Jan:9–10.
[20] Brumm MC. Water as a predictor of tomorrow's pig performance. Available at: http://pork central.unl.edu/water%20predict.pdf. Accessed June 29, 2005.
[21] Wattiaux MA. Fine-tuning test-day MUN records for DHI-related variables. In: Proceedings of the Four-State Dairy Nutrition and Management Conference. Dubuque (IA): Iowa State University; 2005. p. 75–83.
[22] Bennett RH. Milk quality and mastitis: the management connection. In: Proceedings of the National Mastitis Council. Orlando (FL): 1987. p. 133–50.
[23] Neave FK, Dodd FH, Kingwill RG. A method of controlling udder disease. Vet Rec 1966; 78:521–5.
[24] Guterbock WM, Blackmer PE. Veterinary interpretation of bulk-tank milk. Vet Clin North Am Large Anim Pract 1984;6(2):257–68.
[25] Pankey JW. Premilking udder hygiene. J Dairy Sci 1989;2:1308–12.
[26] Bodoh GW, Battista WJ, Schultz LH. Variation in somatic cell counts in dairy herd improvement milk samples. J Dairy Sci 1976;59:1119–23.
[27] Barkema HW, Van der Ploeg JD, Schukken YH, et al. Management style and its association with bulk tank somatic cell count and incidence of clinical mastitis. J Dairy Sci 1999;82:1655–63.
[28] Lukas J, Kinsel ML, Reneau JK. Consistency index as a dynamic field measure of BTSCC variation [abstract]. In: ADSA ASAS PSA Joint Meeting Abstracts. Savoy (IL): American Dairy Science Association 2004. p. 375. Abstract W248.
[29] Ruegg P. Pre-milking cow preparation—secret methods of producing high quality milk. In: Proceedings of the National Mastitis Council Regional Meeting. Verona (WI): National Mastitis Council; 2004. p. 34–40.
[30] Stone WC. What is acceptable variation in the nutrition program and how can it be managed? In: Proceedings of the Southwest Nutrition Conference. Verona (WI): National Mastitis Council; 2005. p. 1–10.
[31] Weiss WP. Variation exists in composition of concentrate feeds. Feedstuffs 2004;May:11–13.
[32] Godden SBR, Reneau JK, Farnsworth R, et al. Field validation of a milk-line sampling device for monitoring milk component data. J Dairy Sci 2002;85(9):2192–6.

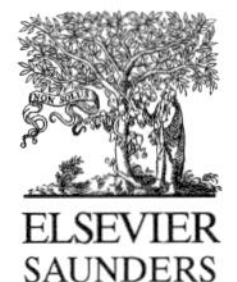
ELSEVIER
SAUNDERS

Vet Clin Food Anim 22 (2006) 195–205

VETERINARY
CLINICS
Food Animal Practice

Using and Interpreting Diagnostic Tests

Shawn L.B. McKenna, DVM, PhD*,
Ian R. Dohoo, DVM, PhD

Department of Health Management, Atlantic Veterinary College, University of Prince Edward Island, 550 University Avenue, Charlottetown, PEI, C1A 4P3, Canada

Diagnostic tests are an integral part of large animal veterinary practice. Typically, we think of a diagnostic test as being applied to a sample (eg, serum, milk, feces) that is sent to a laboratory for testing (eg, a milk sample for blood calcium levels or a milk sample for mastitis pathogen culture). Any information-gathering procedure, however, can be viewed as a diagnostic test. For example, history taking, clinical examination, rectal palpation, and evaluation of an animal's environment can all be considered diagnostic tests. The issues related to the use and interpretation of diagnostic tests described in this article apply equally to these procedures.

Diagnostic tests can be used to identify disease risk factors (eg, Does a dairy herd have excessive teat-end vacuum fluctuations in their milking machines?), disease states (eg, Is a cow hypocalcemic?), infection status (eg, Is a steer infected with *Mycobacterium avium* subsp *paratuberculosis* [MAP]?), or evidence of exposure (eg, a serologic titer). The distinction between disease, infection, and exposure is important to keep in mind when dealing with tests for infectious diseases. Throughout this article, the authors use examples of tests designed to detect infection or exposure to MAP, but given the persistent nature of these infections, the authors consider exposure indicative of infection.

Diagnostic tests can be applied to an individual or a group of individuals to look for evidence of disease or infection. In the latter case, the test is sometimes referred to as a "screening test," but the principles involved in using screening tests are the same as those for a diagnostic test on an individual animal, so the authors refer to tests as diagnostic tests throughout this article. Tests can also be applied at the animal or herd level (or at other levels of organization). For example, milk cultures can be

* Corresponding author.
E-mail address: slmckenna@upei.ca (S.L.B. McKenna).

doi:10.1016/j.cvfa.2005.12.006 *vetfood.theclinics.com*

performed at the quarter, cow (composite sample), or herd (bulk tank) levels. For simplicity, throughout this article, the authors focus their discussion at the animal level, but all of the principles described also apply to the other levels.

Two important facts need to be kept in mind when considering using a diagnostic test:

1. Tests are not infallible. They will sometimes give the wrong answer, and understanding the implications of those wrong answers is the focus of much of the material in this article.
2. Tests should only be used if the result will influence the course of action. Using tests on the basis of "Well, it would be nice to know," or "Let us test and see what we get" is likely going to be a waste of money. Before applying a test, the practitioner should have a clear idea of how the test result will impact on his or her decision regarding the animal or herd.

Sensitivity and specificity

In a laboratory, the sensitivity (Se) of a test relates to the ability of a test to detect very small quantities of a substance, which is called the **analytic Se**. For a laboratory, the specificity (Sp) of a test relates to its ability to react to a single compound (chemical, infectious agent, and so forth), which is called the **analytic Sp**.

As clinicians, we are more interested in how well a test is able to classify whether an animal is diseased (or infected or exposed). These measures are called the **diagnostic Se** and the **diagnostic Sp**, but for the sake of brevity, the authors simply call them the Se and the Sp of the test.

The Se of a test is the ability of the test to correctly classify an infected (or diseased or exposed) animal as being infected (or diseased or exposed). If a fecal culture is done on 165 animals that are known to be infected (D+), and 36 come up as culture positive (T+), then the Se of the test is

$$\mathrm{Se} = \frac{\text{Number of test-positive animals}}{\text{Number of truly infected animals}} = \frac{\mathrm{T+}}{\mathrm{D+}} = \frac{36}{165} = 22\%$$

Infected animals that produce a negative test result (T−) are called **false negatives**, and the proportion of disease-positive animals that give a give a negative test result is known as the **false negative rate**, which is equal to (1 − Se).

The Sp of a test is its ability to correctly classify noninfected animals. If the same fecal culture is done on 823 noninfected animals and all 823 come up culture negative, then the Sp of the test is

$$\text{Sp} = \frac{\text{Number of test-negative animals}}{\text{Number of truly noninfected animals}} = \frac{\text{T}-}{\text{D}-} = \frac{823}{823} = 100\%$$

Noninfected animals that produce a positive test result (T+) are called **false positives**, and the proportion of disease-negative animals that give a positive test result is known as the **false positive rate**, which is equal to (1 – Sp).

Determining the Se and the Sp of a test implies that the true status of the animal is known, but this knowledge is possible only when there is a "**gold standard**" test—or a combination of tests—that always gives the correct answer. Rarely is there a true gold standard test, but in some circumstances, practitioners can come up with a method of determining the true status that they believe is close enough to be considered "gold." For instance, in the Johne's disease examples used in this article, the gold standard was based on culturing or recovery of the causative organism (MAP). The authors believe that this test gives a good indication of whether an animal is infected. The accuracy of a test refers to a combination of its Se and Sp but is not a very useful term because ultimately, you need to know both the Se and the Sp of a test.

Data for the evaluation of a diagnostic test are often laid out in a 2 × 2 table as shown in Table 1. For the MAP example [1], the data for the evaluation of the fecal culture compared with tissue culture (gold standard) are shown in Table 2. Based on these data, the Se of the test is 36/165 = 22% and the Sp is 823/823 = 100%.

Many tests (eg, serum calcium, MAP ELISA) produce results on a continuous scale (ie, they can have many values) instead of as a dichotomous (positive/negative) result. Practitioners, however, often want to classify animals as positive or negative (eg, hypocalcemic or not, MAP infected or not), so they must choose a cutpoint. If the test result is over the cutpoint, then the animal is considered T+; if the test result is under the cutpoint, then the animal is classified as T–. The distribution of possible test results from infected and noninfected animals often overlap, however, so there is no cutpoint that provides completely correct classification (Se = 100% and Sp = 100%). As can be seen in Fig. 1, increasing the cutpoint reduces the number of false positives (increased Sp) but increases the number of false negatives (reduced Se). Lowering the cutpoint has the opposite effect.

Table 1
A 2 × 2 table of test results versus "gold standard" disease classification

	Test result		
True disease status (gold standard)	T+	T–	Total
D+	a	b	a + b
D–	c	d	c + d
Total	a + c	b + d	n

Table 2
A 2 × 2 table of *Mycobacterium avium* Subsp *paratuberculosis* fecal culture results versus disease classification based on tissue cultures[a]

Tissue culture (gold standard)	Fecal culture T+	Fecal culture T−	Total
D+	36	129	165
D−	0	823	823
Total	36	952	988

[a] Five animals that were fecal culture positive but tissue culture negative were classified as infected on the basis that it is very unlikely that a fecal positive animal is not truly infected.

The decision of where to set the cutpoint can be based on whether it is more important to minimize false positives or false negatives. If a MAP ELISA was being used and positive cattle were to be culled, then a very high cutpoint would be needed to ensure that very few noninfected cattle were culled. If, however, the ELISA was to be used only as a screening test to determine which cattle should have fecal cultures done, then a lower threshold could be used so that very few infected animals would be missed.

The Se and Sp of a test are not something that the practitioner is likely to determine in practice. One must rely on research studies to provide this information. When evaluating a research report, the following two questions should be asked:

1. How good was the gold standard used in the study? Evaluating a test against a poor gold standard will provide misleading results. In some studies, the standards are not "gold," "silver," or "bronze"—"tin" would be a better description.
2. How representative of the population are the animals that will be tested? This question is particularly relevant with regard to the stage of disease

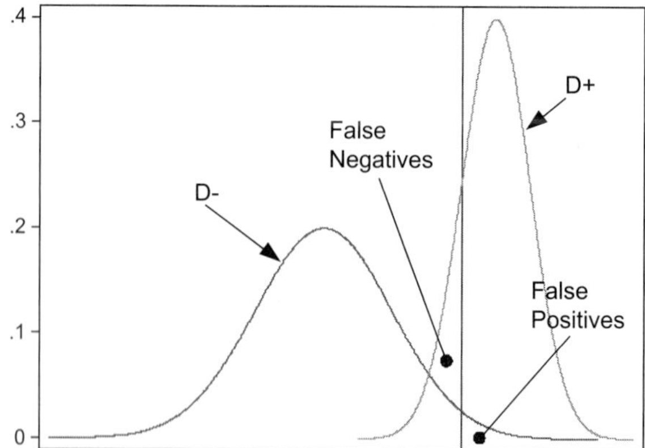

Fig. 1. Effect of changing cutpoint on Se and Sp of a diagnostic test.

of the animals. Evaluating a test for MAP in a population in which the D+ cows have clinical signs will grossly overestimate the Se of the test compared with an evaluation that includes many animals in early stages of the disease.

Apparent prevalence and predictive values

Although it is important to know the Se and Sp of a diagnostic test, knowing these is not adequate to effectively use a test in a clinical setting. Both are based on the assumption that the true infection status of the animal is known, but in practice, this status is not known. Clinicians need to know

- How likely it is that an animal is truly infected if it has a positive test result. This value is called the **positive predictive value** (PPV).
- How confident they can be that an animal is truly noninfected if it has a negative test result. This value is called the **negative predictive value** (NPV).
- How close the **apparent prevalence** (AP; an estimate of the prevalence of infection based on the number of positive test results) will be to the **true prevalence** of infection in the population when testing a group of animals.

Based on the data in Table 2, the PPV is 36/36 = 100%. (Note: the only reason that the PPV is 100% is that the Sp of the test is 100%, which only occurs with culture-based procedures). The NPV is 823/952 = 86%. The AP of MAP is 36/988 = 3.6%, which is much lower than the true prevalence of MAP (165/988 = 16.7%).

Because predictive values and AP depend not only on the Se and Sp of the test but also on the true prevalence of infection in the population in which the test is being used, diagnostic tests perform differently in different populations. What a positive test result means in one herd is not the same as what it means in another herd.

The following example demonstrates this concept: an ELISA for bovine viral diarrhea (BVD) was evaluated using a virus neutralization test as a gold standard [2]. The evaluation was performed in 1000 animals, of which 521 were positive on the virus neutralization test (Table 3, left panel). The Se of this test is 98% and the Sp is 99%. In this study population, the PPV is 510/514 = 99% and the NPV is 475/486 = 94%. If an animal from this population has a positive test result, it is almost certainly infected (PPV = 99%).

In a low-prevalence (1%) population (see Table 3, right panel), the PPV is now only 99/199 = 50%, whereas the NPV is 9890/9891 = 100%. Even though this ELISA has a very high Se and Sp, there is only a 50:50 chance that an animal with a positive test result is truly infected. In the low-prevalence population, half of the test-positive animals are false positives. Certainly, a positive test result in this population has a completely different meaning than a positive test result in the study population.

Table 3
Evaluation of a bovine viral diarrhea ELISA compared with a virus neutralization test as the "gold standard" in two populations with high (52%) and low (1%) prevalence

Virus neutralization test (gold standard)	Study population ELISA T+	T−	Totals	Low-prevalence population ELISA T+	T−	Totals
D+	510	11	521	99	1	100
D−	4	475	479	100	9890	9990
Total	514	486	1000	199	9891	10000

In the study population, the AP is 514/1000 = 51.4%, which is very close to the true prevalence of 52.1%. In the low-prevalence population, however, the AP is 199/10,000 = 2%, which is double the true prevalence (1%). In most cases, the AP overestimates the true prevalence in low-prevalence populations (unless the Se of the test is very poor).

The effect of prevalence on the predictive values for this BVD ELISA can be seen in Fig. 2. In this case, because the Se and the Sp of the test are very high, the predictive values fall off by a large degree only when the prevalence goes low or high. In general, PPVs are always low when a test is used in a low-prevalence population, unless the test has perfect Sp (100%). Because of the strong connection between prevalence and PPVs, reports in the literature of predictive values are of very limited use: they only apply to the population in which the study was conducted.

Agreement among tests

In some situations, clinicians want to determine how well two tests agree, without regard for their Se or Sp (eg, comparing two ELISAs for MAP). In

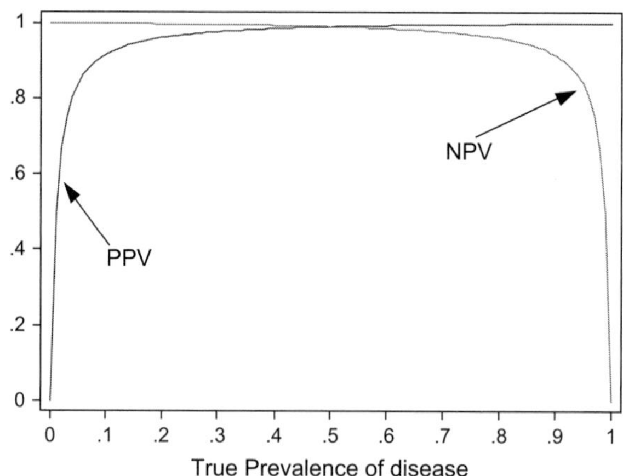

Fig. 2. Effect of prevalence on predictive values.

other cases, because it is not possible to come up with a suitable gold standard for evaluating Se and Sp, we can only see how well a new test compares with a test that is currently being used. The **observed agreement**, which is the proportion of animals in which two tests agree, could be computed; however, some of that agreement is just going to be due to chance. (If a coin is flipped twice, some of the time it will show 2 heads or 2 tails, but that does not mean there is any connection between the two coin tosses).

Consequently, a measure of agreement is needed that adjusts for the amount of agreement that could be attained by chance alone. For this calculation, clinicians use **kappa** (κ), which measures the amount of agreement above and beyond what one would expect from chance alone. (For method of calculation, see Dohoo and colleagues [3]). A κ value of 1 indicates perfect agreement between tests, whereas a value of 0 indicates no agreement beyond what would be expected by chance.

For an example, the authors compared two ELISAs (from different test kit manufacturers) for MAP in 160 cows that were tissue culture positive (ie, all of these animals were truly infected) [4]. The data are shown in Table 4. Although all of the animals were infected, neither test produced many positive test results. The observed agreement, however, is $(6 + 141)/160 = 92\%$. On the surface, this agreement seems good, but most of it is due to there being many infected animals that neither test was able to detect. Of the 19 animals that one or both tests found to be positive, only 6 were found to be positive by both tests. The κ value for this comparison is only 0.45, suggesting poor agreement beyond what would be expected by chance alone. (Note, when disease prevalence is low [<20%] or high [>20%], κ values are negatively biased, so the estimate of 0.45 in this situation will be a bit of an underestimation, but it is clear that the two tests do not agree very well). If tests are measured on a continuous scale, then their agreement can be evaluated by computing a concordance correlation. This calculation, however, is beyond the scope of this article (see Dohoo and colleagues for details [3]).

Measures of test agreement can be used to compare laboratories. When duplicate samples are sent to the same laboratory, the agreement between the two sets of test results is a measure of within-laboratory agreement and is called the **repeatability** of a test. When duplicate samples are sent to different laboratories, the between-laboratory agreement is called the **reproducibility** of the test (assuming that the two laboratories are running the

Table 4
A 2 ×2 table for comparing two ELISAs for *Mycobacterium avium* subsp *paratuberculosis* using samples taken from 160 cows that were tissue culture positive

	ELISA B		
ELISA A	T+	T−	Total
T+	6	8	14
T−	5	141	146
Total	11	149	160

same test). Most practitioners do not evaluate the repeatability or reproducibility of tests within or between laboratories, but it is important to determine whether the laboratory is monitoring their own performance routinely as part of the quality assurance program.

Using multiple tests

Practitioners are often in a position in which they have multiple tests to choose from, and it may be to their advantage to use two or more tests when dealing with a clinical problem. For this discussion, the authors consider the use of ELISA and fecal culture in a herd of dairy cows to determine which cows have MAP. Table 5 shows the results of the two tests when applied to the same 988 cows presented in Table 2.

A pair (or more) of tests can be interpreted in two ways. If an animal is considered positive if it tests positive on either test, then **parallel** interpretation is being used. Based on the data in Table 5, this interpretation results in an Se of (6 + 30 + 8)/165 = 27%. Only animals negative on both tests are considered negative, so the Sp is 803/823 = 98%. Parallel interpretation maximizes Se but reduces Sp. The tests might be interpreted this way if the practitioner wanted to identify all cows for which special care should be taken to minimize contact with calves in the herd.

Two tests are interpreted in **series** if an animal is considered positive only if it is positive on both tests. In this case, the inexpensive test (eg, ELISA) is often applied first and then the more expensive test (eg, fecal culture) is carried out only on animals that were positive on the first test. Using this interpretation, the Se of the combined tests is 6/165 = 3.6%, whereas the Sp is 823/823 = 100%. Series interpretation maximizes Sp. This approach would be appropriate if the practitioner was going to cull test-positive animals but wanted to minimize the number of noninfected cows culled.

Herd-level testing

In many situations, practitioners want to determine whether a herd is positive or negative for a disease of interest. If the herd status is determined

Table 5
Classification of cows according to fecal culture, ELISA, and true infection status for Johne's disease

	Number of cows by test-result category				Total
Fecal culture	+	+	−	−	
ELISA	+	−	+	−	
D+	6	30	8	121	165
D−	0	0	20	803	823
Series interpretation	+	−	−	−	
Parallel interpretation	+	+	+	−	

by testing a single sample that already represents the whole herd (eg, bulk tank milk culture), then all of the principles described previously can be applied directly. Often, however, a herd's status can be determined by testing multiple individual animals and then drawing a conclusion about the herd from those test results.

The herd-level Se (HSe) and the herd-level Sp (HSp) of a testing program depend on four factors:

- Se of the test applied at the individual animal level
- Sp of the test applied at the individual animal level
- Number of animals tested (and possibly the size of the herd)
- Number of positive test results required to declare the herd as infected

Assuming that a single positive test result is all that is required to declare the herd as infected and that the number of animals to be tested is relatively small compared with the size of the herd, in this case, an infected herd will be misclassified as noninfected only if all test results are negative. The probability of one animal being test negative is (1 − AP), so the probability of all animals being test negative is $(1 - AP)^n$, where *n* is the number of individual animal tests performed. Consequently, $HSe = 1 - (1 - AP)^n$.

A negative herd will be considered negative if all test results are negative—the chance of this happening is Sp^n, so $HSp = Sp^n$.

For other situations, it is much easier to use freely available software such as Herdacc (© Dave Jordan, 1995) [5] to perform the calculations. If the objective is specifically to be able to declare a herd free of a disease, then the program FreeCalc (© Angus Cameron) [6] can be used to determine the number of animals that need to be tested. Both of these programs are available through access of the Internet [7].

To illustrate the implications of herd-level testing, an example using the BVD ELISA (Se = 98% and Sp = 99%) on two fictitious 200-cow herds (one free of disease and one with 10% prevalence) using the Herdacc program is presented in Table 6. The point illustrated for the negative herd is

Table 6
Herd-level sensitivity and specificity calculations for two herds (one negative and one positive with 10% of cows infected with bovine viral diarrhea) tested with a bovine viral diarrhea ELISA

Herd	Sample size	Cutpoint	HSe (%)	HSp (%)
Negative	10	1	na	90.1
	20	1	na	81.2
	10	2	na	99.8
	20	2	na	99.0
Positive	10	1	67.9	na
	20	1	90.4	na
	10	2	28.3	na
	20	2	65.3	na

Abbreviation: na, not applicable.

that one does not need to test the whole herd to be relatively certain that the herd is negative, especially when using a test with a high Sp. This example illustrates that because no tests are perfect, it is better to allow for two positive tests before a herd is called positive to maximize the HSp because if enough animals are tested, there will be some false positives. For the positive herd, using a cutpoint of one positive test will maximize the HSe, but this impact is highly influenced by prevalence in the herd.

Other issues

There are a number of other issues related to the use and interpretation of diagnostic tests but they are beyond the scope of this article. The authors, however, provide a brief introduction to each of these areas and references for further reading.

Evaluating tests in the absence of a gold standard

There has been much recent research into the development of methods for evaluating tests when there is no gold standard available. These methods were recently reviewed by Enoe and colleagues [8]; here, the authors just summarize the requirements for this approach. To carry out this type of analysis, one must have test results from two or more tests from two or more populations that have distinctly different prevalences of disease. The methods are based on several key assumptions. The first assumption is that the tests are independent (ie, the result on the first test does not influence the likelihood of a given result on the second test). This situation is most likely to be true if the tests are biologically independent (eg, a culture procedure and a polymerase chain reaction). Second, it assumes that the Se and the Sp of the test are the same in the two populations. These assumptions can be relaxed when data are available on more than two tests or more than two populations. As these methods become more widely used, it is inevitable that practitioners will see more good evaluations of diagnostic tests in the veterinary literature.

Using pooled samples

In many cases, it is desirable to pool samples (eg, milk, blood, feces) before testing the sample to keep down the cost of testing. The Se and the Sp of pooled samples are affected by the analytic Se and Sp of the test, the concentration of the agent in the individual samples, the number of animals combined into each pool, and the prevalence (and concentration) of cross-reacting agents in the samples. The Se and the Sp of pooled sampling procedures need to be evaluated in much the same way that individual sample diagnostic tests need to be determined. These studies should also determine the optimal pool size to minimize overall testing costs.

Likelihood ratios

If a test produces results on a continuous scale or an ordinal scale (multiple categories such as very low, low, moderate, high, very high), then reducing the test result to a simple positive/negative classification may be a waste of useful information. For example, if it is preferred to use a somatic cell count (from a composite milk sample) to predict whether a cow has an intramammary infection, then a cutpoint of 200,000 cells per milliliter could be used and the cow could be considered positive if her cell count is over that level. A cow with a count of 950,000 cells per milliliter, however, is much more likely to be infected than a cow with a count of 201,000 cells per milliliter. Likelihood ratios can be computed for various levels of cell count and used to help estimate the actual probability that a cow will have an infection. For details of likelihood ratios, see Dohoo and colleagues [3].

Summary

Diagnostic tests are invaluable to the practice of veterinary medicine. Using them correctly and interpreting the results appropriately, however, depend on having a good understanding of the basic principles outlined here. The most important principle is recognition that the interpretation of test results (predictive values) varies across populations (eg, herds) and requires an estimate of the prevalence of the infection (or disease) in the population being studied.

References

[1] McKenna SL, Keefe GP, Barkema HW, et al. Evaluation of three ELISAs for *Mycobacterium avium* subsp. *paratuberculosis* using tissue and fecal culture as comparison standards. Vet Microbiol 2005;110(1–2):105–11.

[2] Kramps JA, Van Maanen C, van de Wetering G, et al. A simple, rapid and reliable enzyme-linked immunosorbent assay for the detection of bovine virus diarrhoea virus (BVDV) specific antibodies in cattle serum, plasma and bulk milk. Vet Microbiol 1999;64(2–3):135–44.

[3] Dohoo IR, Martin SW, Stryhn H. Screening and diagnostic tests. In: McPike SM, editor. Veterinary epidemiologic research. Charlottetown, PEI, Canada: AVC; 2003.

[4] McKenna SL, Barkema HW, Keefe GP, et al. Agreement between three ELISAs for *Mycobacterium avium* subsp. *paratuberculosis* in dairy cattle. Vet Microbiol, in press.

[5] Jordan D. Aggregate testing for the evaluation of Johne's disease herd status. Aust Vet J 1996; 73(1):16–9.

[6] Cameron AR, Baldock FC. A new probability formula for surveys to substantiate freedom from disease. Prev Vet Med 1998;34(1):1–17.

[7] Epi Vet Net. The Web site for veterinary epidemiologists. 2004. Available at: http://www.vetschools.co.uk/EpiVetNet/Sampling_software.htm. Accessed December 12, 2005.

[8] Enoe C, Georgiadis MP, Johnson WO. Estimation of sensitivity and specificity of diagnostic tests and disease prevalence when the true disease state is unknown. Prev Vet Med 2000; 45(1–2):61–81.

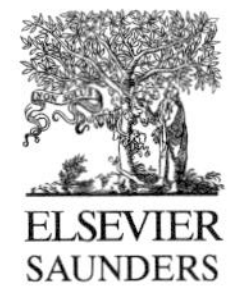

ELSEVIER
SAUNDERS

Vet Clin Food Anim 22 (2006) 207–227

VETERINARY
CLINICS
Food Animal Practice

Economic Assessment of Animal Health Performance

David Galligan, VMD, MBA

Center for Animal Health and Productivity, School of Veterinary Medicine, University of Pennsylvania, 382 West Street Road, Kennett Square, PA 19348, USA

The purpose of this article is to describe the fundamental principles of economic assessment of animal health performance in the modern animal production environment. In the early 1900s, veterinary services were focused on the national control of devastating animal diseases that could decimate animal populations quickly and over a wide geographic area [1]. Formal economic analysis was not needed given the obvious magnitude of the economic effects of these diseases relative to their control cost. In modern animal agriculture, many of these disease threats have been controlled to the point that they pose little risk to the average producer in most developed countries. Most production-limiting diseases now involve a complex dysfunction that encompasses biology, management, environment, economic, and social factors, and hence, therapeutic interventions must deal with all of these aspects to be effective [2]. Now the emerging threat to the survivability of a modern animal production system is the sociologic/technologic/economic changes in the industry that have resulted in decreasing profit margins for producers despite dramatic increases in production per animal over time. In response to these changes, herds have increased in scale, the use of resources (labor/facilities) has intensified, and new technologies and management practices are being embraced [3]. To remain economically sustainable in the future, producers must ensure that animal production and health are at optimal profit-making levels; any deviation from this level is a lost economic opportunity, which depending on the magnitude, might very well sink the operation.

Animal health performance can be affected by many management decisions and by unexpected disease events. Management has a direct effect on production performance, with and without the presence of infectious or metabolic diseases, through decisions regarding housing, nutrition,

E-mail address: galligan@vet.upenn.edu

doi:10.1016/j.cvfa.2005.11.007 *vetfood.theclinics.com*

reproduction, and so forth. Because of the dynamic and influential role that management plays in animal production and the progression of disease processes, deviations in animal health performance should be measured from the profit-maximizing levels of production efficiency attained by implementation of proven industry practices. Failure to successfully implement new technologies is a "disease" of management and can threaten the viability of the operation in the same manner as highly infectious disease. The lack of animal health performance is a departure from this level, which may be caused by inefficient management, by infectious/metabolic diseases, or more commonly, by both.

Some diseases lend themselves to managerial interventions at the preventative level (effective vaccines, ventilation, animal segregation/culling, bedding management, and so forth) or the treatment level after a disease has occurred. Good management often takes advantage of these opportunities for disease prevention/control and treatment, whereas poor management does not. Diseases or investment opportunities differ in the degree to which management has the potential to intervene and exert its influence. Thus, the managerial responses (or the failure to respond) to disease prevention/occurrence opportunities can mitigate or exacerbate their economic consequences.

Economic assessments are used to understand the value of diseases or management inefficiencies and the benefits of corrective actions. The assessment measures must capture the total economic value of the attributes of the disease or management issue being studied to define opportunities for improved profitable production. The most common attributes include the magnitude of the benefits and cost, the time at which they occur, and any risk or uncertainty they might have. When appropriate, the economic metric must also recognize and place value (real option value) on the potential role that managerial interventions can play in influencing the economic consequence of a disease or decision process.

Animal production systems

Animal production systems involve the use of resources (eg, animals, feed, labor, capital, and management skills) in a production process to create products that are valued by consumers [4]. The production process involves the complex interaction of management with the extraction of animal products (milk, eggs, work, wool) throughout the animals' lives, the meat and carcass products harvested at the end of their lives (eg, beef, fish, pork, chicken), or both (eg, beef cows, sows, poultry). This production process can be modulated by animal diseases and poor management practices that alter dimensions of the production process, require a greater use of resources, or result in decreased production (Fig. 1) [5].

At the consumer level, animal diseases can create food safety concerns (real or perceived) that can influence the demand for an animal product and, thus,

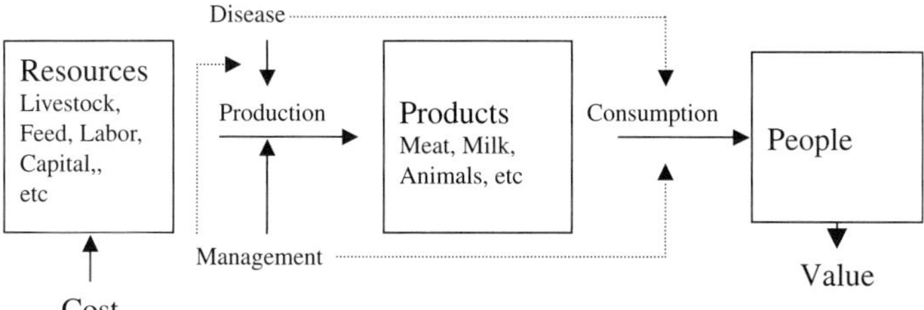

Fig. 1. The basic model of an animal production system. (*Adapted from* Howe KS, McInerney JP. Disease in livestock: economics and policy. Brussels, Belgium: Commission of the European Communities; 1987. Publication #EUR 11285 EN; with permission.)

affect product value. The recent bovine spongiform encephalopathy and foot-and-mouth disease outbreak in England demonstrated this level of impact [6]. These diseases caused direct losses to the producer (slaughter of clinical and suspect animals) and decreases in demand for the products.

Management practices can also affect consumer preferences for animal products. Some consumers place additional value on animal products produced in a certain way (eg, organically raised products, special cheeses based on pastured animals, bovine somatotropin–free milk, swine housing facilities). The advent and scope of global markets has increased consumer choices for food products in general and indirectly challenged animal food production to be safe and competitively priced and marketed.

Definition of disease/lack of health or production

The very definition of disease in an animal production setting has changed over time as veterinary medicine has evolved with the animal industries. Initially, disease was easily defined when overt clinical signs occurred such as the immediate death or severe debilitation of livestock, often due to a bacterial or viral infection. These diseases acutely affected the production system and resulted in very direct and visible losses (eg, death, abortion, dramatic decreased production). As the knowledge of animal physiology and metabolism improved, the definition of disease was broadened to include noninfectious diseases such as metabolic diseases that influence animal production through primarily nutrition (eg, ketosis and postparturient paresis in dairy cattle).

The term *subclinical disease* was embraced to define diseased animals in which overt clinical signs of disease (in terms of immediate death or aberrant physiologic measures such as elevated temperature or increased heart rate) were absent but production attributes (eg, milk per day, milk quality, piglets per year, reproductive efficiency) were debilitated. The term *herd health* was used to describe veterinary approaches to these infectious/metabolic problems confronting production facilities. Epidemiology emerged as a veterinary science by providing the metrics in which to measure disease occurrence and to understand the risk factors associated with production failure. This transition was important because the definition of health was broadened to include not only the maintenance of appropriate physiologic measures (eg, temperature, heart rate) but also production expectations. Management was also recognized as playing an influential role on the causation of diseases. The production benchmark by which disease cost was estimated was based on the production deviations from prior levels (Fig. 2), the goal being to prevent the disease (to prevent any departure from current production levels) or, in the case of diseased animals, to bring their production back to at least prior levels.

More recently, *suboptimal production performance* was also recognized as a direct consequence of poor management that fails to adopt effective technologies or practices (eg, nutritional advice, reproductive services) that ensure profitable production [2,7]. *Production medicine* emerged as a term used to describe veterinary approaches to diseases and management inefficiency. Failure to implement proven technologies or management practices for a given industry was recognized and treated as a "disease." In addition, production medicine recognized that part of the effects of an infectious/metabolic disease process could be influenced directly by management practices. Part of the "solution" often involved changing management to adopt a new technology (eg, breeding system, housing plan) that might alleviate some of the production losses associated with the disease. There was a need for a holistic approach to problem/disease solving that addressed disease and management factors simultaneously.

Table 1 illustrates this interaction between management and disease, showing the effects of postpartum metritis on first-service conception rates in well-managed and poorly managed dairy herds. Good and poor management is defined on the basis of first-service estrus detection rates (percentage of cows first bred who are eligible). In this simple illustration, biology dictates that healthy cows in both herds will have a first-service conception rate (percentage of cows conceiving on first breeding) of 30%. During the first 21 days, after the start of the breeding window, the well-managed herd (using a systematic breeding technology to ensure breeding) will have 95% of the eligible cows first serviced, whereas the poor herd (using visual estrus detection technology) will have only 50% of the eligible cows first serviced. At the herd

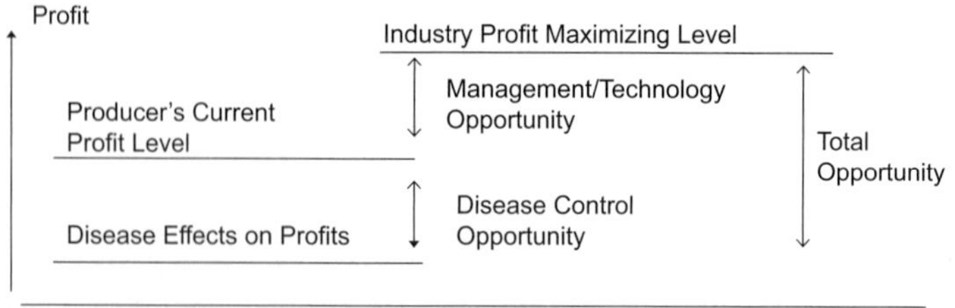

Fig. 2. Opportunity areas for improved profits in animal production systems.

Table 1
Management effects on pregnancy rates

Management	First-service estrus detection	Healthy conception	Diseased conception	Healthy PR[a]	Diseased PR[a]
Good	95%	30%	20%	29%	19%
Poor	50%	30%	20%	15%	10%

Abbreviation: PR, pregnancy rate.
[a] Percentage of cows becoming pregnant during the first 21 days of the breeding window.

level, the herd with good management will have 29% (0.95 × 0.30) of the healthy cows conceiving over the 21-day period, whereas the poorly managed here will have only 15% (0.50 × 0.30) of healthy cows conceiving. The production technology gap between herds is 14% fewer cows becoming pregnant over a 21-day period on the poorly managed operation.

The metritis cows in each herd will have reduced pregnancy rates due to the direct disease effects on conception; affected cows in both herds will have a conception rate of 20%. The resulting first-service pregnancy rate on the diseased animals will be 19% (0.95 × 0.20) on the good herd and 10% (0.50 × 0.20) on the poor herd. The well-managed herd dropped the pregnancy rate by 10% (29%−19%), whereas the poorly managed herd dropped by 5% from the previous healthy levels (15%−10%).

Both herds could (and should) try to take corrective actions to improve conception rates in cows with metritis (reducing its occurrence by better calving practices, nutritional interventions, and other methods). In addition, the poorly managed herd could mitigate the effect of metritis by adopting first-service breeding technologies (taking advantage of the technology opportunity), resulting in the metritis cows (even with their lower conception rate) having a higher pregnancy rate (19%) than the "healthy cows" in this herd on the old breeding system (15%). A production health consultant to this herd would be remiss if he or she did not encourage the producer to adopt the new breeding technologies before attempting to correct the conception rate issue.

In summary, production-limiting diseases do not often have the direct catastrophic effects of the highly infectious/viral diseases of the past but exert their influence more subtly in many dimensions that have economic consequences. Economically, it is prudent to control these to low levels of occurrence rather than pursue the expensive "eradication" campaigns used for highly infectious and debilitating diseases. Furthermore, these production-limiting diseases often allow management to compensate for productive losses in other dimensions.

Common effects evaluated in animal production systems

Animal production systems share many common attributes that are typically affected by a disease process or by poor management decisions. In the normal healthy state, an animal unit produces products over time at a favorable rate of economic efficiency. The nature of that production process varies across and even within species but ultimately results in some net accumulated economic value to the producers per animal unit per unit of time. For a dairy operation, this economic value might be total milk sold per cow per year, whereas for a swine or beef operation, it might be total pounds of meat sold per sow or cow per year. In addition to the product production function, there is typically an ongoing process to generate replacement animals, which has value in its own right. This process can be completed along with the production unit, as a separate enterprise, or by the sale of young stock and the external purchase of replacement animals.

At the producer level, the production process can be negatively affected by (1) altered production value as a consequence of lower production of the products or a lowering of their prices, (2) altered replacements patterns of animal units, and (3) direct changes in input cost. Each of these negative effects is discussed individually.

Altered product value

Two elements determine total product value: the physical amount of product (eg, pounds of milk, pounds of meat) and the market price for that product (eg, dollars per hundred weight of milk, dollars per hundred weight of meat). An animal production system may produce a spectrum of products (eg, milk, calves, and cull cows in a dairy operation) and receive a range of prices. Diseases and management inefficiencies decrease the productive yield or the amount of one or more of these products (eg, milk per day, offspring per year, meat per animal, wool per animal, eggs per week) that are harvested from the animal process over time [5]. At this point, the animal is not replaced but is still in the herd, producing at a lower level of efficiency. Fundamentally, the daily maintenance cost of the animal is still occurring at a relatively constant level even though a lower production yield is being realized.

Production can be affected in many biologic ways [8]. Gastrointestinal infestations can alter protein metabolism by first causing losses into the bowel, which must then be replaced using energy and protein that could have been used for a productive purpose [9]. Feed intake can be altered by a disease process (eg, sores in the mouth, general malaise) or by management providing a ration of low palatability or improper management of feed delivery. Poor facilities such as inadequate bunk space or the failure to separate lactation groups for dairy cows can directly affect production levels through altered intakes. Feed digestibility, although not commonly affected by diseases [8], can be affected by management's formulation of rations.

Production can be altered indirectly through poor reproductive management in the dairy. Basically, the cow's normal lactation curve is extended into the periods of lower yields by the increase in days open. Average milk per lactation day is reduced by the extended days open, with the extent of the reduction being dependent on the persistency (flatness) of the lactation curve.

Infectious diseases have the potential to not only affect production of the currently infected animal but also to infect other animals and influence their production. How quickly the disease is spread, its ultimate production effects on animals, and the mitigating steps that management can take to limit its spread or influence on production determines the magnitude of this effect [10].

Composition of the product and, therefore, its value (price received) can also be affected by a disease or management factor. Outright visible lesions dramatically lower slaughter value due to increased condemnation (eg, *Fasciola hepatica* can increase liver condemnations). Warble fly infestation and sheep lice may reduce the market value of the products [8]. Milk fat and milk protein content are directly influenced by ration formulations in dairy cows and thereby affect milk prices received.

In summary, within each species, the amount of physical product produced per unit time or the product quality can be affected in numerous ways by a disease process or management intervention. Any economic assessment of altered production value (physical amounts and price value) must quantify these effects over time, recognizing their unique species-specific attributes. When multiple dimensions are affected, they must be aggregated. For example, in the assessment of the economic cost of a day open in a dairy operation, the parity differences in milk yield, the shapes of lactation curves, and the parity distributions of cows within a herd must be part of the calculation [11].

Animal removal from a production system

Within any production system, each productive animal unit has an optimal time at which replacement should occur to maximize profits. This replacement occurs for a number of reasons, including increased health cost with age, reduced production, improved replacement unit characteristics (genetic progress), or increased risk of reproductive failure. Economically, this time point is defined when expected future returns of the animal being removed go below the expected returns of an average replacement animal [12]. The future net returns of the animal to be removed are marginal values in the sense that they represent the future variable revenues minus the future variable cost. The average returns of the replacement animal are also marginal values in the sense that they represent the future earning potential of the replacement animal. Management can influence the average returns of the replacement animal by reducing the cost of rearing relative to the future production value. In dairy cow operations, reducing the age at first calving can substantially reduce the feed cost per heifer and the ultimate number of heifers needed to meet culling needs [13].

Premature death is commonly the most identifiable, immediate, and intuitive loss associated with diseases that have high mortality rates. In a sense, overt mortality precludes management from having to make culling decisions: the replacement decision has been made (assuming the operation is ongoing). These costs are very high when the affected animal's production is substantially higher than herdmates' or when the rearing cost of replacements is high. Management can control the cost of diseases that have an associated premature culling component by ensuring that replacements are reared or purchased as efficiently as possible.

Tempered diseases and management inefficiencies (eg, reproductive inefficiencies in dairy cows) can also result in the premature removal of an animal from the production system. The timing of the removal might not be immediate but at a future point. For example, dairy cows that had successfully corrected for left displaced abomasums were twice as likely to be culled from the herd as cows not experiencing the disease [14]. Any delay in the timing of when the replacement animal is brought into the production process can result in additional losses due to the temporary underuse of production capacity (Fig. 3).

Additional future losses can occur that result from the loss of genetic progress due to the premature removal of productive animals and, therefore, their future offspring. Diseases that affect production can potentially influence or distort the ability to select animals on production metrics [8].

A number of computer models have been developed to structure and quantify the effects of removing an animal from the production process [12,15–19]. In general, the early removal of animals (before the optimal point), whatever the cause, is a lost opportunity cost to the producer.

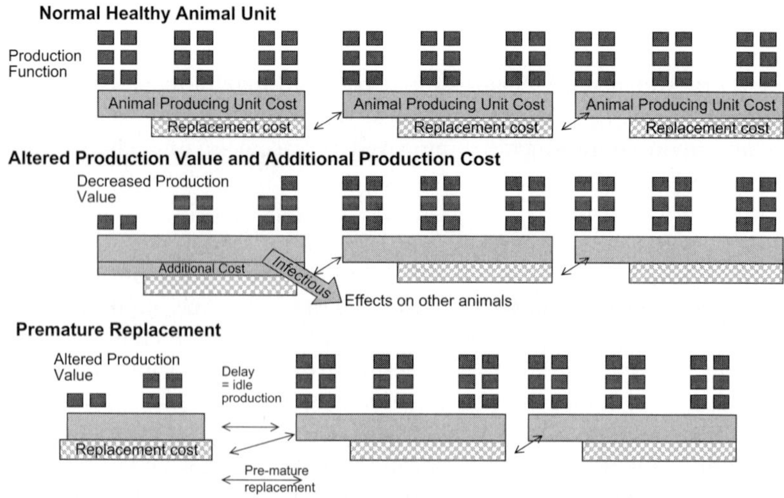

Fig. 3. Simple visual representations of disease effects on animal production.

The economic yield of these animals would have been higher than the returns of the average replacement. This loss is higher for higher-producing animals, in that they have a greater deviation from average production levels.

Several of these models use dynamic programming methodologies to the structure the problem [12,15,17,18] and represent the sequence of optimal replacement decisions. Although there are many implicit assumptions (constant milk prices and production parameters, constant availability of replacement stock, and so forth), these models have identified a less obvious loss associated with animal replacement. This loss occurs when the economically inefficient cow is retained in the herd beyond the point of optimal replacement, thus causing the producer to forgo the better returns on the average replacement. In a disease situation, losses can occur when an animal's production has decreased to the point that it has become an economic cull but management fails to remove the animal. Tempered diseases that influence production parameters and yet do not directly "signal" management with an obvious clinical sign (overt death) can also have an economic effect on this dimension. Thus, managerial efficiency in culling decisions directly influences the estimated cost of any disease issue.

Altered input cost

In many disease processes or management decisions, there is a direct change in input costs. In the disease scenario, veterinary expenditures increase dramatically (as a consequence of the disease condition) through increased therapy and disease control cost. In the case of managerial decisions to improve production, an initial investment must be made to adopt a new technology. This new technology might be in the form of physical items like ventilation fans, production-promoting pharmaceuticals, or a mixer wagon or might be in the form of expert advice such as nutritional consulting or reproductive and culling consulting.

Economic concepts

Animal systems as production functions

A food animal operation is fundamentally a production system that transfers many inputs into several outputs valued by society. The conversion of inputs to outputs defines a theoretic response curve (ie, a production curve) that portrays the current state of technologic knowledge for that industry. It is theoretic in the sense that it is difficult to exactly calculate such a relationship with so many inputs in a typical animal production system. The principles of a production curve, however, define many important fundamental concepts in economics that warrant its study and understanding.

The shape of the production curve can vary within the industry because producers effectively use various combinations or resources to produce a given product. For example, a successful milk production operation can be based on a total-confinement, fully fed system or be entirely or partially pasture based. Both of these approaches might be successfully operational in the same geographic region but would have differently shaped production curves reflecting the different technologies being used.

The shape of the production curve also changes over time as new knowledge emerges or new combinations of inputs are discovered. New knowledge might be in the form of a better understanding of nutrition, better veterinary services, or in the availability of new products (eg, bovine somatotropin to improve milk production) or animal husbandry practices (eg, systematic breeding technologies in the dairy industry). The curve defines the potential opportunity of production and thus represents the benchmark by which opportunity cost can be estimated. Opportunity cost, from this perspective, can be simply defined as not doing the right thing, the right thing being using the current state of knowledge of the production system that maximizes profits.

Fundamental to a defined production system is understanding which inputs should be used and to what level should they be used. Inputs can be in the form of all-or-nothing decisions (eg, milking three times per day versus two times per day; treatment 1 versus treatment 2 for a disease condition) or the decisions can have a graduated aspect (eg, five doses of anthelmintic versus four doses; 4 lb of soybean meal in a ration rather than 3 lb; the exact number of veterinary health care visits per year). A basic rule of production curve economics is that an input should be used if the marginal cost of using that input (implementing or not implementing the decision in an all-or-nothing situation or moving from one level of input to the next in a graduated situation) is less than or equal to the marginal value of the additionally produced product (marginal revenue).

In the illustrative production curve in Fig. 4, a technical relationship between a single input and output is shown in terms of value. In reality, there are many inputs into an animal production system; however, in this example, only one input is considered. Fixed costs that occur irrespective of the decision at hand are represented by the horizontal line and square makers. These costs stay at a constant level over a wide range of input levels. Included in this type of cost might be the mortgage for the farm, long-term debt payments, or labor if it will not change over the level of input being considered.

In addition, there are variable costs that vary directly with production and are associated with the decision at hand (ie, what level of input) (see Fig. 4, triangular makers). The summation of the fixed and variable costs form the total cost for a given level of input. Note that the slope of the line tangential to the variable cost or total cost line at any point is the marginal cost of adding one more unit of input. Hence, this marginal value can be determined solely from the variable factors, ignoring the fixed values. In

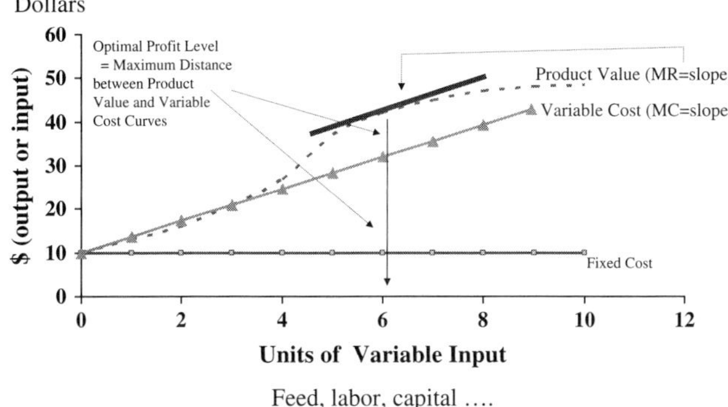

Fig. 4. A simple production curve demonstrating the principle of marginality. MC, marginal cost; MR, marginal revenue.

this example, the variable cost curve is linear, so the marginal cost is constant across all input levels.

The production response level (see Fig. 4, dotted curve) is typically curvilinear and composed of three basic types of relationships: (1) constant productivity—for each increased level of input there is a constant, linear increase in production; (2) increasing production—for each level of input there is an increasing or accelerating amount of product produced; and (3) diminishing returns—for each level of input there is a decreasing or decelerating level of product produced. The response curve can be shown in physical amounts of product produced (pounds of milk or meat, number of pregnancies, and so forth) or in terms of the product value (dollars); however, the fundamental shape remains the same because the value is simply the physical amount of product multiplied by the price. The slope of lines tangent to any point on the response curve represents the marginal physical production produced or the marginal value of the product produced for each increased level of input (see Fig. 4, solid line). When the marginal revenue exceeds the marginal cost for a given level of input, the profit from that decision increases (distance between production value and total cost curve). Profits are maximized up to the point where the marginal cost equals the marginal return (slopes of the tangential lines to the revenue curve and cost line are equal and thus parallel). At this point, the production value is maximally distant from the total cost curve. If inputs are used beyond this level, then the additional revenue received is less than the marginal cost and profits start to decline. It is important to observe that the marginal cost can be calculated by looking at the variable cost only (easy to do) or the total cost (difficult to do). The fixed costs do not alter the marginal cost but only shift the total cost upward; the point of optimal production does not change. It is this principle that allows the partial budget to ignore fixed cost and to be used in the analysis of animal performance or in an investment opportunity.

Partial budget—economic outcome of production curve analysis

To understand the economic impact of a disease or management decision, a partial budget analysis is performed that embraces the fundamental principle of marginality observed in production curve analysis. This marginal approach is used to capture the essential elements and to eliminate extraneous factors (fixed elements) that do not influence the ultimate estimate of economic impact. Marginal physical changes are identified that are associated with the disease occurrence or decision choice. Lowered production, higher input cost (veterinary cost before disposal), reduced slaughter value, idle production cost, and lost future income due to premature culling are common factors that are aggregated in estimating losses at the production system level for many diseases and management problems [11].

The formulation of a partial budget involves the identification of changes in cost and revenue associated with the condition or decision of interest. A partial budget is constructed to calculate the net of these marginal changes (Fig. 5).

With a simple application, the mere direction (positive/negative) and the magnitude of the net changes can be used to rank decisions. Identification and quantification of the changes in revenues and cost can be complex. In many disease situations, numerous facets of the production process might be affected and, thus, must all be aggregated by economic weights and summed. Furthermore, the varied temporal nature of these impacts adds complexity to the analysis in several ways. First, the aggregate effects need to be measured over same time dimension and expressed on a per-animal basis if appropriate. Second, because of the temporal nature of the impacts, discounting (discussed in the Economic valuation section) must be used to account for timing differences of when cash flows are actually realized. Further valuation complications can occur when the issue being evaluated allows the management to potentially intervene and influence the outcome as more information becomes available (see later discussion on managerial flexibility).

Economic valuation

Present value calculations

Valuation of disease cost and managerial decisions or investments in general share common attributes. The issues all deal with a stream cash flow in time that varies in direction (revenue versus cost) and magnitude (Fig. 6). In a disease situation, various physical aspects of the production system (milk production, piglets per litter, eggs per day, and so forth) are affected and, thus, have a negative

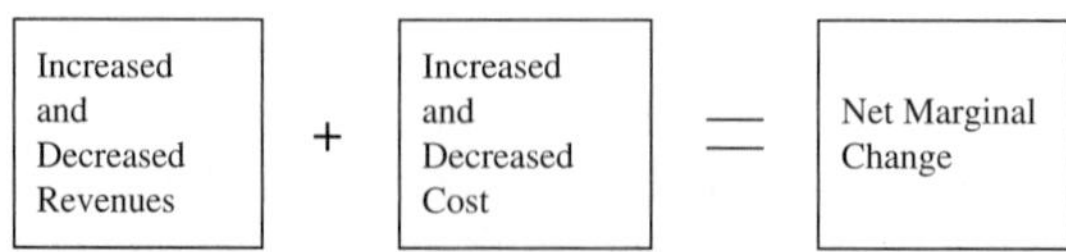

Fig. 5. Basic partial budget format for marginal analysis.

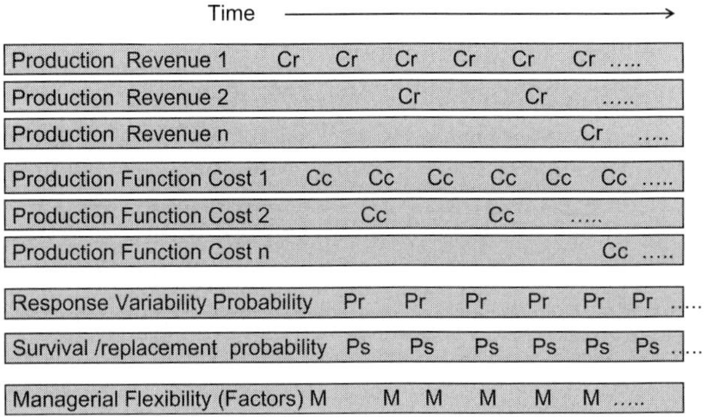

Time ⟶

Production Revenue 1 Cr Cr Cr Cr Cr Cr .....
Production Revenue 2 Cr Cr .....
Production Revenue n Cr .....
Production Function Cost 1 Cc Cc Cc Cc Cc Cc .....
Production Function Cost 2 Cc Cc .....
Production Function Cost n Cc .....
Response Variability Probability Pr Pr Pr Pr Pr Pr .....
Survival /replacement probability Ps Ps Ps Ps Ps Ps .....
Managerial Flexibility (Factors) M M M M M M .....

Fig. 6. Figurative illustration of basic concepts in valuation. Cr, cash revenue; Cc, cash cost; Ps, probability of survivability; Pr, probability of response level; M, option value due to management interventions.

incremental effect on revenue streams. In addition, there are consequential changes in cost (eg, the feed intake might go down, thereby decreasing cost; treatment/preventative cost might increase). Animal units may be culled (generating revenue) at a certain probability and replaced (incurring cost). The net effect of these changes in revenues and cost (ie, partial budget over time) is a net projected cash flow over time. The magnitude and timing of these cash flows differ with the various disease processes that are possible.

Similarly, when management makes a change in the production system, there might be an incremental increase in a production characteristic (eg, improved milk production per day, improved reproductive efficiency) that results in a positive cash flow, and usually, there is an associated implementation cost with the change. To deal with the time dimensions at which these changes in revenues and cost occur, future cash flows are discounted into present values to take into account the time value of money. A future cash flow is worth less than a cash flow today, in that cash today has opportunity value for immediate investment. The following is the general formula for calculation of the net present value (NPV) [20]:

$$\mathrm{NPV} = \mathrm{C_o} + \Sigma \mathrm{C_t}/(1 + \mathrm{r})^{\mathrm{t}}$$

where C_o is cash outflow or inflow occurring in time period 0 (today); t is time period; C_t is investment or cash outflow in time period t; and r is discount rate per time period.

The present value represents the amount of money today one would have to realize C_t at time t in the future. The discount rate (r) represents the opportunity cost of money and can take on different meanings. When used at the level of the returns on a t-bill, the discounting is said to represent the risk-free rate of return or the pure time value of money. It is considered low risk (ie, it is unlikely that the government would default on its obligations and the future cash flow would most likely occur) and, therefore, offers a lower rate of return.

Discount rates higher than the t-bill represent additional risk inherent to a stream of cash flows in addition to purely time. Higher rates of return are expected from investments with higher risk. Therefore, a stream of cash flows from a risky "investment" is worth less in today's dollars (requires a high discount rate) than a less risky opportunity (low discount rate). In animal production systems, most investments that are linked to animal survival are subject to the risk (competitive risk) that the animal might die from other causes before returns on the investment can be harvested. Galligan and colleagues [21] proposed an approach to increase the discount rate based on the underlying mortality rate to reflect this increase of risk.

In a typical investment scenario, the first cash flow (C_o) might be a cost that represents the initial investment, whereas following cash flows represent the effects on the production process. The discount rate that is used should reflect the inherent risk of the investment and be based on opportunities with similar risk. If the NPV is equal to 0, then the decision/investment is known to have a rate of return that is equal to the discount rate (r) used in the analysis. If the NPV is greater than 0, then the rate of return of the investment is greater than the discount rate and the investment is seen as favorable. In other words, for the level of risk being considered, the investment offers greater value. Conversely, if there is a negative NPV, then the rate of return of the investment is less than the discount rate. One would do better pursuing the opportunity represented by the discount rate.

To control risk, investors mix investments using portfolio theory in such a manner to ensure the highest return for a given level of risk [20,22,23]. By diversifying the investment combination, the risk of the mix of investment can be substantially reduced. For example, a portfolio of bulls to be used in a breeding program has considerably less risk than the use of one or two sires alone for a given production trait.

Annuity values

In the comparison of investment opportunities or disease effects, a different time horizon often emerges that can influence the magnitude of an NPV calculation. This is particularly true in animal production systems in which the life spans of the animals can vary across intervention opportunities. It is convenient to express the NPV in the form of a constant cash flow value per time period (an annuity) for the life span of the investment that is equivalent in value. The following formula is used to calculate an annuity [20]:

$$C_{\text{Annuity}} = \frac{\text{NPV}}{\frac{1}{r-1}/[r(1+r)^t]}$$

where t is lifespan of the investment; $C_{Annuity}$ is the constant cash flow for t periods; NPV is the net present value of the cash flows over t periods; and r is discount rate per period.

For example, consider investment opportunities A and B in Table 2. Opportunity A is a series of cash flows that occurs over a 5-year period, whereas B occurs over a 6-year time horizon. At the end of each investment, the producer has the opportunity to reinvest. When discounted at 5%/y using equation 1, investment B has a higher NPV ($302 versus $276) and is ranked superior on this basis alone; however, it is an investment with a longer life span and would tend to have a higher NPV. When the NPVs are converted to annuity values (dollars per year) using equation 2, investment A is superior to investment B; investment A offers a higher flow of value per period than investment B. When investments have different time horizons, annuity values, rather then NPV, should be considered.

Methods to deal with variation

General

Production systems are biologic systems that have considerable sources of variation. There is a range of production (eg, milk per day, piglets per litter, eggs per day) that could be described by a normal distribution with parameters consisting of the mean and standard deviation. The number of disease events within a herd could follow a Poisson distribution defined by the lambda (average number of events observed in a given time period). The time to a disease event is not set in stone but might follow a gamma distribution to represent the different times to events typically observed. Variation adds complexity to the economic evaluation of disease processes and investment opportunities. To facilitate the modeling of these aspects of an investment, one can use spreadsheet add-ons such as @Risk [24] and BASECOW [25] that allow the user to specify distributions and randomly sample the distributions within a spreadsheet environment.

Table 2
Net present value and annuity values for investments with different life spans

	Year							
Investment	1	2	3	4	5	6	NPV[a]	Annuity[b]
Annual cash flows at the end of each year								
A	–$600	–$400	$425	$525	$525	—		
B	–$500	–$400	$300	$375	$375	$375		
Discounted cash flows								
A	–$571	–$363	$367	$432	$411	—	$276	$64/y
B	–$476	–$363	$259	$309	$294	$280	$302	$60/y

[a] NPV values were calculated using equation 1 (see text) and an annual discount rate of 5%.
[b] NPV values were converted to annuity values using equation 2 (see text).

Type 1 and 2 error analysis

Variation in responses to products can create a dilemma to understanding their true value. Type I and type II error analysis can be used to look at the expected cost of using a product and having it fail (a response below breakeven; type I error) compared with the expected cost of not using the product when it would have worked (type II error) [26]. The underlying response variation observed across herds is used to probabilistically weight the partial budgets of varying response levels. The probabilistically weighted partial budgets are summed below (type I error cost) and above (type II error cost) the breakeven level of production.

Stochastic dominance curves

When several choices are available that differ in their mean value and variation, the decision maker must make a selection based on two criteria: the mean and standard deviation (risk). Fig. 7 shows the distribution of the partial budgets of the responses for three separate products used to enhance milk production in dairy cows. The three partial budgets of the products differ in their mean and variation attributes. When ranked on their mean values, product 3 leads, followed by product 2 and then product 1. When ranked on their risk (variability), product 1 is the lowest, followed by product 3 and then product 2.

To facilitate decision making, frequency distribution curves can be converted to their cumulative form (Fig. 8). Cumulative curves laying to the right have a higher partial budget value for the same level of cumulative frequency and are said to dominate curves to the left. When one curve is completely to the right of another, it is said to have first-order stochastic dominance over the other. Product 1 is almost first-order stochastic dominant to product 2 (there is a slight crossover). When cumulative curves cross, as is the case here, the curves are ranked based on the magnitude of the area under them, with the smallest area being dominant to the others. Product 1 is second-order stochastically dominant to products 2 and 3. Product 3 is second-order dominant to product 2.

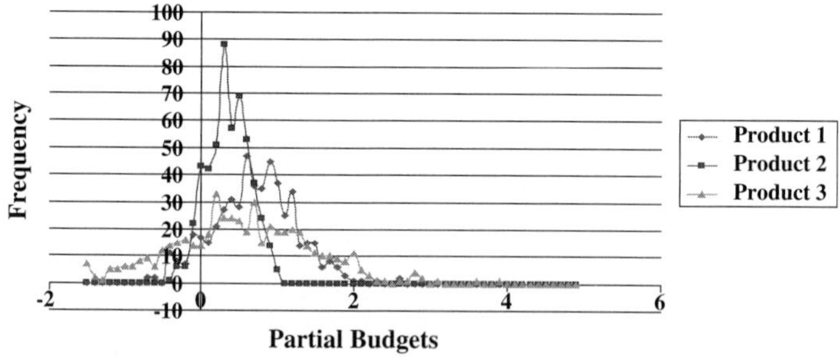

Fig. 7. Frequency distribution of partial budgets for three products.

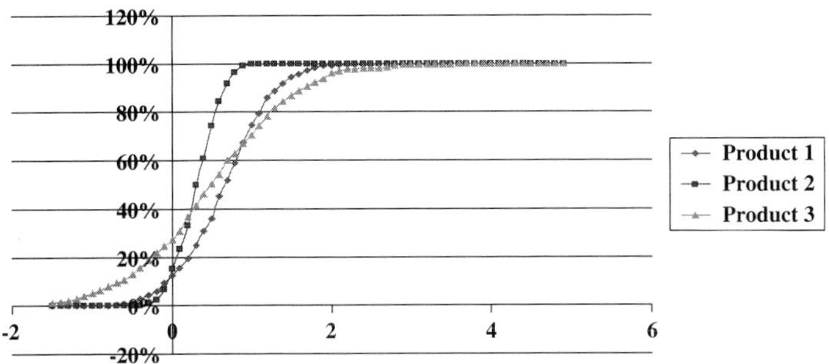

Fig. 8. Cumulative distribution curves of the partial budgets for three products.

Simulation

An animal production system is essentially a complex web of elements that follows various probability distributions [27]. The production ranking within a herd, the likelihood of being bred, the likelihood of conception, and the likelihood of having a disease and being culled are all sources of variation that exist within a typical production system. Monte Carlo simulation is a method that randomly samples an observation from a given distribution, whereby the frequencies of the sampled levels reflect the distribution. Dairy Oracle [27] is a simulation model of a dairy herd in which each cow in a defined herd is represented by random selection from a set of distributions used to define the life cycle of a cow. The user enters parameters of the probability distributions (normal, binomial, Poisson, gamma, and so forth) to define the management of a herd and the inherent biologic variability. The individual cow scenarios are aggregated for the entire herd over time, and generated revenues and cost are calculated. The approach allows the exploration of the economic effects of disease processes or management changes that affect multiple dimensions (eg, production, longevity, reproduction efficiency) of the system over time. This modeling approach was used to explore the potential economic impact of using bovine somatotropin in a dairy operation over a 6-year period [28]. For each herd simulation over time, an NPV was calculated that captured the change in value of the herd composition from the start to the end and the net profits generated within the 6-year period. NPVs for herds using the technology can be compared with those not using it to estimate its potential value. Simulation has been used to investigate the cost and benefits of Johne's disease control programs in dairy cows [29].

Decision-tree analysis

In simple situations in which a frequency distribution is used to describe possible outcomes, a decision-tree analysis can be done. Decision-tree analysis articulates the temporal attributes and the probabilities of various outcomes for a given decision choice (eg, to treat or not to treat) [30–32]. Expected values are calculated for a decision choice by summing the probabilistically weighted outcome values, yielding an expected value. Decisions with a higher expected value would then be selected. In essence, a decision tree deals with variation by calculating an expected value and, therefore, assumes the decision maker is risk neutral in making decisions [33].

Managerial flexibility in dealing with risk

Risk can be divided into two broad categories: variability and uncertainty [34]. Variability is risk that is inherent to the production process and is only changed if the production/biology process is changed. For example, a herd's conception rate might be 40%. As a consequence, there is variation in the number of cows pregnant from a given breeding pool that follows a binomial distribution. There is even a small risk that all cows in the breeding pool are not pregnant; this risk becomes smaller as the breeding population increases. This risk is only changed by a change in the process (eg, improving the conception rate by better nutrition). Even an improved higher conception rate will follow the binomial distribution and, thus, have a risk component.

Uncertainty on the other hand, is risk that can be reduced with further knowledge. The uncertainty about the true conception rate of a herd can be reduced by observing more cows and will follow a beta distribution. The beta distribution narrows as more observations are made on the number of cows pregnant and can be used to define confidence intervals regarding one's understanding of the true conception rate.

In an investment opportunity, many things that are unknown initially become resolved (or partially resolved) over time. Next year's market price of milk or feeder pigs is uncertain today but will be known with 100% certainty next year. The potential yield of forages for next year is unknown today but becomes resolved when harvest is underway. As more cows are inseminated within a herd and the outcomes recorded, one will better understand the conception rate of that herd. Although there still will be variation that might increase or decrease following a binomial process, it will be better understood.

Opportunities that have resolution of an uncertainty give management the potential to use the improved knowledge to make better decisions and, thus, improve the value of the opportunity [35–37]. Consider two hypothetic products that can be used to improve dairy cow milk production per day. One product (A) is added to the silage at the annual harvest to improve its digestibility, whereas the second product (B) is added to the ration on a daily basis. Let us assume that the products improve milk production by 10 lb and the variation (risk) in response is 4 lb (SD), and that the cost per cow is the same for both products. Over time, management will know whether either product works. Traditional economic assessment (NPV analysis) states that the value of these two investments and their risk of failure are identical; however, product B, which is added to the feed daily, allows management to intervene and respond to resolved information (ie, the resulting production response), whereas product A does not share this attribute. For example, if the response to product B is below the breakeven level needed to pay for the product, then management can stop using it and abandon it as a poor investment. In the situation of a poor response (below breakeven) to product A, however, management must live with the outcome and feed out the silage for the remainder of the year; it has no flexibility opportunity. Product B has greater value (flexibility value) to management, in that it has an option for management to abandon the investment if is does not work:

$$\text{Value of product A} = \text{NPV}$$
$$\text{Value of product B} = \text{NPV} + \text{value of an option to abandon}$$

Good management would avail itself of the opportunity to abandon the product should it arise, whereas poor management would continue to pursue a failing investment. Good management would take advantage of resolved uncertainty. Traditional economic assessment (NPV analysis) makes the implicit assumption on such expected scenarios that management will be passive and follow a static policy (continue to use a product that has failed) and not make changes as things unfold [37]. In reality, management cultivates investments as they mature to improve their yields. In the financial world, the value of flexibility has been captured in its purist form in the valuation of puts and calls (options). A call option allows the purchaser the right to purchase a stock at a set fee (strike price) in the future. At the time of purchase of a call option, the future stock price is uncertain (like the product response on the dairy) but will be completely resolved at the time of maturity in the future when management can exert flexibility. If the resolved market price of the stock is higher than the strike price agreed on at the purchase of the call, then management will purchase the stock at the lower strike price and sell it at the market price, harvesting the net difference in prices minus the cost of the call option. Black and Scholes [38] developed a method that is used to place value (the price to sell a call option for) on such an investment opportunity and indirectly captured the value of managerial flexibility.

The concept of managerial flexibility has been recognized as a potential attribute of many investment opportunities, and these investments are considered to have "real option value" [37]. Furthermore, a number of methods have been developed to value these real options in addition to the Black-Scholes approach used to value puts and calls. The application of managerial flexibility to animal production systems is just emerging [39,40].

Summary

Animal health economics is an emerging discipline in veterinary medicine that provides a framework of concepts and methodologies to support decision making in optimizing animal health management [41]. Animal production is a complex system of combined inputs (eg, physical inputs, managerial decision choices) into a production process that produces products valued by society. Perturbations to this system are varied in nature, including disease processes and management inefficiencies. Economic valuation of these perturbations must account for all attributes, including the marginal changes in revenues and cost, the time dimensions of occurrence, and the inherent risk characteristics of biologic systems. In addition, the economic valuation metric must capture the opportunity value that exists in some perturbations (but not all) that allows management to intervene within the process and make economically influencing decisions. It has been recognized that improving animal health, in all its dimensions, can play a major role in achieving efficient and economically rewarding production.

References

[1] Martin SW, Meek AH, Willeberg P. Veterinary epidemiology: principles and methods. Ames (IA): Iowa State University Press; 1987.

[2] Galligan DT. The economics of optimal health and productivity in the commercial dairy. The economics of animal disease control. Rev Sci Tech 1999;18(2):512–9.

[3] Fetrow J, Cady R, Jones G. Dairy production medicine in the United States. Bovine Pract 2004;38(2):113–20.

[4] Howe KS, McInerney JP. Disease in livestock: economics and policy. Brussels, Belgium: Commission of the European Communities; 1987. Publication # EUR 11285 EN.

[5] Dahoo IR, Martin SW. Disease, production and culling in Holstein-Friesian cows. IV. Effects of disease on production. Prev Vet Med 1984;2:755–70.

[6] Buzby JC. Effects of food-safety perceptions on food demand and global trade. Changing structure of global food consumption and trade. ERS/USDA; 2001. Publication #WRS-01–1.

[7] Ferguson J, Galligan DT, Ramberg C, et al. Veterinary nutritional advisory services to dairy farms. Compend Continuing Educ 1987;9:192–201.

[8] Morris RS. How economically important is animal disease and why? In: Dijkhuizen AA, Morris RS, editors. Animal health economics, principles and applications. Sydney: Post Graduate Foundation in Veterinary Science, University of Sidney; 1997. p. 1–10.

[9] Brown MD, Poppi DP, Sykes AR. The effect of post-ruminal infusion of protein or energy on the pathology of *Trichostrongylus culubriformis* infection on body compositions in lambs. Proc N Z Soc Anim Prod 1986;46:27–30.

[10] Groenendaal H, Galligan DT. Economic consequences of control programs for paratuberculosis in midsize dairy farms in the United States. J Am Vet Med Assoc 2003;223:1757–63.

[11] Dijkhuisen AA, Huirne RBM, Jalvingh AW, et al. Economics impact of common health and fertility problems, principles and applications. In: Dijkhuizen AA, Morris RS, editors. Animal health economics, principles and applications. Sydney: Post Graduate Foundation in Veterinary Science, University of Sidney; 1997. p. 41–5.

[12] Van Arendonk JAM. Studies on the replacement policies in dairy cattle [dissertation]. Wageningen, The Netherlands: Departments of Animal Breeding and Farm Management, Wageningen Agricultural University; 1985.

[13] Mourits MCM, Huirne RBM, Dijkhuizen AA, et al. Economic optimization of dairy heifer management decisions. Agric Syst 1999;61:17–31.

[14] Galligan DT, Ferguson JD, Ramberg CF, et al. Postsurgical survival to culling of dairy cows with left displaced abomasum. J Dairy Sci 1993;76(Suppl 1):297.

[15] Huirne RBM. Computerized management support for swine breeding farms [dissertation]. Wageningen, The Netherlands: Department of Farm Management, Wageningen Agricultural University; 1990.

[16] Huirne RBM, Dijkhuizen AA, van Beek P, et al. Dynamic programming to optimize treatment and replacement decisions. In: Dijkhuizen AA, Morris RS, editors. Animal health

economics, principles and applications. Sydney: Post Graduate Foundation in Veterinary Science, University of Sidney; 1997. p. 85–97.
[17] Houben EHP. Economic optimization of decision with respect to dairy cow health management [dissertation]. Wageningen, The Netherlands: Department of Farm Management, Wageningen Agricultural University; 1995.
[18] Kristensen AR. Markov decision programming techniques applied to the animal replacement problem [dissertation]. Copenhagen, Denmark: The Royal Veterinary and Agricultural University; 1993.
[19] Groenendaal H, Galligan DT, Mulder HA. An economic spreadsheet model to determine optimal breeding and replacement decisions for dairy cattle. J Dairy Sci 2004;87:2146–57.
[20] Brealey RA, Myers SC. Principles of corporate finance. 6th edition. 2000.
[21] Galligan DT, Ramberg C, Curtis C, et al. Financial evaluation of animal health programs adjusting for competitive risk. Prev Vet Med 1993;16:15–20.
[22] Galligan DT, Marsh W. An application of portfolio theory for optimal choice of veterinary management programs. Prev Vet Med 1988;5:251–61.
[23] Galligan DT, Ramberg C, Curtis C, et al. Application of portfolio theory in decision tree analysis. J Dairy Sci 1991;74:2138–44.
[24] @Risk advanced risk analysis for spreadsheets, Version 4.5. Newfield (NY): Palisade Corp; 2004.
[25] Galligan DT, Groenendaal H, Munson R, et al. BASECOW: an Excel add-in specific for the dairy production consultant. J Dairy Sci 2001;84(Suppl 1):71.
[26] Galligan DT, Chalupa W, Ramberg C. Application of type 1 and type 2 errors in dairy farm management decision making. J Dairy Sci 1991;74:902–10.
[27] Marsh WE. Economic decision making on health and management in livestock herds: examining complex problems through computer simulation [dissertation]. St. Paul (MN): University of Minnesota; 1986.
[28] Marsh W, Galligan DT, Chalupa W. Economics of recombinant bovine somatotropin use in individual dairy herds. J Dairy Sci 1988;71:2944–58.
[29] Groenendaal H, Nielen M, Jalvingh A, et al. A simulation of Johne's disease control. Prev Vet Med 2002;54:225–45.
[30] Madison J, Fetrow J, Galligan DT. Economic decisions in food animal practice: to treat or not to treat. J Am Vet Med Assoc 1984;185:520–3.
[31] Fetrow J, Madison J, Galligan DT. Economic decisions in veterinary practice: a method for field use. J Am Vet Med Assoc 1985;186:792–7.
[32] Parsons TD, Smith G, Galligan DT. Economics of porcine parvovirus vaccination assessed by decision analysis. Prev Vet Med 1986;4:199–204.
[33] Galligan DT, Marsh W, Madison J. Economic decision making in veterinary practice: expected value and risk as dual utility scales. Prev Vet Med 1987;5:79–86.
[34] Vose D. Risk analysis: a quantitative guide. New York: John Wiley and Sons; 2000.
[35] Hull JC. Options, futures & other derivatives. Fourth edition. Upper Saddle River (NJ): Prentice Hall; 2000.
[36] Luehrman TA. Capital projects as real options: an introduction. Boston (MA): Harvard Business School Publishing; 1995. p. 1–12.
[37] Trigeorgis L. Real options, managerial flexibility and strategy in resource allocation. Cambridge (MA): MIT Press; 1999.
[38] Black F, Scholes M. The pricing of options and corporate liabilities. J Political Econ 1973;81: 637–59.
[39] Groenendaal H, Galligan DT. Real options analysis applied to dairy cow breeding and replacement decisions. J Dairy Sci 2001;84(Suppl 1):26.
[40] Galligan DT, Groenendaal H, Ferguson JD, et al. Real options analysis to evaluate products used in dairy production. J Dairy Sci 2002;85(Suppl 1):180.
[41] Dijkhuisen AA. Modelling animal health economics [inaugural speech]. Wageningen Agricultural University; 1992.

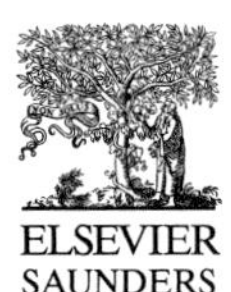
ELSEVIER
SAUNDERS

Vet Clin Food Anim 22 (2006) 229–261

VETERINARY
CLINICS
Food Animal Practice

Use of Molecular Epidemiology in Veterinary Practice

Ruth N. Zadoks, DVM, PhD*,
Ynte H. Schukken, DVM, PhD

Quality Milk Production Services, College of Veterinary Medicine, Cornell University, 22 Thornwood Drive, Ithaca, NY 14850-1263, USA

Epidemiology is the study of determinants of health, disease, and productivity in populations of humans, plants, or animals. Epidemiologic studies often use field observations, laboratory tests for diagnosis of disease, measures of productivity, statistical or mathematic analyses, and other quantitative methods. Molecular methods are another set of tools that can be used in epidemiologic studies. Molecular epidemiology is the study of distribution and determinants of health and disease through the use of molecular biology methods [1]. The term *molecular epidemiology* is sometimes used for studies in molecular taxonomy and phylogeny. Although these scientific disciplines use molecular techniques and provide valuable tools for use in epidemiologic studies, they focus on the classification of organisms into naturally related groups and the study of the line of evolutionary descent rather than the study of determinants of disease and disease transmission [1]. Use of the misnomer "molecular epidemiology" for taxonomic and phylogenetic studies has given rise to the misconception that molecular epidemiology is not epidemiology in the true sense of the word, earning molecular epidemiology the dubious nickname "stamp collection." The goal of molecular epidemiology, however, is not merely to classify organisms into taxonomic or phylogenetic groups but to "identify the microparasites responsible for infectious diseases and determine their physical sources, their biological relationships, and their route of transmission and those of the genes responsible for their virulence, vaccine-relevant antigens and drug resistance" [2].

Applications of molecular epidemiology in human health care, veterinary medicine, and food safety are manifold. Some applications and examples are

* Corresponding author. QMPS Molecular Laboratory, 22 Thornwood Drive, Ithaca, NY 14850-1263.

E-mail address: rz26@cornell.edu (R.N. Zadoks).

doi:10.1016/j.cvfa.2005.11.005 ***vetfood.theclinics.com***

listed in Table 1. Several reviews address applications of molecular epidemiology in specific disciplines or to specific organisms or virulence characteristics. Examples include reviews of molecular epidemiology as pertaining to foodborne pathogens [3], parasitology [4], virology [5,6], mycobacteria [7], foot-and-mouth disease [8], *Theileria parva* [9], *Giardia* [10], antimicrobial resistance [11], and endemic infections [12]. This anthology is by no means exhaustive and is only meant to give the reader an idea of the range of fields in which molecular epidemiology is used and to give suggestions for additional reading. In the remainder of this article, most attention is given to the molecular epidemiology of bacterial infections, although examples from

Table 1
Examples of applications of molecular epidemiology in veterinary medicine

Application	Example	Reference
Determination of the dynamics of disease transmission in geographically widespread areas	Global spread of foot-and-mouth disease; spread of Newcastle disease virus in Asia	[8,38]
Distinction between pathovars and nonpathovars	Pathogenic and nonpathogenic *Escherichia coli* in petting zoos	[47]
Addressing hospital and institutional infectious disease problems	Methicillin-resistant *Staphylococcus aureus* in veterinary teaching hospitals	[120]
Identification of genetic determinants of disease and disease transmission	Lineage-specific pathogenicity of *Listeria monocytogenes* in humans and ruminants	[35]
Confirmation of epidemiologically suspected transmission	Transmission of *Staphylococcus aureus* mastitis by flies	[121]
Detection of epidemiologically unsuspected outbreaks	Multiresistant *Salmonella* in animals and humans	[122]
Support for mathematic modeling	*Streptococcus uberis* mastitis outbreak; local spread of *Campylobacter* spp	[63,64,67,123]
Identification of risk factors and environments where transmission occurs	*Mycobacterium bovis* control schemes	[7]
Challenging of accepted dogmas	Origin of high bacteria counts in bulk tank milk	[55]
Identification of sources and reservoirs	*Staphylococcus aureus* in milk processing plants	[124]
Differentiation between persistence and reintroduction	Recurrent episodes of clinical *E coli* mastitis	[77]
Development of future control strategies	Identification of vaccine candidates	[113]
Host adaptation of strains	Human and bovine *Streptococcus agalactiae*	[92]
Differentiation between zoonotic, waterborne, and anthroponotic transmission	*Cryptosporidium* in cattle and humans; *Giardia* in humans, livestock, and pets	[10,125]

virology and other disciplines are included. First, a brief overview of terminology and molecular methodology is provided, followed by examples of applications of molecular epidemiology in veterinary medicine.

Molecular terminology

Internationally, attempts have been made to use standard definitions of a few key terms. These definitions are adhered to in this article and are explained in the following paragraphs. The reader should be aware that not all investigators and journals use the same definitions. In particular, the word "strain" is often used as a synonym for "isolate." When using, discussing, or reading results from molecular epidemiologic studies, it is important that all parties have the same understanding of what is meant by these terms. The definitions of isolate, strain, and clone used in this article are in line with those used by the Molecular Typing Working Group of the Society for Healthcare Epidemiology of America [13], the European Study Group on Epidemiological Markers [14], and the recent book, *Molecular Epidemiology of Infectious Diseases*, published by the American Society for Microbiology [1].

An **isolate** is a population of microbial cells in pure culture derived from a single colony on an isolation plate and identified to the species level. For example, when *Staphylococcus aureus* is obtained from a milk sample, and a pure subculture from one colony of *Staphylococcus aureus* is used for storage or further study, this would be referred to as an isolate. A **strain** is an isolate or a group of isolates exhibiting characteristics that set it apart from other isolates belonging to the same species. For example, isolates belonging to the species *Staphylococcus aureus* can be subdivided into penicillin-sensitive and penicillin-resistant strains. This distinction can be made with **phenotypic** methods (expression of visible characteristics, such as growth on Mueller-Hinton agar with antibiotic-impregnated discs) or with **genotypic** methods (DNA-based methods, such as detection of a penicillin-resistance gene). Penicillin resistance is a determinant of health and disease because cows with mastitis caused by penicillin-resistant isolates are less likely to cure in response to antibiotic treatment than cows with penicillin-sensitive isolates, even when treatment choices are based on the antimicrobial sensitivity of the isolate [15]. A **clone** is the progeny of a common ancestor and the result of a direct chain of replication of that ancestor. Identification of clones is based on the monitoring of multiple genetic markers of sufficient discriminatory power. In human medicine, many infections with methicillin-resistant *Staphylococcus aureus* are caused by a limited number of clones that have spread internationally. For example, there is an Iberian clone and a New York clone of methicillin-resistant *Staphylococcus aureus* [16]. The terms *isolate*, *strain*, and *clone* form a hierarchic series (ie, our knowledge of the organism's characteristics is increasingly detailed at every step in the series) (Fig. 1). For some organisms, descriptive groupings are used that are based on their geographic origin or

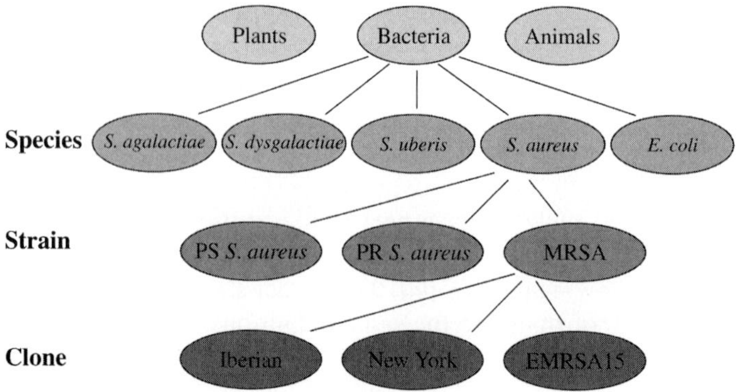

Fig. 1. Hierarchic ordering of species, strains, and clones of bacteria. Note that an isolate can belong to a species, a strain, or a clone depending on how much is known about its phenotype and genotype. PS, penicillin sensitive; PR, penicillin resistant; MRSA, methicillin-resistant *Staphylococcus aureus*; EMRSA15, epidemic MRSA clone number 15.

pathogenicity. Examples of such descriptive groupings include **topotypes** (for groups of foot-and-mouth disease viruses that are genetically and geographically related) [8], and **pathovars** (pathogenic variants of an organism) [1].

When discussing molecular epidemiology or strain typing with producers or others, it can be helpful to compare the concept of strains within infectious organisms with the concept of breeds or cultivars within animal or plant species. Within the species "sheep," we can distinguish breeds kept for milk production, for meat, or for fiber. The animals have enough in common to belong to the same species but they have enough differences to belong to different breeds. Similarly, bacteria may have enough in common to belong to the same species, say *Escherichia coli*, yet they may have enough differences to belong to different strains. Strains of *E coli* that produce shiga-like toxins, such as *E coli* O157:H7, have very different characteristics than strains that do not produce these toxins. The toxins are a determinant of health and disease, and the response to detection of *E coli* O157:H7 in well water on a farm would be very different than the response to detection of a non–shiga toxin-producing strain of *E coli.* A major difference between the breed concept and the strain concept is that breeds are well defined through breed standards and breeding organizations, whereas no such standardization exists for the naming of microbial strains. Some naming systems allow for a degree of standardization, such as the identification of *E coli* by presence of shiga toxins, the identification of *Salmonella* DT104 by means of phage typing, or the use of DNA sequenced–based strain typing methods. Many strain typing systems, however, are not universally meaningful.

Typing methods that are not universally meaningful are called **comparative typing** methods. They can be used to study organisms within a defined context. An example of such a context is the comparison of *Staphylococcus aureus* isolates within herds (eg, from teat skin and from milk). This comparison allows us to determine whether skin and milk within these herds harbor the same or different strains of *Staphylococcus aureus* [17]. When a milk sample is submitted to a diagnostic laboratory and found to contain *Staphylococcus aureus*, however, there is no possibility of determining whether this particular isolate belongs to a skin strain or a milk strain using the same methodology. Do to so, a **library typing** method is needed. Library typing methods are methods that generate results with universal meaning, irrespective of when, where, or by whom the results were generated. Using a library typing method, it should be possible to identify an isolate from a single milk sample as belonging to a skin strain or a milk strain of *Staphylococcus aureus*. Indeed, it is now possible to do this using multilocus sequence typing (MLST), which is a library typing method based on DNA sequencing [18]. Comparative typing methods and library typing methods have a place in veterinary molecular epidemiology, and examples of applications of both types of methods are provided throughout this article.

Diagnostic tests are characterized by their sensitivity and specificity and by practical aspects such as cost, ease of use, and turn-around times. Cost, ease of use, and turn-around times also play a role in selection of suitable molecular tools in epidemiology. Other important characteristics of molecular methods are typeability, discriminatory power, reproducibility, and concordance [14,19]. **Typeability** is the proportion of isolates that are assigned a type by the typing system [14]. Some techniques that were developed for typing of human pathogens do not work well for typing of animal isolates belonging to the same pathogen species. For example, serotyping is commonly used to classify *Streptococcus agalactiae* in humans, but it does not work well for bovine isolates of *Streptococcus agalactiae* [20]. Similarly, a proportion of bovine strains of *Staphylococcus aureus* are not typeable using phages developed for typing of human *Staphylococcus aureus* [21]. **Reproducibility** is the ability of the test to generate the same results every time that the test is applied to an isolate. Streptococci and enterococci can be speciated based on combinations of multiple phenotypic characteristics. Commercial test systems based on this principle are on the market and are used in veterinary diagnostic laboratories. Some of these systems produce results that are not reproducible. For example, an isolate that is identified as *Enterococcus faecium* the first time it is tested may be identified as *Enterococcus faecalis* at other times [22]. **Discriminatory power** is the ability of a method to differentiate between strains. The discriminatory power can be quantified using Simpson's Index of Discrimination, which is the probability that the typing system will assign a different type to two strains that are not related [23]. The outcome of molecular epidemiologic studies can be highly dependent on the discriminatory power of the typing method that is used. Comparisons of skin and milk isolates of *Staphylococcus aureus* were initially performed using phenotyping. Phenotyping did not differentiate between isolates from skin and milk, and it was concluded that bovine teat skin was an important reservoir of *Staphylococcus aureus* causing intramammary infections [24]. When the same isolates were re-examined with more discriminatory genotypic methods, it became apparent that the isolates did not belong to the same strains, and that teat skin is not as important as a source of intramammary *Staphylococcus aureus* as initially thought [17]. The discriminatory power of phenotypic methods can be improved by addition of more biochemical tests, phages, antibodies, and so forth, or through a change in interpretation criteria for test results. Such an increase in discriminatory power is often accompanied by a decrease in reproducibility of results [25], and a balance between the two characteristics may need to be struck, similar to the balance between sensitivity and specificity of diagnostic methods. **Concordance** can be assessed in two ways. Typing system concordance is a taxonomic interpretation of the concordance concept. It is the agreement between results of two independent typing systems. One could think of it as a kind of kappa-statistic for typing methods. Epidemiologic concordance is a purely epidemiologic concept and refers to the ability of a typing method to identify strains in agreement with the epidemiologic origin of the isolates. When a new typing method is developed, the epidemiologic origin of the isolates is the "gold standard" for evaluation of the typing system [14]. After the typing technique has been validated, it can subsequently be used to investigate epidemiologic questions.

By and large, phenotypic tests have lower typeability, reproducibility, and discriminatory power than genotypic methods, although exceptions to that rule certainly exist [1]. The popularity of phenotypic methods stems from their low cost, ease of use, and short turn-around time, which makes them the method of choice for many diagnostic applications. The term *molecular methods* is commonly used to refer to techniques that rely on the characterization of an organism according to its genetic material (ie, genotypic method) [1]. In this article, the same interpretation of molecular methods is used and the focus is henceforth on genotypic characterization of microorganisms.

Molecular methods

It would require more than a whole textbook to introduce all of the genotypic methods currently in use in molecular epidemiology, and such a textbook would be outdated before it could be published. A short introduction to some widely used techniques and the "alphabet soup" of acronyms used for molecular methods is given here to facilitate reading of this and other texts. More comprehensive introductions to conventional and molecular techniques used in molecular epidemiology can be found elsewhere [1,26].

Most comparative genotyping methods are based on modifications of two principles: the "cutting" (restriction) of specific points in the DNA by means of restriction enzymes or the amplification of specific parts of DNA by means of polymerase chain reaction (PCR). The DNA fragments that are obtained through amplification, restriction, or combinations thereof have a negative charge and will move through an electrical field, with small pieces of DNA moving faster than large pieces, allowing for separation of the fragments. The separated fragments appear as a banding pattern or "DNA fingerprint." Because it is difficult to standardize sample processing and gel electrophoresis completely, slight variations in patterns between runs or even within runs are difficult to avoid. As a result, comparison of isolates that are run on the same gel or in the same laboratory is useful, giving rise to the name "comparative methods," whereas comparison of results between laboratories, studies, or countries is difficult. Even within studies, pattern interpretation can be debatable. One article that claims environmental transmission of *E coli* O157:H7 from a cow to a pasture and then to children shows riboprinting results as evidence that the cow shed the strain with which the children became infected [27]. Although these investigators interpret banding patterns as being the same, the authors interpret them as being different and as evidence that the cow was not the source of infection. This example demonstrates the ambiguity of banding pattern based strain characterization and the potential for conflicting interpretations. To overcome difficulties with interpretation of banding patterns generated by comparative methods, standard protocols for strain characterization have been developed and implemented (eg, by the Centers for Disease Control and Prevention) [28].

Some commonly used comparative methods that are based on restriction (cutting) of DNA include restriction enzyme analysis (REA) or random fragment length polymorphism (RFLP), pulsed-field gel electrophoresis (PFGE), and ribotyping. In REA, the microbial genome is digested with a restriction enzyme, and DNA fragments of different lengths are visible on a gel after electrophoresis. The term RFLP refers to the fact that there is polymorphism (differences between isolates) in the size and number of fragments that are generated. The number of fragments generated by REA is often so large that it can be difficult to interpret results. This problem is overcome in PFGE by the use of restriction enzymes that cut less frequently. As a result, fewer and larger DNA fragments are generated (Fig. 2). DNA fragments generated by PFGE are so large that they barely move through a gel unless their ability to move is enhanced by use of specialized equipment that uses changing electric fields or pulsed fields. The need for specialized equipment and training limits the availability of this method for diagnostic laboratories. Specialized equipment is also needed for automated ribotyping. Ribotyping is based on the enzymatic digestion of DNA, followed by capture of the digested fragments on a membrane, and detection of the fragments through hybridization of DNA probes to ribosomal genes in the fragments. The method can be used with or without automation. Automation and use of prefabricated reagents reduces run-to-run variability and contributes to ease of use and short turn-around times. Ribotyping increases standardization of typing results, allowing for comparison of typing results to libraries of banding patterns (Fig. 3). It also

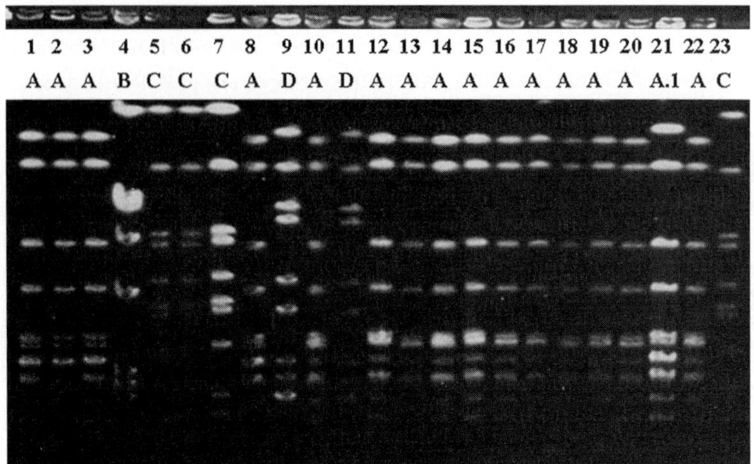

Fig. 2. Example of PFGE typing results. *Staphylococcus aureus* from bulk tank milk (lanes 18 and 19) and quarter milk samples. Numbers and letters indicate sample and strain assignment, respectively. Samples 1 through 8 originate from herd I, samples 9 through 20 from herd II, and samples 21, 22, and 23 from herds III, IV, and V, respectively. Variability in intensity of banding patterns can be seen for strain A (eg, lane 18 is weaker than others) and for strain C (lane 7 is stronger than others). Imperfect standardization of band intensity may affect reproducibility of results. (*Adapted from* Zadoks R, van Leeuwen W, Barkema H, et al. Application of pulsed-field gel electrophoresis and binary typing as tools in veterinary clinical microbiology and molecular epidemiologic analysis of bovine and human *Staphylococcus aureus* isolates. J Clin Microbiol 2000;38(5):1933; with permission.)

increases the cost of strain typing. As a very rough rule of thumb, one could say that "you get what you pay for" with strain typing. Generally, higher discriminatory power, speed, standardization, and ease of use are associated with a higher cost. All of these factors, the availability of equipment and trained personnel, and most important, the epidemiologic question determine the suitability of a typing technique for any given situation [29,30].

Many PCR-based methods are used in molecular epidemiology for DNA fingerprinting and in other applications. PCR can be used for diagnostic or epidemiologic applications and it is the goal and the context rather than the method that makes it a molecular diagnostic tool or a molecular epidemiologic tool. The primers used in PCR determine which complementary sequence in the target DNA is recognized and, hence, what characteristic is detected or which product is generated. The primers can be specific for bacterial species such as *Salmonella* or *Listeria monocytogenes* in milk or beef [31,32]. Primers can also be selected to detect virulence genes or antimicrobial resistance genes, which may or may not be species specific. PCR can be used to generate amplicons (copies of DNA fragments) for subsequent DNA sequencing. This process is the starting point for MLST and can be used to track horizontal transmission of antimicrobial resistance genes [33] or other virulence genes [34]. A plethora of PCR-based strain typing

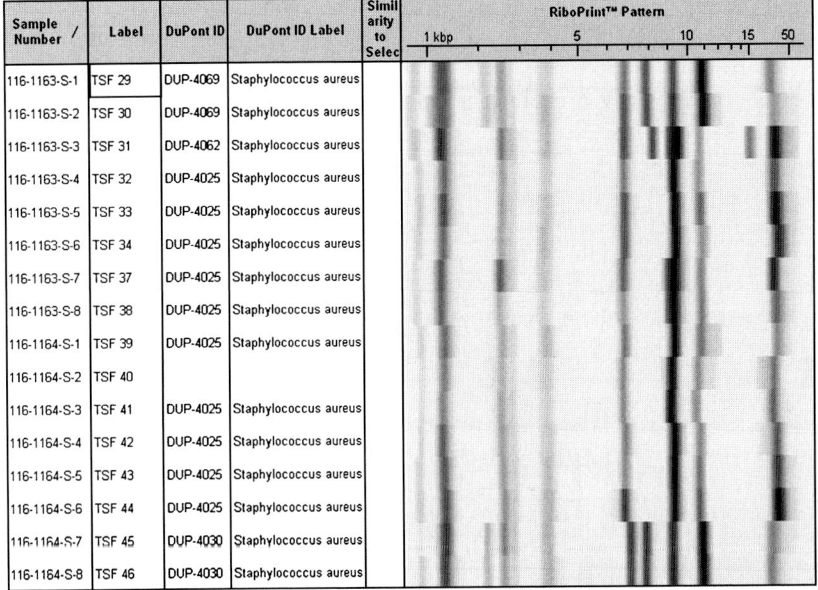

Sample Number /	Label	DuPont ID	DuPont ID Label	Similarity to Selec	RiboPrint™ Pattern 1 kbp 5 10 15 50
116-1163-S-1	TSF 29	DUP-4069	Staphylococcus aureus		
116-1163-S-2	TSF 30	DUP-4069	Staphylococcus aureus		
116-1163-S-3	TSF 31	DUP-4062	Staphylococcus aureus		
116-1163-S-4	TSF 32	DUP-4025	Staphylococcus aureus		
116-1163-S-5	TSF 33	DUP-4025	Staphylococcus aureus		
116-1163-S-6	TSF 34	DUP-4025	Staphylococcus aureus		
116-1163-S-7	TSF 37	DUP-4025	Staphylococcus aureus		
116-1163-S-8	TSF 38	DUP-4025	Staphylococcus aureus		
116-1164-S-1	TSF 39	DUP-4025	Staphylococcus aureus		
116-1164-S-2	TSF 40				
116-1164-S-3	TSF 41	DUP-4025	Staphylococcus aureus		
116-1164-S-4	TSF 42	DUP-4025	Staphylococcus aureus		
116-1164-S-5	TSF 43	DUP-4025	Staphylococcus aureus		
116-1164-S-6	TSF 44	DUP-4025	Staphylococcus aureus		
116-1164-S-7	TSF 45	DUP-4030	Staphylococcus aureus		
116-1164-S-8	TSF 46	DUP-4030	Staphylococcus aureus		

Fig. 3. Example of ribotyping results. *Staphylococcus aureus* from dairy cows. Through comparison to the reference database of the Riboprinter Microbial Identification System (DuPont Qualicon, Wilmington, Delaware), species and strain identification is possible. Four strains were identified in this set of samples (DUP-4025, -4030, -4062, and -4069).

methods exists, ranging from random amplified polymorphic DNA (RAPD) typing (Fig. 4), which is highly versatile and can be used for nearly all known bacterial, fungal, viral, and parasitic pathogens, to insertion element PCR assays that are used only for typing of a specific bacterial subspecies (eg, IS*900* typing of *Mycobacterium avium* subsp *paratuberculosis* [MAP]) [1]. PCR can be performed with one set of primers at a time, also known

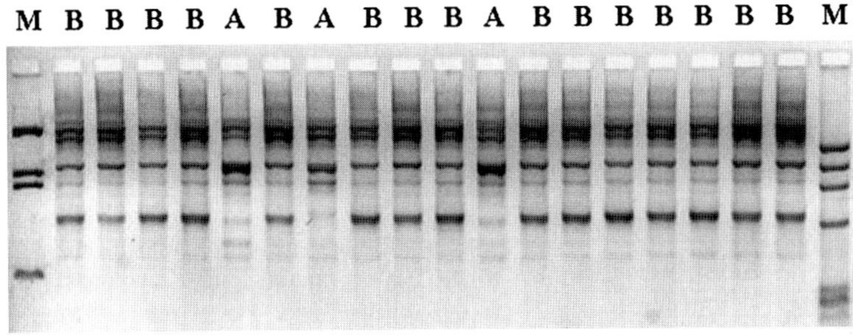

Fig. 4. Example of RAPD PCR. *Streptococcus uberis* isolates from a bovine dairy herd collected during an outbreak of mastitis. Two strains (A and B) were identified among samples from 10 cows. M, molecular marker.

as uniplex PCR, or with multiple primer sets in one reaction vial, known as multiplex PCR. PCR can be followed by gel electrophoresis for detection of PCR products or take place in "real time," that is, with detection of PCR products while they are being generated in the PCR machine, usually by means of a fluorescence-based method. Restriction methods can be combined with PCR methods. PCR can be the first step, followed by restriction of the amplified product, as in hemolysin typing of *Listeria monocytogenes* [35] or PCR-RFLP of *Cryptosporidium parvum* [36]. Alternatively, restriction can be followed by PCR, as in amplified fragment length polymorphism typing. In this last method, the ends of the fragments that are generated by restriction (similar to RFLP) are recognized by PCR primers that subsequently amplify the fragments, resulting in a higher sensitivity of detection [1].

DNA sequencing has been used for more than a decade to study the molecular epidemiology of viral infections. For RNA viruses, use of reverse transcriptase PCR (RT-PCR; not to be confused with real-time PCR, which is also abbreviated RT-PCR) may be necessary. In this process, viral RNA is reverse transcribed into copy-DNA (cDNA), which is subsequently amplified by PCR. The method is used to trace the geographic origin of FMD outbreaks in cattle [37] and Newcastle disease (NCD) in poultry [38]; to determine the transmission potential of avian influenza viruses that jump the species barrier from poultry to humans, and to identify the origin of newly emerged or emerging viruses including HIV and severe acute respiratory syndrome [6]. In molecular epidemiology of bacterial diseases, the use of DNA sequencing was popularized by the introduction of MLST in the late 1990s. With MLST, isolates are identified by sequencing of multiple genes or loci in the organism's DNA (Fig. 5). In a narrow sense, MLST has been defined as the sequencing of 450 to 500 base pair fragments of seven housekeeping genes [39]. Housekeeping genes encode essential cell functions. Their DNA sequence is mostly highly conserved because any change in DNA or in the proteins encoded by the gene's DNA might be

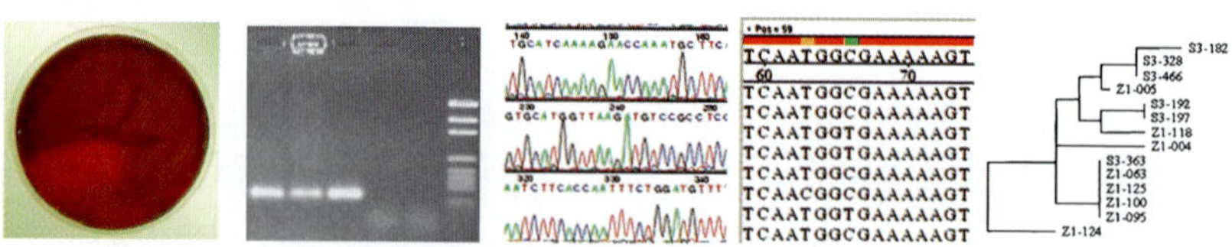

Fig. 5. Producing and using DNA sequence data. Bacteria are grown in pure culture (*left*) to generate material for DNA isolation. Target DNA is amplified by PCR and detected (in this case) using gel electrophoresis (*second from left*). DNA is sequenced using a fluorescence-based detection system that generates electopherograms (*center*). Sequence data are aligned so that similarities (*shown in red*) and dissimilarities (*shown in other colors*) become visible (*second from right*). Dendrograms display the extent of similarity between sequences (*right*). This information can be used for species identification, MLST, and other applications.

detrimental to the cell's survival. In a broader sense, MLST comprises any method that identifies strains based on sequencing of any type or number of loci, including virulence genes [34,40], hypervariable genes [41], and stress-response genes [42]. The DNA sequence of such genes is not highly conserved. On the contrary, changes in the DNA of virulence genes and in the proteins encoded by these genes may help an organism to adapt to adverse circumstances and may thus contribute to its survival. MLST is a library typing method, irrespective of the kind of gene that is included in the typing scheme. Databases with unambiguous strain typing results are accessible on-line (eg, http://www.mlst.net/ and http://pubmlst.org/) for a number of bacterial species [43]. The combination of MLST or other strain typing methods with the sequencing of virulence factor genes or antimicrobial resistance genes allows for the study of evolution of pathogenic strains (eg, shiga-toxin producing *E coli* [STEC]) [34] and the monitoring of the spread of antimicrobial resistance (eg, *Salmonella*) [33]. DNA sequencing of housekeeping genes can be used for species identification, especially when phenotypic methods for species identification are not fully reliable, as for example, in the case of enterococci of animal origin [44].

Source tracing

Source tracking or tracing is no doubt one of the most common applications of molecular epidemiologic methods in veterinary medicine, food safety, and public health. Much of the current emphasis on on-farm food safety (eg, efforts to control *E coli* O157:H7 in feedlots) is due to the fact that molecular epidemiologic tools incriminated live animals as the primary sources of foodborne pathogens. Source tracing can be helpful at many levels, ranging from the detection of on-farm sources of infection or contamination to tracing of multistate or multinational outbreaks of foodborne or animal disease. It can be used to trace animal-to-human or animal-to-animal transmission of pathogens, to monitor spread of antimicrobial resistance determinants in pathogens and commensals of animals and people, to detect sources of pathogens or contaminants in animal products, and to detect products or environmental niches that may act as a source of infection for animals. It is beyond the scope of this article to summarize the wealth of studies on source tracing of foodborne pathogens and antimicrobial resistance determinants. Reviews of both topics have recently been published elsewhere [11,45–47]. The authors focus on examples of source tracing that veterinarians may encounter in large animal practice.

For clinicians, it is important to be aware of the possibility of on-farm animal-to-human transmission of disease, through direct or indirect contact. Veterinarians, family members, farm workers, and visitors to a farm may be at risk. When disease is diagnosed in farm animals, with a possibility of zoonotic pathogens playing a role, herd managers must be alerted so that preventive measures can be taken. Keep in mind that healthy animals may carry and shed foodborne pathogens too, posing a risk that is even harder to identify. Healthy goats and sheep in petting zoos have caused *E coli* O157:H7 disease in children on numerous occasions, as proved by epidemiologic investigations and PFGE typing of isolates [47,48]. Healthy dairy cows have also caused infections in children. A 16-month-old girl on a dairy farm in Ontario contracted *E coli* O157:H7 although she had not been in contact with the cattle and had not consumed raw milk. Molecular investigations showed that cattle, well water, and the child were contaminated or infected with the same strain of *E coli* O157:H7. Subsequent hydrogeologic investigation revealed that the design and location of the well allowed manure-contaminated surface water to flow into the well [49]. In Pennsylvania, a class of school children developed diarrhea after a visit to a dairy and petting farm. Fifty-one patients were confirmed with or suspected of *E coli* O157:H7 and 8 developed hemolytic uremic syndrome [50]. The opening of farms to visitors may help people from nonagricultural communities to develop more appreciation for farming but when visits result in disease, the good intentions may backfire. Hemolytic uremic syndrome can also be associated with enterohemorrhagic *E coli* other than O157:H7 (eg, *E coli* O26:H−). Two children from different families came down with the disease. The families had stayed at the same hotel, and both children had consumed raw cow's milk. The strain that caused hemolytic uremic syndrome in the children was identified in cows on the farm that supplied the raw milk [51]. It is not just *E coli* that we need to worry about. Children attending a farm day camp in Minnesota contracted numerous animalborne infections, including *Cryptosporidium parvum*, a variety of STECs, *Salmonella*, and *Campylobacter jejuni*. PFGE of STECS and PCR-RFLP of *Cryptosporidium parvum* confirmed that calves that were bottle-fed by children shed the strains that infected the children. The risk of infection was increased for children that cared for a sick calf, failed to wash hands after calf contact, or had visible manure present on their hands [36].

Raw milk can be a source of numerous foodborne pathogens. Molecular epidemiologic studies have identified raw milk as the source of several outbreaks of disease, including disease due to *Campylobacter jejuni* in Wisconsin [52] and *Salmonella enterica* serotype Typhimurium in Illinois, Indiana, Ohio, and Tennessee [53]. Especially for a multistate outbreak, it would have been difficult to confirm a common origin without the use of molecular methods. The list gets much longer when raw milk cheeses or other raw milk products are included. A nice example (from an epidemiologic perspective) is an outbreak of *Salmonella enterica* serotype Typhimurium DT104 in Yakima County in Washington State, where investigations resulted in identification of the cause of the problem, and subsequent measures to prevent repeat occurrences were taken. This outbreak was associated with consumption of queso fresco (fresh cheese) made from raw milk, a traditional food in the Hispanic diet, and sparked an intervention in the human population.

A pasteurized-milk queso fresco recipe with taste and texture acceptable to the Hispanic community was developed. Trained Hispanic volunteers conducted safe-cheese workshops, which were attended by more than 225 persons. Workshop participants' acceptance of the new recipe was excellent, and positive behavior changes were maintained over 6 months [54].

Strain typing is not only used to identify sources of foodborne pathogens. It can also be used to trace the source of nonpathogenic bacteria contaminating a product. Recently, the authors worked on a case of *Lactobacillus* contamination of a dairy product that compromised product quality. A specific farm was thought to be the source of the contaminant, and shipment of raw milk from the farm to the plant was suspended. A combination of selective culture methods, DNA sequencing (following the process outlined in Fig. 5) and automated ribotyping was used to determine the presence of *Lactobacillus* in raw milk from the suspected farm and other farms and to compare isolates from raw milk to those from processed product. Other farms were included because detection of the product strain in raw milk of the suspected farm would not mean much if that strain is commonly present in raw milk of most farms. Several raw milk samples contained *Lactobacillus* or related species, as shown by culture and DNA sequencing, but none of the DNA fingerprint patterns from raw milk isolates matched the fingerprint of an isolate from processed product. Based on results from the molecular investigation, herd inspections, and management changes, shipment of milk from the farm to the processing plant could be resumed.

Another example of the use of molecular epidemiologic methods to address on-farm milk quality issues concerns identification of sources of high bacteria counts in bulk tank milk (BTM). In New York State, streptococci are the most common group of bacteria identified in BTM, with 98% of BTM samples testing positive for streptococci. Streptococci also surpass staphylococci and coliform bacteria as contaminants of BTM in terms of the number of colony-forming units per milliliter of milk [55]. Streptococci other than *Streptococcus agalactiae* are commonly thought to be of environmental origin, and their presence in BTM is attributed to poor cow hygiene or poor milking-time hygiene [56]. *Streptococcus uberis*, in particular, which was the most common species of *Streptococcus* found in BTM [57], is thought to be of environmental origin. The environment harbors a wide variety of *Streptococcus uberis* strains. A few grams of soil may contain as many as five or more different strains [58]. Thus, if environmental contamination is the source of high *Streptococcus uberis* counts in milk, one would expect a large variety of strains to be present in the BTM sample. Comparison of multiple *Streptococcus uberis* isolates within BTM samples showed that the opposite was true: all samples tested (n = 5) contained one predominant strain of *Streptococcus uberis*, pointing to a single source rather than the environment as the source of contamination. In each herd, a cow shedding this predominant *Streptococcus uberis* strain was identified, showing that mastitic cows rather than poor cow hygiene or poor milking hygiene were the mostly likely cause of high *Streptococcus uberis* counts in BTM. The same approach (ie, the comparison of multiple isolates from a BTM sample to assess strain diversity and comparison to cow isolates to determine whether a cow could be the source of a predominant strain) has been used to troubleshoot a high *E coli* count problem. Contrary to prevailing paradigm, a cow was identified as the source of a high coliform count. The farm's BTM bacteria count problem was remedied by dry-off of the cow. No changes were made to milking routines, equipment cleaning, or BTM cooling, and yet BTM counts dropped from 37,000 colony-forming units per milliliter to below 10,000 colony-forming units per milliliter.

Molecular epidemiologic investigations may also be helpful when animals are the recipients rather than the sources of pathogens. Outbreaks of bovine mastitis due to *Pseudomonas aeruginosa* are uncommon but have been reported from Ireland and the Netherlands. In both countries, outbreaks occurred on multiple farms, often resulting in severe clinical disease or death [59,60]. Epidemiologic findings suggested that the infection was associated with the use of certain teat wipes. Bacteriology confirmed presence of *Pseudomonas aeruginosa* in the wipes. The wipes had been provided free with the purchase of dry cow therapy as part of a sales promotion. Ironically, the purpose of the wipes was to clean and sterilize the teat end before the infusion of dry cow therapy antibiotic into the mammary gland by way of the teat opening. Molecular typing of isolates from the Irish herds confirmed that all outbreaks had been caused by the same *Pseudomonas aeruginosa* strain [58]. This example not only serves to show how preventive measures can go bad but also demonstrates that presence of the same strain in multiple animals does not necessarily prove contagious transmission. When multiple animals are infected with the same environmental strain, predominance of one strain is the result. It is easy to prove that infection in multiple animals is not the result of contagious transmission. Detection of different strains in each animal proves that. The opposite, proving that contagious transmission causes the spread of a disease, is much harder to do. Usually, a combination of molecular and epidemiologic data is needed to support the likelihood that infection of multiple animals with the same strain was due to common source exposure or contagious transmission, respectively.

Transmission dynamics

The distinction between transmission dynamics and source tracing is somewhat arbitrary. For the sake of this article, the authors consider the focus of transmission dynamics to be how organisms spread, as opposed to where they come from. Transmission dynamics can be studied at the international, regional, local, and farm level. International studies are often necessary to understand transmission dynamics of viral diseases such as classical swine fever [62], foot-and-mouth disease [8], avian influenza [61], or NCD [38]. Sequence analysis of NCD virus in Korea showed that five outbreaks of NCD, occurring in 1949, 1982 to 1984, 1988 to 1997, and 1995 to 2002 had been caused by five different strains of NCD virus that had replaced each other serially. It also showed that the strains causing the epidemics were closely related to those causing NCD outbreaks in other parts of the world. The early outbreaks were caused by strains that were related to a European NCD virus. From 1988 onward, outbreak strains resembled genotypes from Japan, Taiwan, and China. The increased trade of agricultural products and poultry among Far East Asian countries is likely to explain this shift in origin of outbreak strains [38]. Stricter sanitary measures and import controls are needed to prevent such transmission in the future.

An example at the regional level is provided by a multistate study of the transmission dynamics of *Corynebacterium pseudotuberculosis* in the United States [62]. Using RAPD typing, the origin of perceived epidemics of *Corynebacterium pseudotuberculosis*, which mostly affected horses, was shown to differ between states. All isolates from Utah belonged to one RAPD type of *Corynebacterium pseudotuberculosis*, consistent with a clonally expanding epidemic in that state. In contrast, the increased number of infections in Colorado, Kentucky, and California was caused by multiple strains of *Corynebacterium pseudotuberculosis* that were not derived from a common source. Possible causes for the perceived increase in *Corynebacterium pseudotuberculosis* incidence include reporting bias due to increased awareness of the disease, environmental factors facilitating infection, or host factors facilitating infection, such as greater herd susceptibility [62]. Although prevention of animal-to-animal transmission through biosecurity measures could halt the outbreak of the clonally expanding epidemic in Utah, different management measures would be needed to reduce the incidence of *Corynebacterium pseudotuberculosis* in the other states.

The transmission dynamics of *Campylobacter* have been studied at the local level in a rural area with a large number of dairy farms and outdoor recreational areas in the United Kingdom [63]. Samples were collected from water, soil, wildlife feces, and livestock feces, all of which could potentially play a role in exposure of humans to *Campylobacter*. Using model-based spatial statistics, the distribution of *Campylobacter jejuni* was shown to be consistent with very localized within-farm or within-field transmission. Thus, the risk of human exposure to *Campylobacter jejuni* is high in areas contaminated with cattle feces, but the risk of transmission from cattle feces to adjacent wildlife territories, watercourses, or other geographic features transcending field and farm boundaries is limited [63]. Results from the spatial analysis were confirmed by MLST. MLST showed that wildlife and water isolates largely belonged to sequence types that were different from those of bovine isolates. It also showed that many wildlife and water isolates belong to strains that have not been associated with human infections [64]. The combined results show how molecular data can support the results from mathematic or statistical analysis.

Poultry is another reservoir of *Campylobacter*. Litter from bird houses is thought to play a role in transmission of *Campylobacter* in poultry operations. Molecular typing was used to explore the role of litter as source of infection. In one study, a flock was raised in a broiler house. This flock, flock 1, had a high prevalence of *Campylobacter jejuni* in cecal droppings (60%). Most isolates from flock 1 belonged to one strain, RAPD type A. After flock 1 had been removed, part of the litter was transported to a different location and chicks were subsequently raised on this used litter. None of these chicks tested positive for *Campylobacter jejuni* during their 7-week growing period. The remainder of the litter from flock 1 stayed in the original broiler house and was subsequently used for flock 2. In flock 2, *Campylobacter jejuni* was detected but its prevalence was lower than in flock 1 (28%). Furthermore, almost none of the isolates from the second flock belonged to RAPD type A. The conclusion of both experiments was that litter does not play a large role in transmission of *Campylobacter jejuni* [65]. Studies like this can also be used to assess how well cleaning and disinfection of broiler houses prevent carryover between sequential flocks [66]. With collection of suitable samples and data, such farm-level studies could be performed in veterinary practice.

Analysis of patterns of transmission in seemingly similar situations does not always yield similar conclusions. Different patterns of transmission (ie, contagious transmission of a specific pathogen strain and environmental transmission of a multitude of strains) can also be identified within one farm operation [67]. The authors have used molecular epidemiology to help dairy herds determine the origin of their mastitis problem and to identify management measures that could improve the udder health situation. One producer consulted the authors because he failed to earn quality premiums for his milk, which would have been paid if BTM somatic cell counts were below 200,000 cells per milliliter. Despite his best efforts, BTM somatic cell counts remained around 300,000 cells per milliliter. The milk inspector suggested that milking time hygiene might be insufficient, resulting in transmission of mastitis pathogens and subsequent elevated BTM somatic cell counts. The producer insisted that he did everything he could in the milking parlor to prevent mastitis in his animals. A herd visit, with inspection of the milking process, analysis of data stored in a management program, bacteriology of milk samples, and molecular identification of bacterial isolates, revealed (1) the milking routine was impeccable; (2) a scatter plot of linear scores (LS) for the most recent milk test day and the preceding test day showed that most animals had low LS on both test days (healthy cows) or high LS on both test days (chronic infections); (3) the number of cures (low LS on most recent test day, high LS on the preceding test days) was low; and (4) the number of new infections (high LS on most recent test day, low LS on preceding test day) was very low, as the parlor inspection suggested (Fig. 6). Milk samples were taken from several animals with chronic high LS. Six animals tested positive for nonagalactiae streptococci. Using primers for identification of *Streptococcus* species [68], two animals

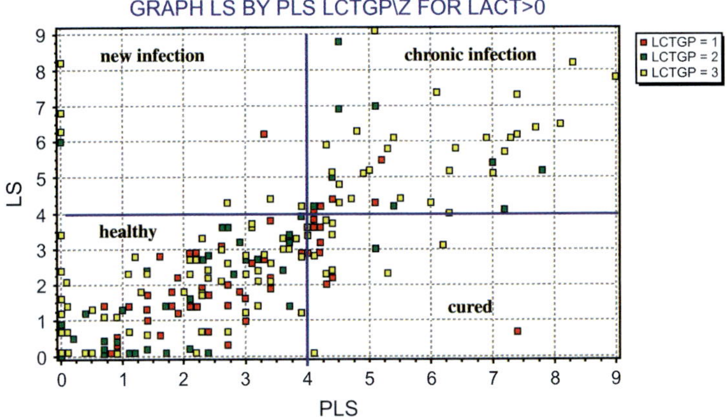

Fig. 6. Scatter plot of most recent LS (vertical axis) and previous LS (horizontal axis) used to determine whether chronic or new infections were the main cause of elevated BTM somatic cell count. LS = 4 is used as cutoff value for elevated somatic cell count at the cow level. Cows from the upper right quadrant were selected for sampling and molecular follow-up.

were shown to be infected with *Streptococcus dysgalactiae*, whereas four others were infected with *Streptococcus uberis*. The presence of two species proves that not all infections had resulted from cow-to-cow transmission. Subsequent RAPD-based strain typing of the *Streptococcus uberis* isolates revealed that each cow was infected with her own strain of *Streptococcus uberis*, confirming again that these cases of mastitis were not due to contagious transmission or poor milking-time hygiene but to infections from environmental sources (Fig. 7). With these data in hand, the producer felt confident that his milking routines were as good as he had thought. The problem was not in the milking parlor but in the close-up and fresh cow pens: animals became infected with streptococci around calving. In the LS

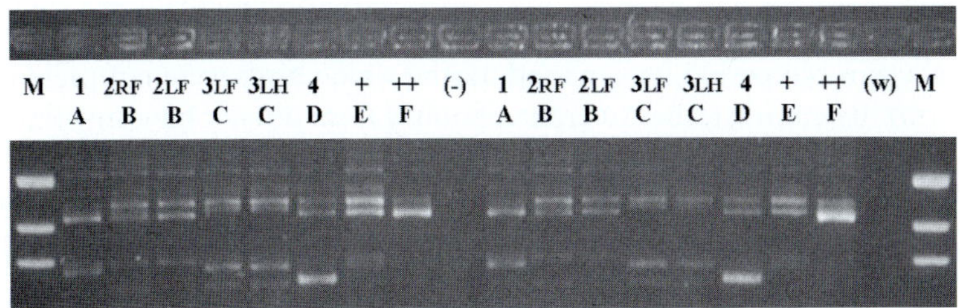

Fig. 7. RAPD fingerprinting results for *Streptococcus uberis* isolates from six quarters of four cows in one herd. Isolates are fingerprinted in duplicate to assess reproducibility of fingerprint patterns. Each cow (identified by a number) has a unique pattern (identified by a letter), whereas multiple quarters within a cow (RF, LF, and LH) are infected with the same strain. Lanes marked + and ++ contain positive controls; lanes marked (−) and (w) contain negative controls. LF, left front; LH, left hind; M, marker; RF, right front.

graph, new infections around calving show up with a previous LS of zero and high LS for the most recent test day (see Fig. 6). In this herd, prevention of new infections through improved hygiene around calving and a reduction in mastitis prevalence through culling or treatment of chronically infected animals were the pathways to achieving the goal of a BTM somatic cell counts worthy of a quality premium.

Persistence, reintroduction, and reinfection

When repeated outbreaks of infection in a farming operation or repeated manifestations of clinical disease in an animal occur, the question arises whether the problem was ever solved or merely "went underground." Molecular epidemiology can be used to distinguish between persistence and reintroduction of a pathogen or between failure to cure and cure followed by reinfection with a different organism.

Series of outbreaks of fowl cholera have been observed, raising the question whether such series were the result of persistence or repeat introductions of the causative agent, *Pasteurella multocida*. In Australia, two outbreaks of fowl cholera on a multiage free-range egg farm were investigated. The outbreaks occurred 8 years apart, in 1994 and 2002. In the 1994 outbreak, only acute fowl cholera was seen. The 2002 outbreak included acute and chronic cases of the disease. Despite the difference in time and manifestation, the same strain of *Pasteurella multocida* caused both outbreaks, as shown by REA typing [69]. In a Danish duck flock, outbreaks of fowl cholera occurred in 1996 and 1997, and asymptomatic carriers of *Pasteurella multocida* were detected in 1998 [70]. In this flock, a different REA type was found for each outbreak and each year. In the Australian example, repeated introduction of the same *Pasteurella* strain cannot be ruled out completely, but endemic persistence of the outbreak strain in healthy birds is a more likely explanation for repeated isolation of the same REA type. In the Danish flock, multiple introductions must have occurred, as evidenced by the diversity of REA types. The difference in epidemiology that was revealed by molecular methods could easily be explained by differences in management. The Danish duck farm had an annual clean-out period (ie, a period during which birds were not present on the farm). By contrast, the Australian poultry farm did not have any time period in which birds were completely absent from the property, not even in the 8 years separating the two observed outbreaks. It is not known why so many years went by without outbreaks, but it is thought that stress factors may precipitate fowl cholera [70]. For both outbreaks in the Australian farm, stress factors were identified. The first outbreak followed an attack on the hen house by dingos, and the second outbreak escalated while the flock owner was away [69]. It should be noted that repeated isolation of the same pathogen strain is not always the result of persistence of infection in the animal population. In feedlots, there is a high turnover of animals. Even so, pathogen strains may persist, as in the case for *E coli* O157:H7. Environmental survival of

O157:H7 strains for 6 months and detection of the pathogen in other animal species could explain such persistence in feedlots [71]. The farm environment may thus be more important as a reservoir of *E coli* O157:H7 than the incoming animals [72].

To complicate matters, repeated isolation of the same pathogen strain does not need to be the result of persistence at all. As an example, consider two series of fowl cholera outbreaks in Hungary. One series of outbreaks occurred in goose flocks kept for eiderdown production and another series of outbreaks occurred in turkey farms. The strains of *Pasteurella multocida* that were isolated differed between host species; however, within each bird species, the outbreaks were caused by a predominant strain [73]. Analysis of epidemiologic data and contact structures indicated that the two series of outbreaks had different underlying causes. The goose flocks were all located in a village but belonged to different owners, and sharing of fodder or animals between flocks did not occur. The turkey flocks were geographically more dispersed but all belonged to the same large-scale breeder. Flock-to-flock transmission was deemed unlikely for the geese. Instead, the fact that multiple outbreaks were caused by the same strain was attributed to the presence of wildlife in the village. Wild animals were thought to have introduced the same strain to each farm. For the turkey flocks, distances and time intervals between outbreaks made transmission by wild animals unlikely. Here, repeated isolation of the same *Pasteurella multocida* strain due intracompany transmission was suspected. Both types of introduction (ie, by wildlife and through intracompany transmission) have also been described for *Pasteurella multocida* and *Mycoplasma gallisepticum* in turkeys in the United States [74–76].

For an animal-level example of distinction between persistence and reinfection, the authors return to mastitis in dairy cattle. In 1999, Döpfer and colleagues [77] described repeated cases of clinical *E coli* mastitis in dairy cows. Back then, infections with *E coli* were generally considered to be acute and of short duration, and repeat cases would be explained by repeat infections of the susceptible cows or quarters. Considering the large variety of *E coli* strains in the environment [78], each infection would be anticipated to be caused by a different strain, just like multiple infections within one dairy herd are caused by different strains [79]. Indeed, 13% of all clinical cases were repeat clinical cases caused by different strains. In those cases, recurrence of clinical episodes was the result of reinfection, and the fact that repeat cases were seen was probably associated with increased susceptibility of individual cows. Five percent of repeat clinical cases, however, were not caused by different strains but by one strain [77]. For those cases, intramammary persistence of the causative strain was the most likely explanation for observation of multiple clinical episodes, although this concept was highly disputed at the time. Since then, intramammary persistence has been proved with daily samplings, culture, and strain typing for cows with chronic *E coli* mastitis, and the existence of chronic *E coli* mastitis is now well accepted

(Fig. 8) [80–82]. Even single cases of clinical *E coli* mastitis during early lactation have been shown to be manifestations of pre-existing, chronic subclinical infections that originated in the dry period [83]. This finding implies that control measures to prevent clinical *E coli* mastitis may need to be taken in the dry period, rather than in lactation. In treatment trials, strain typing can be used to determine whether apparent failures to cure are true failures or cures followed by reinfection. Oliver and colleagues [84] showed that cows that test positive for *Streptococcus uberis* or *Streptococcus dysgalactiae* before and after the dry period can be persistently infected with the same strain (failure to cure) or infected with different strains at dry-off and at calving (cure and reinfection). If a dairy producer wants to assess the efficacy of the dry cow treatment used on a farm, strain typing is a tool that would allow him or her to do so. One caveat is that for strains that spread in a contagious manner, predominance of that contagious strain is expected, and repeat isolation of that strain from an animal could signify failure to cure or cure followed by reinfection with the predominant strain. It is only when different strains are isolated before and after treatment that one can be reasonably certain that reinfection occurred. Typing of multiple isolates from a sample may be necessary to assess strain diversity within samples and to identify mixed infections and partial cures [85]. Herd-level and animal-level examples of differentiation between persistence

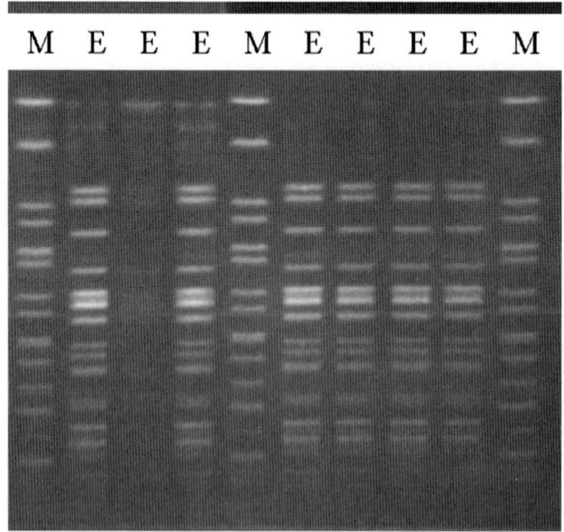

Fig. 8. PFGE fingerprints of *E coli* isolates from seven sequential milk samples collected from one udder quarter at weekly intervals. All isolates have the same PFGE fingerprint, showing that recurrent clinical episodes were the result of persistent infection with one strain rather than the result of repeated cure and reinfection with *E coli* strains from the environment. E, *E coli*; M, molecular marker. (Courtesy of Dr. B. Dogan, Cornell University, Ithaca, New York).

and reintroduction re-emphasize that molecular data cannot be interpreted in a meaningful manner without knowledge of the epidemiologic context in which the strain typing data were collected.

Host specificity and niche adaptation

Molecular epidemiologic studies have provided a wealth of insight regarding niche adaptation of strains. Niche adaptation can be interpreted as adaptation to survival in a host (as opposed to the environment), as adaptation to a specific host species, or even as adaptation to an organ system of the host. Examples for all types of niche adaptation can be found among bovine mastitis pathogens.

In bovine mastitis, a distinction is commonly made between environmental and contagious mastitis. Environmental mastitis pathogens are adapted to environmental survival. They do not need a host for survival but can cause opportunistic infections in animals. When the immune system is compromised by negative energy balance, the risk of infection with environmental *E coli* is increased [86]. During the dry period, when udders are not "flushed out" by milking and the composition of mammary secretions changes, the risk of *Streptococcus uberis* mastitis is increased. There is a large variety of *E coli* and *Streptococcus uberis* strains in the environment [57,78], and a large variety of strains may cause mastitis [79,85]. In recent years though, several outbreaks of *Streptococcus uberis* mastitis have been described that were not caused by a variety of environmental strains but by a predominant strain (see Fig. 4) [67,87]. Infection of multiple cows or quarters with the same strain has also been reported in nonoutbreak situations [84,88]. In some cases, there is evidence to suggest that contagious transmission by way of the milking machine took place, similar to the transmission that is known to occur for *Staphylococcus aureus* [67]. In two herds, the strains that predominated caused infections that were more chronic than those caused by other strains. This observation gives rise to the ideas that certain strains may be more host adapted than others and that they may provide themselves with a longer window of opportunity for transmission to other animals in the population [67]. Differences in the ability of strains to spread within a herd have also been described for *Staphylococcus aureus* [89] and for *Streptococcus agalactiae* [90]. Between-cow transmission of *E coli* has not been documented, but adaptation of some pathogen strains to survival in the mammary gland, resulting in chronic infections and within-cow transmission, appears to occur [80].

Streptococcus agalactiae, also known as group B streptococci in human medicine, provides us with a nice example of adaptation to host species. Differences in the clinical manifestation and epidemiology of intramammary infections caused by *Streptococcus agalactiae* isolates of human and bovine origin were documented in the early 1980s [90,91]. Comparison of human and bovine isolates of *Streptococcus agalactiae* of temporally and geographically matched origins in New York State showed that compared with mastitis in dairy cows, clinical disease in humans was caused by different strains of *Streptococcus agalactiae* [92]. On occasion, *Streptococcus agalactiae* has been isolated in the authors' diagnostic laboratory from milk samples originating from a closed herd thought to be free of *Streptococcus agalactiae*. Such isolates, which did not seem to spread in the herd or were found in BTM only, were shown to belong to a human type of *Streptococcus agalactiae* on a number of occasions. Opportunistic transmission to cattle and lack of spread in the bovine population has also been reported in the United Kingdom [93]. It is interesting to note that companion animals that carry *Streptococcus agalactiae* tend to harbor human rather than bovine strains of the organism [94]. Many humans are asymptomatic carriers of *Streptococcus agalactiae*, and several molecular epidemiologic studies have shown that most cases of severe clinical disease is associated with a limited number of specific strains only. MLST recently confirmed this finding. What is more, MLST showed that a neonatal invasive clone, which can be fatal to newborns, evolved from bovine rather than human subtypes of *Streptococcus agalactiae* [95]. Although evidence for direct bovine to human transmission had not been published at the time this article was written, the evolutionary relation between bovine and human *Streptococcus agalactiae* infections is seen by some as a reason to call for mandatory eradication of *Streptococcus agalactiae* from the dairy cattle population [96].

The third type of niche adaptation of interest is adaptation to organ systems within a host. Again, a mastitis pathogen can be used as an example. Several studies have shown that mammary isolates from different countries tend to belong to a limited number of strains [97], and that teat skin and milk harbor different strains [17]. MLST of *Staphylococcus aureus* isolates from North and South America and Europe confirmed the predominance of a limited number of clones—grouped together in a so-called "clonal complex"—as causative agents of mastitis, and differentiated this clonal complex from clones found on teat skin [18]. This organ specificity seems to hold across host species because mastitis isolates from cows, goats, and sheep have more in common with each other than skin and udder isolates within the bovine host species [98]. Existence of host-adapted or udder-specific strains as opposed to environmental strains has also been suggested based on clinical and epidemiologic observations. Precalving heifers in a dairy herd would not have been in contact with the milking machine and infected herd mates, so epidemiologic data would suggest that infections in heifers have a different origin. Strain typing confirmed this notion. In addition, the strains found in heifers were associated with very severe clinical disease, resulting in loss of life or loss of the affected udder quarters [99]. Loss of life or productivity removes the infected host or quarter from the dairy population that is milked and, hence, from the opportunity for contagious transmission. For a host-adapted pathogen, such severe damage to the host would not be a smart survival strategy.

The niche adaptation of mastitis pathogens implies that traditional classifications of pathogen species as contagious (host adapted) or environmental (non–host adapted) are too simplistic. Some species, for example *Staphylococcus aureus*, tend to be contagious, whereas other species such as *Streptococcus uberis* are commonly of environmental origin. Depending on management conditions and strains, however, environmental *Staphylococcus aureus* and contagious *Streptococcus uberis* may occur. Even *Streptococcus agalactiae*, which can be considered the prototype of contagious pathogens, can on rare occasions originate from environmental sources (human, companion animal). At the other end of the spectrum, *E coli*, the prototype of environmental pathogens, appears to be adapting to long-term survival in the bovine host. Thus, a black-and-white dichotomy does not do the epidemiology of mastitis justice and fails to provide dairy producers with adequate management advice in all circumstances. Rather, a sliding scale with *Streptococcus agalactiae* at the contagious end and *E coli* at the environmental end should be used to represent the epidemiology of mastitis (Fig. 9).

In veterinary practice, molecular typing data from milk isolates can be used to differentiate between contagious and environmental transmission, as discussed elsewhere in this article. In the absence of typing data, epidemiologic and clinical data on infected animals (new infections predominantly in heifers and dry cows versus new infections predominantly in lactating cows), herd hygiene (bedding, milking routine), and management information (implementation of postmilking teat disinfection, segregation of infected animals) can be used to assess the most likely mode of transmission. If people are reluctant to let go of the old mastitis paradigm,

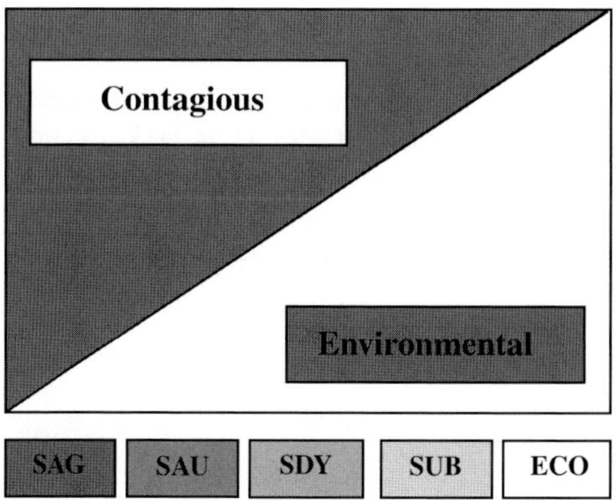

Fig. 9. Sliding scale for contagious and environmental origin of mastitis pathogens, based on insights from molecular epidemiology. Vertical axis indicates to what extent species behave as contagious (*orange*) or as environmental (*white*) pathogens. The transmission pattern in a specific herd depends on bacterial species and strains and on management conditions. ECO, *E coli*; SAG, *Streptococcus agalactiae*; SAU, *Staphylococcus aureus*; SDY, *Streptococcus dysgalactiae*; SUB, *Streptococcus uberis*.

then molecular typing can be helpful to clarify the herd-specific situation. A last interesting twist to the mastitis story was revealed by the study on MLST of *Staphylococcus aureus* [18]. Among the isolates typed was the Newbould 305 strain. This strain was originally used to induce intramammary infections as part of a method to study intramammary treatments [100]. Strain Newbould 305 has since been used to study the effect of antibiotics [101], vaccines [102], and teat-dips [103] and to study the pathogenesis of *Staphylococcus aureus* mastitis [104], the role of minor pathogens [105], and host-level risk factors for infection [106]. MLST showed that Newbould 305 does not belong to the clonal complex of mammary *Staphylococcus aureus* strains. It is a skin strain. Thus, all the studies listed here (and many others) were done with a strain of *Staphylococcus aureus* that is not representative of most mastitis cases that occur naturally in our dairy herds.

An example of less clear-cut host adaptation is provided by MAP. Comparison of MAP isolates from sheep, goat, and cattle herds from Morocco, South Africa, the United States, and Germany showed that all sheep isolates grouped together in one cluster, whereas all cattle and goat isolates grouped together in a different cluster [107]. This finding means that sheep do not pose a risk of MAP infection for cattle. An Australian study also differentiated ovine MAP from bovine MAP and put MAP from goats, alpacas, a rhinoceros, and two humans into the same group as bovine MAP [108]. Later studies, however, showed that contact of calves with paratuberculous sheep can result in presence of ovine MAP in cattle. Under extensive grazing conditions, transmission of ovine MAP among cattle appeared uncommon [109]. Very different results were obtained in a study of MAP isolates from multiple host species, including wildlife, humans, sheep, and cattle in the United States [110]. In that study, MAP isolates from bovine and ovine sources from the same state were more closely associated with each other than isolates from the same host species but from different geographic regions. These results suggest that there is a lack of host adaptation and that strains are shared between ruminant species. A subsequent study confirmed that some strains of MAP are host specific, whereas others can be shared been domestic animals and wildlife [111].

Molecular epidemiology and vaccines

Molecular epidemiology is useful in the development of vaccines, in monitoring of intentional or unintentional spread of vaccine strains, and when predicting vaccine efficacy. Molecular methods are used to determine whether disease is predominantly caused by one strain of a pathogen or by a multitude of strains. In the case of bovine rotavirus diarrhea in France, most isolates were shown to belong to one genotype, G6. Consequently, a monovalent vaccine based on G6 antigen should be sufficient to elicit good protection [112]. For other diseases, a monovalent vaccine would not be useful. Multiple serotypes of bovine *Staphylococcus aureus* can cause mastitis, and a multivalent vaccine would be needed to protect against all main serotypes. To complicate matters, the distribution of serotypes differs between countries. A vaccine that could be useful in France would be only marginally effective in the United States because of differences in the distribution of the most common serotypes [113]. Even when vaccines do not induce antibodies against surface antigens of the infectious agent, an understanding of molecular epidemiology can be important. For several years, the possibility of a vaccine that targeted the plasminogen activator of *Streptococcus uberis*, PauA, was explored. The idea behind this vaccine target was that the immune response of the cow fails to clear the mammary gland of *Streptococcus uberis*, even though antibody levels can be boosted [114]. PauA is used by *Streptococcus uberis* to acquire nutrients when growing in milk. The aim of the vaccine was to prevent bacterial growth by depriving the bacteria of essential nutrients through inactivation of its nutrient-acquisition system with vaccine-induced antibodies against PauA [115]. Not all *Streptococcus uberis* isolates harbor *pau*A, the gene that codes for the protein PauA, and MLST showed that there is a *pau*A-negative subpopulation of *Streptococcus uberis* that also differs from most *Streptococcus uberis* isolates in presence and composition of several other genes [40]. A *pau*A-based vaccine would not provide protection against such strains. In the population of *Streptococcus uberis* isolates that does contain the *pau*A gene, the gene experiences positive selection, which implies that the gene may have the ability to change over time in response to selective pressures in the environment [40]. Other virulence genes and vaccine targets are currently sought after, and molecular tools facilitate that search dramatically [116]. While genomic and proteomic studies provide a rational basis for selection of vaccine candidates, MLST of the bacterial population provides a rational framework for selection of strains that represent relevant subgroups of the species that will be targeted with the vaccine.

Sometimes, administration of vaccines results in unintentional transmission of vaccine strains or contaminants. In Italy and the Netherlands, modified live-marker vaccine was used for active immunization of cattle against infectious bovine rhinotracheitis, caused by bovine herpesvirus 1 (BHV1). Ten to 15 days after vaccination, drop in milk yield, diarrhea, abortion, and death were reported from some farms. All case farms had been vaccinated with batches derived from the same stock materials. Serum neutralization tests and real-time PCR showed that the batches were contaminated with a highly virulent strain of bovine viral diarrhea virus type II. To prevent spread of this bovine viral diarrhea virus strain, which had not been detected in Europe before this outbreak, all contaminated product was recalled and all vaccinated cattle that had not yet died were slaughtered [117]. Vaccine contamination was also suspected when outbreaks of scrapie were observed in sheep and goats that had been vaccinated against *Mycoplasma agalactiae* in Italy. Iatrogenic scrapie in the vaccinated flocks was attributed to the presence of prions in mammary gland and brain homogenates used for vaccination [118]. Although prions do not have DNA, and molecular typing in the sense of DNA-based typing does not apply, the investigators described their study as a molecular analysis of scrapie strains. This example shows the risks involved in use of vaccines derived from animal tissues.

Spread of vaccine strains is not limited to vaccine contaminants. It can also result from the use of live vaccines. *T parva* is a tickborne protozoa that causes East Coast fever in cattle. To prevent the disease, which is often fatal, vaccination is used. Vaccines can be based on a so-called "local" strain approach or a "cocktail" approach. In Zambia, the local strain approach has been used on a large scale, whereas vaccination with a trivalent cocktail of exotic strains has been used on a limited geographic scale and for a limited time only. Comparison of RFLP-PCR data for *T parva* isolates from Kenya and Zambia showed that most Zambian isolates belonged to one stock, which contrasted with the variety of stocks found among Kenyan strains [9]. Zambian field isolates collected in 1996 to 1997 were subsequently compared with Zambian isolates from the prevaccination era and with vaccine stocks used for preparation of local and cocktail vaccines. The field data strongly suggested that one of the exotic vaccine stocks became widely disseminated in the country. For a full discussion of the interaction of protozoa, ticks, and bovine hosts in the epidemiology of this *T parva* strain, the reader is referred to the original publication [9]. Unintentional transmission of a viral vaccine strain was suspected in a Dutch herd, where replacement heifers on a dairy farm had been erroneously vaccinated with a live-virus infectious bovine rhinotracheitis vaccine. More than 18 months later, serology of the herd showed that more than 70% of the animals had developed an antibody response toward BHV1, interfering with the serology-based disease-free certification program. To determine whether the vaccine strain had caused seroconversion in the herd, two vaccinated and two unvaccinated animals (all seropositive) were treated with corticosteroids to reactivate latent BHV1. Virus isolates were obtained from the animals and analyzed by REA. At least one isolate was clearly distinct from the vaccine strain. It was concluded that there was no indication that the vaccine strain had circulated and that a BHV1 field virus had most likely been introduced into the farm despite the herd being closed and having biosecurity measures in place [119].

Summary

The advent of molecular or DNA-based typing methods for microorganisms has opened up a new world of possibilities in veterinary epidemiology. Molecular epidemiology deals with the detection of sources and transmission dynamics of microorganisms using molecular methods and with the identification of determinants of health, disease, spread, and control. Examples of such determinants include virulence genes, antimicrobial resistance genes, and potential vaccine targets. Using molecular epidemiologic methods, it is possible to monitor global spread of pathogens, to identify highly virulent or highly contagious strains of pathogens, to differentiate between persistence and reintroduction of infectious agents in the farm environment, to distinguish between chronic and recurrent infections at the animal level, to detect transmission of vaccine strains, and to classify the epidemiology of an infectious disease as contagious or environmental. The use of molecular tools provides a level of detail and insight that is not available with traditional culture methods or species-level identification of viruses, bacteria, protozoa, or parasites. Molecular epidemiology can pinpoint not only sources of infection or contamination in humans, animals, farm environments, and animal products but also environmental or host factors that contribute to the introduction and spread of microorganisms. As a result, old paradigms can be reassessed, specific targets for intervention and control can be identified, and the effectiveness of control measures can be monitored. Molecular epidemiologic methods have been used with incredible success in global, national, regional, local, farm-level, and animal-level studies. Now that techniques are becoming increasingly user friendly and affordable, they have started to make their way into veterinary diagnostic laboratories. Although their routine implementation still faces challenges (eg, in terms of cost recovery and turn-around times), it is inevitable that in another few years, molecular methods will be among the routine tools that are used in veterinary epidemiology to promote veterinary public health and to improve production-animal health management.

Acknowledgments

The authors thank Dr. Linda L. Tikofsky and Dr. Frank L. Welcome for helpful discussions and critical reading of the manuscript and Dr. Belgin Dogan for providing Fig. 8.

References

[1] Riley LW. Molecular epidemiology of infectious diseases. Principles and practices. Washington, DC: ASM Press; 2004.

[2] Levin BR, Lipsitch M, Bonhoeffer S. Population biology, evolution, and infectious disease: convergence and synthesis. Science 1999;283(5403):806–9.

[3] Lukinmaa S, Nakari UM, Eklund M, et al. Application of molecular genetic methods in diagnostics and epidemiology of food-borne bacterial pathogens. APMIS 2004; 112(11–12):908–29.

[4] Thompson RC, Constantine CC, Morgan UM. Overview and significance of molecular methods: what role for molecular epidemiology? Parasitology 1998;117(Suppl):S161–75.

[5] Haas L. Molecular epidemiology of animal virus diseases. Zentralbl Veterinarmed B 1997; 44(5):257–72.

[6] Hungnes O, Jonassen TO, Jonassen CM, et al. Molecular epidemiology of viral infections. How sequence information helps us understand the evolution and dissemination of viruses. APMIS 2000;108(2):81–97.
[7] Skuce RA, Neill SD. Molecular epidemiology of *Mycobacterium bovis*: exploiting molecular data. Tuberculosis (Edinb) 2001;81(1–2):169–75.
[8] Knowles NJ, Samuel AR. Molecular epidemiology of foot-and-mouth disease virus. Virus Res 2003;91(1):65–80.
[9] Geysen D, Bishop R, Skilton R, et al. Molecular epidemiology of *Theileria parva* in the field. Trop Med Int Health 1999;4(9):A21–7.
[10] Thompson RC. The zoonotic significance and molecular epidemiology of Giardia and giardiasis. Vet Parasitol 2004;126(1–2):15–35.
[11] Boerlin P. Molecular epidemiology of antimicrobial resistance in veterinary medicine: where do we go? Anim Health Res Rev 2004;5(1):95–102.
[12] Blanc DS. The use of molecular typing for epidemiological surveillance and investigation of endemic nosocomial infections. Infect Genet Evol 2004;4(3):193–7.
[13] Tenover FC, Arbeit RD, Goering RV. How to select and interpret molecular strain typing methods for epidemiological studies of bacterial infections: a review for healthcare epidemiologists. Molecular Typing Working Group of the Society for Healthcare Epidemiology of America. Infect Control Hosp Epidemiol 1997;18(6):426–39.
[14] Struelens M. Members of the European Study Group on Epidemiological Markers (ESGEM) of the European Society for Clinical Microbiology and Infectious Diseases (ESCMID). Consensus guidelines for appropriate use and evaluation of microbial epidemiologic typing systems. Clin Microbiol Infect 1996;2:2–11.
[15] Sol J, Sampimon OC, Barkema HW, et al. Factors associated with cure after therapy of clinical mastitis caused by *Staphylococcus aureus*. J Dairy Sci 2000;83(2):278–84.
[16] Crisostomo MI, Westh H, Tomasz A, et al. The evolution of methicillin resistance in *Staphylococcus aureus*: similarity of genetic backgrounds in historically early methicillin-susceptible and -resistant isolates and contemporary epidemic clones. Proc Natl Acad Sci U S A 2001;98(17):9865–70.
[17] Zadoks RN, van Leeuwen WB, Kreft D, et al. Comparison of *Staphylococcus aureus* isolates from bovine and human skin, milking equipment, and bovine milk by phage typing, pulsed-field gel electrophoresis, and binary typing. J Clin Microbiol 2002;40(11): 3894–902.
[18] Smith EM, Green LE, Medley GF, et al. Multilocus sequence typing of intercontinental bovine *Staphylococcus aureus* isolates. J Clin Microbiol 2005;43:4737–43.
[19] Maslow JN, Mulligan ME, Arbeit RD. Molecular epidemiology: application of contemporary techniques to the typing of microorganisms. Clin Infect Dis 1993;17(2):153–62.
[20] Dogan B, Schukken YH, Santisteban C, et al. Distribution of serotypes and antimicrobial resistance genes among *Streptococcus agalactiae* isolates from bovine and human hosts. J Clin Microbiol 2005;43:5899–906.
[21] Aarestrup FM, Wegener HC, Jensen NE, et al. A study of phage- and ribotype patterns of *Staphylococcus aureus* isolated from bovine mastitis in the Nordic countries. Acta Vet Scand 1997;38(3):243–52.
[22] Hudson CR, Fedorka-Cray PJ, Jackson-Hall MC, et al. Anomalies in species identification of enterococci from veterinary sources using a commercial biochemical identification system. Lett Appl Microbiol 2003;36(4):245–50.
[23] Hunter PR, Gaston MA. Numerical index of the discriminatory ability of typing systems: an application of Simpson's index of diversity. J Clin Microbiol 1988;26(11):2465–6.
[24] Fox LK, Gershman M, Hancock DD, et al. Fomites and reservoirs of *Staphylococcus aureus* causing intramammary infections as determined by phage typing: the effect of milking time hygiene practices. Cornell Vet 1991;81(2):183–93.
[25] Hunter PR. Reproducibility and indices of discriminatory power of microbial typing methods. J Clin Microbiol 1990;28(9):1903–5.

[26] Van Belkum A. High-throughput epidemiologic typing in clinical microbiology. Clin Microbiol Infect 2003;9(2):86–100.
[27] Grif K, Orth D, Lederer I, et al. Importance of environmental transmission in cases of EHEC O157 causing hemolytic uremic syndrome. Eur J Clin Microbiol Infect Dis 2005; 24(4):268–71.
[28] Swaminathan B, Barrett TJ, Hunter SB, et al. PulseNet: the molecular subtyping network for foodborne bacterial disease surveillance, United States. Emerg Infect Dis 2001;7(3): 382–9.
[29] Olive DM, Bean P. Principles and applications of methods for DNA-based typing of microbial organisms. J Clin Microbiol 1999;37(6):1661–9.
[30] van Belkum A, Struelens M, de Visser A, et al. Role of genomic typing in taxonomy, evolutionary genetics, and microbial epidemiology. Clin Microbiol Rev 2001;14(3): 547–60.
[31] Van Kessel JS, Karns JS, Perdue ML. Using a portable real-time PCR assay to detect *Salmonella* in raw milk. J Food Prot 2003;66(10):1762–7.
[32] Nguyen LT, Gillespie BE, Nam HM, et al. Detection of *Escherichia coli* O157:H7 and *Listeria monocytogenes* in beef products by real-time polymerase chain reaction. Foodborne Pathog Dis 2004;1(4):231–40.
[33] Alcaine SD, Sukhnanand SS, Warnick LD, et al. Ceftiofur-resistant *Salmonella* strains isolated from dairy farms represent multiple widely distributed subtypes that evolved by independent horizontal gene transfer. Antimicrob Agents Chemother 2005;49(10):4061–7.
[34] Reid SD, Herbelin CJ, Bumbaugh AC, et al. Parallel evolution of virulence in pathogenic *Escherichia coli*. Nature 2000;406(6791):64–7.
[35] Wiedmann M, Bruce JL, Keating C, et al. Ribotypes and virulence gene polymorphisms suggest three distinct *Listeria monocytogenes* lineages with differences in pathogenic potential. Infect Immun 1997;65(7):2707–16.
[36] Smith KE, Stenzel SA, Bender JB, et al. Outbreaks of enteric infections caused by multiple pathogens associated with calves at a farm day camp. Pediatr Infect Dis J 2004;23(12): 1098–104.
[37] Stram Y, Chai D, Fawzy HE, et al. Molecular epidemiology of foot-and-mouth disease (FMD) in Israel in 1994 and in other Middle-Eastern countries in the years 1992–1994. Arch Virol 1995;140(10):1791–7.
[38] Lee YJ, Sung HW, Choi JG, et al. Molecular epidemiology of Newcastle disease viruses isolated in South Korea using sequencing of the fusion protein cleavage site region and phylogenetic relationships. Avian Pathol 2004;33(5):482–91.
[39] Enright MC, Spratt BG. Multilocus sequence typing. Trends Microbiol 1999;7(12):482–7.
[40] Zadoks RN, Schukken YH, Wiedmann M. Multilocus sequence typing of *Streptococcus uberis* provides sensitive and epidemiologically relevant subtype information and reveals positive selection in the virulence gene *pau*A. J Clin Microbiol 2005;43(5):2407–17.
[41] Meinersmann RJ, Phillips RW, Wiedmann M, et al. Multilocus sequence typing of *Listeria monocytogenes* by use of hypervariable genes reveals clonal and recombination histories of three lineages. Appl Environ Microbiol 2004;70(4):2193–203.
[42] Nightingale KK, Windham K, Wiedmann M. Evolution and molecular phylogeny of *Listeria monocytogenes* isolated from human and animal listeriosis cases and foods. J Bacteriol 2005;187:5537–51.
[43] Aanensen DM, Spratt BG. The multilocus sequence typing network: mlst.net [Web server issue]. Nucleic Acids Res 2005;1(33):W728-33.
[44] Loch IM, Glenn K, Zadoks RN. Macrolide and lincosamide resistance genes of environmental streptococci from bovine milk. Vet Microbiol 2005;111(1–2):133–8.
[45] Guardabassi L, Schwarz S, Lloyd DH. Pet animals as reservoirs of antimicrobial-resistant bacteria. J Antimicrob Chemother 2004;54(2):321–32.
[46] Torrence ME. Epidemiology and food safety. Foodborne Pathog Dis 2005;2(1):2–11.

[47] Heuvelink AE, van HC, Zwartkruis-Nahuis JT, et al. *Escherichia coli* O157 infection associated with a petting zoo. Epidemiol Infect 2002;129(2):295–302.

[48] David ST, MacDougall L, Louie K, et al. Petting zoo-associated Escherichia coli 0157:h7—secondary transmission, asymptomatic infection, and prolonged shedding in the classroom. Can Commun Dis Rep 2004;30(20):173–80.

[49] Jackson SG, Goodbrand RB, Johnson RP, et al. *Escherichia coli* O157:H7 diarrhoea associated with well water and infected cattle on an Ontario farm. Epidemiol Infect 1998;120(1): 17–20.

[50] Crump JA, Sulka AC, Langer AJ, et al. An outbreak of *Escherichia coli* O157:H7 infections among visitors to a dairy farm. N Engl J Med 2002;347(8):555–60.

[51] Allerberger F, Friedrich AW, Grif K, et al. Hemolytic-uremic syndrome associated with enterohemorrhagic *Escherichia coli* O26:H infection and consumption of unpasteurized cow's milk. Int J Infect Dis 2003;7(1):42–5.

[52] Anonymous. Outbreak of *Campylobacter jejuni* infections associated with drinking unpasteurized milk procured through a cow-leasing program—Wisconsin, 2001. MMWR Morb Mortal Wkly Rep 2002;51(25):548–9.

[53] Mazurek J, Salehi E, Propes D, et al. A multistate outbreak of *Salmonella enterica* serotype typhimurium infection linked to raw milk consumption—Ohio, 2003. J Food Prot 2004; 67(10):2165–70.

[54] Bell RA, Hillers VN, Thomas TA. The Abuela Project: safe cheese workshops to reduce the incidence of *Salmonella* typhimurium from consumption of raw-milk fresh cheese. Am J Public Health 1999;89(9):1421–4.

[55] Zadoks RN, Gonzalez RN, Boor KJ, et al. Mastitis-causing streptococci are important contributors to bacterial counts in raw bulk tank milk. J Food Prot 2004;67(12):2644–50.

[56] Farnsworth RJ. Microbiologic examination of bulk tank milk. Vet Clin North Am Food Anim Pract 1993;9(3):469–74.

[57] Zadoks RN, Tikofsky LL, Boor KJ. Ribotyping of *Streptococcus uberis* from a dairy's environment, bovine feces and milk. Vet Microbiol 2005;109:257–65.

[58] Daly M, Power E, Bjorkroth J, et al. Molecular analysis of *Pseudomonas aeruginosa*: epidemiological investigation of mastitis outbreaks in Irish dairy herds. Appl Environ Microbiol 1999;65(6):2723–9.

[59] Sol J, Barkema HW, Berghege IM, et al. [Mastitis following drying up associated with teat wipes contaminated with *Pseudomonas aeruginosa*.] Tijdschr Diergeneeskd 1998;123(4): 112–3.

[60] Greiser-Wilke I, Fritzemeier J, Koenen F, et al. Molecular epidemiology of a large classical swine fever epidemic in the European Union in 1997–1998. Vet Microbiol 2000;77(1–2): 17–27.

[61] Suarez DL, Spackman E, Senne DA. Update on molecular epidemiology of H1, H5, and H7 influenza virus infections in poultry in North America. Avian Dis 2003;47(3 Suppl): 888–97.

[62] Foley JE, Spier SJ, Mihalyi J, et al. Molecular epidemiologic features of *Corynebacterium pseudotuberculosis* isolated from horses. Am J Vet Res 2004;65(12):1734–7.

[63] Brown PE, Christensen OF, Clough HE, et al. Frequency and spatial distribution of environmental *Campylobacter* spp. Appl Environ Microbiol 2004;70(11):6501–11.

[64] French NP, Barrigas M, Brown P, et al. Spatial epidemiology and natural population structure of *Campylobacter jejuni* colonizing a farmland ecosystem. Environ Microbiol 2005;7:1116–26.

[65] Payne RE, Lee MD, Dreesen DW, et al. Molecular epidemiology of *Campylobacter jejuni* in broiler flocks using randomly amplified polymorphic DNA-PCR and 23S rRNA-PCR and role of litter in its transmission. Appl Environ Microbiol 1999;65(1):260–3.

[66] Shreeve JE, Toszeghy M, Ridley A, et al. The carry-over of *Campylobacter* isolates between sequential poultry flocks. Avian Dis 2002;46(2):378–85.

[67] Zadoks RN, Gillespie BE, Barkema HW, et al. Clinical, epidemiological and molecular characteristics of *Streptococcus uberis* infections in dairy herds. Epidemiol Infect 2003; 130(2):335–49.

[68] Phuektes P, Mansell PD, Browning GF. Multiplex polymerase chain reaction assay for simultaneous detection of *Staphylococcus aureus* and streptococcal causes of bovine mastitis. J Dairy Sci 2001;84(5):1140–8.

[69] Zhang P, Fegan N, Fraser I, et al. Molecular epidemiology of two fowl cholera outbreaks on a free-range chicken layer farm. J Vet Diagn Invest 2004;16(5):458–60.

[70] Muhairwa AP, Christensen JP, Bisgaard M. Investigations on the carrier rate of *Pasteurella multocida* in healthy commercial poultry flocks and flocks affected by fowl cholera. Avian Pathol 2000;29:133–42.

[71] Hancock D, Besser T, Lejeune J, et al. The control of VTEC in the animal reservoir. Int J Food Microbiol 2001;66(1–2):71–8.

[72] Lejeune JT, Besser TE, Rice DH, et al. Longitudinal study of fecal shedding of *Escherichia coli* O157:H7 in feedlot cattle: predominance and persistence of specific clonal types despite massive cattle population turnover. Appl Environ Microbiol 2004;70(1):377–84.

[73] Kardos G, Kiss I. Molecular epidemiology investigation of outbreaks of fowl cholera in geographically related poultry flocks. J Clin Microbiol 2005;43(6):2959–61.

[74] Carpenter TE, Snipes KP, Kasten RW, et al. Molecular epidemiology of *Pasteurella multocida* in turkeys. Am J Vet Res 1991;52(8):1345–9.

[75] Snipes KP, Hirsh DC, Kasten RW, et al. Use of an rRNA probe and restriction endonuclease analysis to fingerprint *Pasteurella multocida* isolated from turkeys and wildlife. J Clin Microbiol 1989;27(8):1847–53.

[76] Charlton BR, Bickford AA, Chin RP, et al. Randomly amplified polymorphic DNA (RAPD) analysis of *Mycoplasma gallisepticum* isolates from turkeys from the central valley of California. J Vet Diagn Invest 1999;11(5):408–15.

[77] Döpfer D, Barkema HW, Lam TJ, et al. Recurrent clinical mastitis caused by *Escherichia coli* in dairy cows. J Dairy Sci 1999;82(1):80–5.

[78] Nemeth J, Muckle CA, Gyles CL. In vitro comparison of bovine mastitis and fecal *Escherichia coli* isolates. Vet Microbiol 1994;40(3–4):231–8.

[79] Lam TJ, Lipman LJ, Schukken YH, et al. Epidemiological characteristics of bovine clinical mastitis caused by *Staphylococcus aureus* and *Escherichia coli* studied by DNA fingerprinting. Am J Vet Res 1996;57(1):39–42.

[80] Bradley AJ, Green MJ. Adaptation of *Escherichia coli* to the bovine mammary gland. J Clin Microbiol 2001;39(5):1845–9.

[81] Döpfer D, Almeida RA, Lam TJ, et al. Adhesion and invasion of *Escherichia coli* from single and recurrent clinical cases of bovine mastitis in vitro. Vet Microbiol 2000;74(4): 331–43.

[82] Schukken YH, Dogan B, Klaessig S, et al. Chronic and recurrent coliforms: implications for lactation therapy. Proceedings of the 43rd Annual Meeting of the National Mastitis Council. Verona (WI): National Mastitis Council; 2004. p. 35–40.

[83] Bradley AJ, Green MJ. A study of the incidence and significance of intramammary enterobacterial infections acquired during the dry period. J Dairy Sci 2000;83(9):1957–65.

[84] Oliver SP, Gillespie BE, Jayarao BM. Detection of new and persistent *Streptococcus uberis* and *Streptococcus dysgalactiae* intramammary infections by polymerase chain reaction-based DNA fingerprinting. FEMS Microbiol Lett 1998;160(1):69–73.

[85] McDougall S, Parkinson TJ, Leyland M, et al. Duration of infection and strain variation in *Streptococcus uberis* isolated from cows' milk. J Dairy Sci 2004;87(7):2062–72.

[86] Suriyasathaporn W, Heuer C, Noordhuizen-Stassen EN, et al. Hyperketonemia and the impairment of udder defense: a review. Vet Res 2000;31(4):397–412.

[87] VanWorth C, Rossitto PV, Wood S, et al. PFGE analysis of Streptococcus uberis recovered from two San Joaquin Valley dairy herds with elevated levels of environmental

streptococcus in California. Proceedings of the 44th Annual Meeting of the National Mastitis Council. Verona (WI): National Mastitis Council; 2005. p. 295–6.

[88] Phuektes P, Mansell PD, Dyson RS, et al. Molecular epidemiology of *Streptococcus uberis* isolates from dairy cows with mastitis. J Clin Microbiol 2001;39(4):1460–6.

[89] Smith TH, Fox LK, Middleton JR. Outbreak of mastitis caused by one strain of *Staphylococcus aureus* in a closed dairy herd. J Am Vet Med Assoc 1998;212(4):553–6.

[90] Jensen NE. Herd types of group-B streptococci. Their prevalence among herds in four Danish mastitis control areas and the relation of type to the spread within herds. Acta Vet Scand 1980;21(4):633–9.

[91] Jensen NE. Experimental bovine group-B streptococcal mastitis induced by strains of human and bovine origin. Nord Vet Med 1982;34(12):441–50.

[92] Sukhnanand S, Dogan B, Ayodele MO, et al. Molecular subtyping and characterization of bovine and human *Streptococcus agalactiae* isolates. J Clin Microbiol 2005;43(3):1177–86.

[93] Leigh JA. Are bovine *Streptococcus agalactiae* (GBS) a leading cause of neonatal death? Proceedings of the 44th Annual Meeting of the National Mastitis Council. Verona (WI): National Mastitis Council; 2005. p. 41–51.

[94] Yildirim AO, Lammler C, Weiss R, et al. Pheno- and genotypic properties of streptococci of serological group B of canine and feline origin. FEMS Microbiol Lett 2002;212(2):187–92.

[95] Bisharat N, Crook DW, Leigh J, et al. Hyperinvasive neonatal group B streptococcus has arisen from a bovine ancestor. J Clin Microbiol 2004;42(5):2161–7.

[96] Hillerton JE, Leigh JA, Ward PN, et al. *Streptococcus agalactiae* infection in dairy cows. Vet Rec 2004;154(21):671–2.

[97] Fitzgerald JR, Meaney WJ, Hartigan PJ, et al. Fine-structure molecular epidemiological analysis of *Staphylococcus aureus* recovered from cows. Epidemiol Infect 1997;119(2): 261–9.

[98] van Leeuwen WB, Melles DC, Alaidan A, et al. Host- and tissue-specific pathogenic traits of *Staphylococcus aureus*. J Bacteriol 2005;187(13):4584–91.

[99] Zadoks R, van Leeuwen W, Barkema H, et al. Application of pulsed-field gel electrophoresis and binary typing as tools in veterinary clinical microbiology and molecular epidemiologic analysis of bovine and human *Staphylococcus aureus* isolates. J Clin Microbiol 2000; 38(5):1931–9.

[100] Newbould FH. The use of induced mammary infections for evaluating dry cow treatment products. I. Development of a method. Can J Comp Med 1979;43(4):426–9.

[101] Owens WE, Washburn PJ, Ray CH. The postantibiotic effect of selected antibiotics on *Staphylococcus aureus* Newbould 305 from bovine intramammary infection. Zentralbl Veterinarmed B 1993;40(9–10):603–8.

[102] Shkreta L, Talbot BG, Diarra MS, et al. Immune responses to a DNA/protein vaccination strategy against *Staphylococcus aureus* induced mastitis in dairy cows. Vaccine 2004;23(1): 114–26.

[103] Watts JL, Boddie RL, Owens WE, et al. Determination of teat dip germicidal activity using the excised teat model. J Dairy Sci 1988;71(1):261–5.

[104] Hensen SM, Pavicic MJ, Lohuis JA, et al. Location of *Staphylococcus aureus* within the experimentally infected bovine udder and the expression of capsular polysaccharide type 5 in situ. J Dairy Sci 2000;83(9):1966–75.

[105] Pankey JW, Nickerson SC, Boddie RL, et al. Effects of *Corynebacterium bovis* infection on susceptibility to major mastitis pathogens. J Dairy Sci 1985;68(10):2684–93.

[106] Schukken YH, Leslie KE, Barnum DA, et al. Experimental *Staphylococcus aureus* intramammary challenge in late lactation dairy cows: quarter and cow effects determining the probability of infection. J Dairy Sci 1999;82(11):2393–401.

[107] Bauerfeind R, Benazzi S, Weiss R, et al. Molecular characterization of *Mycobacterium paratuberculosis* isolates from sheep, goats, and cattle by hybridization with a DNA probe to insertion element IS*900*. J Clin Microbiol 1996;34(7):1617–21.

[108] Whittington RJ, Hope AF, Marshall DJ, et al. Molecular epidemiology of *Mycobacterium avium* subsp. *paratuberculosis*: IS*900* restriction fragment length polymorphism and IS*1311* polymorphism analyses of isolates from animals and a human in Australia. J Clin Microbiol 2000;38(9):3240–8.

[109] Whittington RJ, Taragel CA, Ottaway S, et al. Molecular epidemiological confirmation and circumstances of occurrence of sheep (S) strains of *Mycobacterium avium* subsp. *paratuberculosis* in cases of paratuberculosis in cattle in Australia and sheep and cattle in Iceland. Vet Microbiol 2001;79(4):311–22.

[110] Motiwala AS, Strother M, Amonsin A, et al. Molecular epidemiology of *Mycobacterium avium* subsp. *paratuberculosis*: evidence for limited strain diversity, strain sharing, and identification of unique targets for diagnosis. J Clin Microbiol 2003;41(5):2015–26.

[111] Motiwala AS, Amonsin A, Strother M, et al. Molecular epidemiology of *Mycobacterium avium* subsp. *paratuberculosis* isolates recovered from wild animal species. J Clin Microbiol 2004;42(4):1703–12.

[112] Vende P, Karoum R, Manet G, et al. Molecular epidemiology or bovine rotaviruses from the Charolais area. Vet Res 1999;30(5):451–6.

[113] Guidry A, Fattom A, Patel A, et al. Prevalence of capsular serotypes among *Staphylococcus aureus* isolates from cows with mastitis in the United States. Vet Microbiol 1997;59(1):53–8.

[114] Leigh JA, Field TR. *Streptococcus uberis* resists the bactericidal action of bovine neutrophils despite the presence of bound immunoglobulin. Infect Immun 1994;62(5):1854–9.

[115] Leigh JA, Finch JM, Field TR, et al. Vaccination with the plasminogen activator from *Streptococcus uberis* induces an inhibitory response and protects against experimental infection in the dairy cow. Vaccine 1999;17(7–8):851–7.

[116] Leigh JA, Ward PN, Field TR. The exploitation of the genome in the search for determinants of virulence in *Streptococcus uberis*. Vet Immunol Immunopathol 2004;100(3–4): 145–9.

[117] Falcone E, Tollis M, Conti G. Bovine viral diarrhea disease associated with a contaminated vaccine. Vaccine 1999;18(5–6):387–8.

[118] Zanusso G, Casalone C, Acutis P, et al. Molecular analysis of iatrogenic scrapie in Italy. J Gen Virol 2003;84(4):1047–52.

[119] van der Poel WH, Rijsewijk FA, Meijer FA, et al. [Identification of an introduced bovine herpesvirus type 1 strain in a closed dairy herd by experimental virus reactivation followed by DNA restriction enzyme analysis.] Tijdschr Diergeneeskd 2000;125(23):714–7.

[120] Middleton JR, Fales WH, Luby CD, et al. Surveillance of *Staphylococcus aureus* in veterinary teaching hospitals. J Clin Microbiol 2005;43(6):2916–9.

[121] Gillespie BE, Owens WE, Nickerson SC, et al. Deoxyribonucleic acid fingerprinting of *Staphylococcus aureus* from heifer mammary secretions and from horn flies. J Dairy Sci 1999;82(7):1581–5.

[122] O'Brien TF, Hopkins JD, Gilleece ES, et al. Molecular epidemiology of antibiotic resistance in salmonella from animals and human beings in the United States. N Engl J Med 1982;307(1):1–6.

[123] Zadoks RN, Allore HG, Barkema HW, et al. Analysis of an outbreak of *Streptococcus uberis* mastitis. J Dairy Sci 2001;84(3):590–9.

[124] Tondo EC, Guimaraes MC, Henriques JA, et al. Assessing and analysing contamination of a dairy products processing plant by *Staphylococcus aureus* using antibiotic resistance and PFGE. Can J Microbiol 2000;46(12):1108–14.

[125] Xiao L, Ryan UM. Cryptosporidiosis: an update in molecular epidemiology. Curr Opin Infect Dis 2004;17(5):483–90.

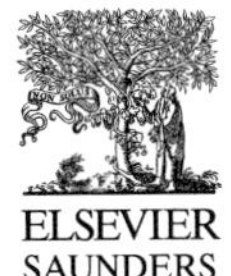

ELSEVIER
SAUNDERS

VETERINARY
CLINICS
Food Animal Practice

Vet Clin Food Anim 22 (2006) 263–270

Index

Note: Page numbers of article titles are in **boldface** type.

0749-0720/06/$ - see front matter
doi:10.1016/S0749-0720(06)00014-4 *vetfood.theclinics.com*

B

C

M

N

O

P

Changing Your Address?

Make sure your subscription changes too! When you notify us of your new address, you can help make our job easier by including an exact copy of your Clinics label number with your old address (see illustration below.) This number identifies you to our computer system and will speed the processing of your address change. Please be sure this label number accompanies your old address and your corrected address—you can send an old Clinics label with your number on it or just copy it exactly and send it to the address listed below.

We appreciate your help in our attempt to give you continuous coverage. Thank you.

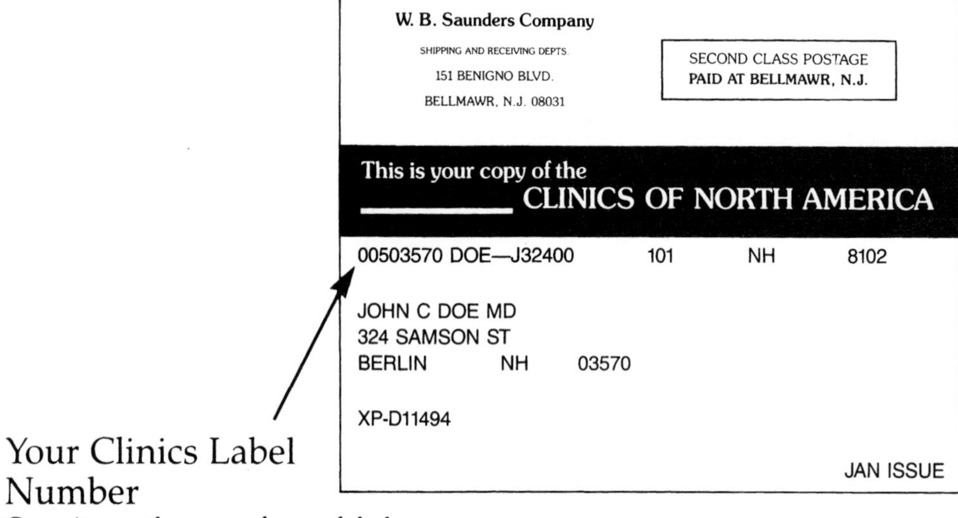

Copy it exactly or send your label along with your address to:
W.B. Saunders Company, Customer Service
Orlando, FL 32887-4800
Call Toll Free 1-800-654-2452

Please allow four to six weeks for delivery of new subscriptions and for processing address changes.